COGNITIVE-BEHAVIORAL THERAPY FOR ADULTS WITH AUTISM SPECTRUM DISORDER

Also Available

Living Well on the Spectrum:
How to Use Your Strengths to Meet the Challenges
of Asperger Syndrome/High-Functioning Autism
Valerie L. Gaus

Cognitive-Behavioral Therapy for Adults with Autism Spectrum Disorder

SECOND EDITION

Valerie L. Gaus

Foreword by Tony Attwood

THE GUILFORD PRESS
New York   London

Library of Congress Cataloging-in-Publication Data

Names: Gaus, Valerie L., author.
Title: Cognitive-behavioral therapy for adults with autism spectrum disorder
    / Valerie L. Gaus.
Other titles: Cognitive-behavioral therapy for adult Asperger syndrome
Description: Second edition. | New York : The Guilford Press, [2019] |
Revision of: Cognitive-behavioral therapy for adult Asperger syndrome.
    c2007. | Includes bibliographical references and index.
Identifiers: LCCN 2018015005 | ISBN 9781462537686 (hardcover)
Subjects: LCSH: Asperger's syndrome—Patients—Rehabilitation. | Asperger's
    ssyndrome—Complications. | Cognitive therapy.
Classification: LCC RC553.A88 G38 2019 | DDC 616.85/8832—dc23
LC record available at *https://lccn.loc.gov/2018015005*

For my parents, June and Ray Gaus

About the Author

Valerie L. Gaus, PhD, is a clinical psychologist in private practice in Long Island and New York City. Her focus is treating mental health problems in adults with autism spectrum disorder, intellectual disability, and other learning and developmental disorders. Since receiving her doctorate in 1992, she has approached her work with a cognitive-behavioral orientation. Dr. Gaus serves on the advisory board of the Asperger Syndrome and High Functioning Autism Association and as the grant review committee of the Organization for Autism Research, and she teaches an advanced training course through the Swedish Psychological Association. She has written numerous articles and chapters on mental health issues in developmental disabilities and has lectured extensively in the United States and internationally. Dr. Gaus is the author of the self-help resource *Living Well on the Spectrum*.

Foreword

Autism is characterized by different ways of perceiving, thinking, learning, and relating that, while positive and advantageous to the individual in some ways, may also contribute to considerable psychological problems throughout the lifespan. Should psychotherapy be required to help the individual cope with and assimilate these differences, it will need to be adapted from the conventional approach in order to accommodate these variations.

The differences in perception can include sensory sensitivity, such that sensory experiences perceived by the neurotypical (nonautistic) person as barely noticeable (e.g., the noise from the fan of an air-conditioning unit or someone coughing) may be perceived as highly distracting or even painful. Sensory sensitivity can be a lifelong problem—with the person experiencing high levels of anxiety throughout the day, fearing that an aversive sensory experience will inevitably occur, and exhaustion from the constant state of apprehension and vigilance.

Another difference in perception can be a difficulty noticing and reading the social information conveyed in facial expressions, gestures, and tone of voice, as well as contextual cues and any associated codes of social conduct. The person who has autism may be able to read some fragments of social information, but not enough to be able to accurately determine what someone is thinking and feeling and thus anticipate what he or she will say or do. This can lead to a sense of belonging to an alien culture, of being overwhelmed and confused in a social context. There may be constant criticism for the frequent social errors, but no guidance in what to do in social situations. The psychological consequences of all of this can be a need for frequent periods of isolation, yet intense loneliness, and the development of overwhelming anxiety in social situations.

Internal states, such as subtle emotions, hunger, and low levels of pain, can also be difficult for the person with autism to both recognize and explain in speech. When a person with autism is asked, "What are you feeling now?" the brief reply may be "I don't know." This is not being obtuse. The actual reply, if only it could be articulated, could well be "I don't know . . . how to grasp one of the many thoughts and feelings swirling in my mind, hold and identify that thought or feeling, then convey that thought or feeling precisely and coherently in speech, so that you will understand." Clearly, this deficit in recognizing and describing emotions can lead to difficulties when conducting psychotherapy, which is based on the ability to accurately communicate internal thoughts and feelings.

The different way of thinking can include having areas of natural cognitive talent, such as an encyclopedic memory, great attention to detail, an ability to perceive patterns and pattern breaks, and originality in problem solving. If the person with autism is not able to rely on an intuitive ability to read people and social situations, he or she may rely on one of his or her thinking strengths to process social information. The person may observe and analyze social situations to determine any patterns or theoretical models of social and interpersonal behavior. The creation of a structure of idiosyncratic rules and theoretical models can, at times, be successful. However, the person can become extremely distressed if his or her rules are broken, or if people do not behave according to their psychological constructs. The psychotherapist will need to engage in autism "archaeology" in order to determine when and how these rules were created, and provide an alternative explanation along with new rules and exceptions.

Another concern in psychotherapy is when the theoretical models of the sense of self are based solely on the bullying, teasing, rejection, humiliation, and criticisms of peers throughout childhood. This, of course, can lead to a very negative sense of self, which is one of the causes of the high levels of depression among adults who have autism. Their tendency to pessimism and reliance on dysfunctional beliefs and cognitive distortions will all need to be addressed during psychotherapy.

The thinking style associated with autism can include cognitive inflexibility and distress when experiencing change. There can be a difficulty conceptualizing an alternative perspective and resistance to changing thoughts, beliefs, and responses. Psychotherapy is based on the recognition that positive change can occur. Unfortunately, the person with autism may resist change, and will need considerable encouragement to embrace an alternative way of thinking and responding. His or her previous coping mechanisms, developed over many years, may work superficially, and the person with autism must allow him- or herself to trust that the alternatives suggested by the psychotherapist could be an improvement on the current coping strategies.

The differences in learning style and information processing of the person with autism also need to be accommodated in psychotherapy. There will need to be an assessment of the most effective and preferred ways of learning the changes in thinking and expressing emotions that are the core components of psychotherapy. There may need to be consideration given to the use of modern technology, such as relevant apps, and an awareness of issues for the person applying the therapy in real-life situations. The person with autism may have cognitively learned what to do from his or her psychotherapist: metaphorically, the information is in a file within the brain's filing cabinet, and during therapy is easily retrievable. However, when the person is stressed or feeling an intense emotion, the "filing cabinet" becomes locked and he or she resorts to previous responses. Hence, there is a need for greater practice in real-life situations than would be expected with someone who is neurotypical, and the focus will need to be on how to remain calm in a crisis in order to access the therapy plan.

There may also be issues resulting from specific learning disabilities in areas such as reading and handwriting, delayed intellectual processing time, organizational and planning deficits, fear of making a mistake, a tendency to be overly literal and pedantic, and a need for guidance in the art of conversation. The psychotherapist needs to be fluent in "Aspergerese"; in other words, to recognize that autism is a different way of thinking—almost a different culture—and be able to translate the concepts and components of the therapy to someone with this different way of thinking. This may have to include accepting the autism characteristic of spotting and correcting errors, such that the psychotherapist must not become distressed when he or she is frequently corrected.

The different way of relating can include difficulties achieving and maintaining friendships and relationships, with a resultant sense of being a social failure. There will be a need for guidance in interpersonal skills, not a usual requirement for someone who is neurotypical in psychotherapy. For example, the person may need guidance in how to perceive and resonate with the feelings of others, and in the development of trust and self-acceptance. One of the causes of stress and depression is having a limited social support network; psychotherapy will probably need to include strategies to improve social abilities, the social network, and social confidence. There may well be a history of social rejection by peers and colleagues, and thus a need for an explanation of the motives of those who appeared to enjoy causing distress. The psychotherapist may need to provide guidance in the motives of others in order to enable the person with autism to have closure regarding past slights and insults.

Thus, there is a need to modify conventional psychotherapy in a number of ways for the differences in abilities associated with autism. This is becoming increasingly important as psychotherapists are observing a surge in referrals of adults with autism. The second edition of *Cognitive-Behavioral Therapy for Adults with Autism Spectrum Disorder* will be the "go-to" resource for psychotherapists treating adults with autism. This second edition provides a review of the recent therapy research and conceptual models of autism. It also includes clear guidelines for assessment, case conceptualization, and development and evaluation of a treatment plan. The revised edition includes the "third wave" of cognitive-behavioral therapy, and addresses how mindfulness and acceptance therapies can be adapted for those with autism. Valerie Gaus has more than 20 years of experience developing and evaluating psychotherapy for adults who have autism, and her wisdom is clear throughout this revision of her original book. Her new edition will be greatly appreciated by psychotherapists, and will contribute to the successful treatment of those who endure the psychological aspects and consequences of having autism.

TONY ATTWOOD, PhD
Chairperson, Minds and Hearts Clinic,
Brisbane, Australia
Adjunct Associate Professor, Griffith University,
Queensland, Australia

Acknowledgments

This second edition, like its predecessor, represents a collection of ideas about adult autism spectrum disorder (ASD) that resulted from countless and varied learning experiences I have had over the years. I am continually influenced by such a diverse network of people, and I could never properly thank all of them. With a focus on the 12 years that have passed between the first and this edition, I highlight the most important relationships in that time frame here.

I will start with the people who taught me the most, and they are my patients. Without their courageous accounts of struggle and survival and articulate descriptions of how they process information, I would have no book to present to you. Their determination to improve their lives is what drove me to look for answers from literature, supervisors, and colleagues.

Because my work setting is a private practice, my colleagues and mentors are found through various network and supervision activities. By regularly attending conferences and meetings related to several different aspects of this book, including autism, developmental disabilities, and cognitive-behavioral therapy, I have thankfully become part of a large network of people who share my interests and goals. I may not have taken on the project of writing this book if not for the leaders within these communities, who each inspired and supported me in some way. They are, in alphabetical order, Michael John Carley, Robert Fletcher, Dena Gassner, Peter Gerhardt, Amy Gravino, Bernice Polinsky, Marcia Scheiner, Pat Schissel, Stephen Shore, Liane Holliday Willey, Michelle Garcia Winner, and Karl Wittig. Hundreds of conversations with other colleagues, supervisors, and supervisees have also been crucial in helping me to solidify my thoughts about working with adult ASD. Some of the people with whom I have had the most meaningful exchanges over the last 12 years are, in alphabetical order, Faith Kappenberg, Jill Krata, Arnetta McKenna, Kristen Memoli, Gina Moravcik, Shana Nichols, Maria Scalley, Lara Scher, Mark Sisti, Alyson Skinner, Dina Vivian, and Monica Wells (Arevalo). Thanks to Lynda Geller, for founding Spectrum Services, and to Rahimeh Andalibian, for keeping it going; this New York City–based cooperative practice brings together a multidisciplinary group of clinicians, all dedicated to serving patients with ASD, and I have been privileged to make it a part-time home for my work. The people at YAI–National Institute for Disabilities, especially Mary Brady and Matthew Sturiale, will always be important to me for helping form my earliest ideas about promoting independence for people with developmental disabilities. My ongoing involvement with the clinical psychology doctoral program at Long Island University, C.W. Post, has also been an important source of inspiration, with David Roll and Eva Feindler among my earliest and continuously influential mentors.

Special thanks to the team at Cognitive Behavioral Associates, where directors Ruth DeRosa and Jill Rathus have been so welcoming to patients with ASD in need of dialectical behavior therapy. If not for their creativity and collaborative approach, some patients would have been at risk for significant crises. Clinicians Gus Kutz and Steven (Shamshy) Schlager were particularly helpful to me for some of my complex cases. I am very grateful to the psychiatrists with whom I have collaborated, including Brian Bonfardin, Peter Della Bella, David Inwood, Robert King, and Jane Perr.

On the international front, I thank Eva Larsson and Sylvia Mellfeldt Milchert for inviting me to design and teach a Web-based specialist course for psychologists in Sweden serving adults with ASD. Because of their initiative and tireless work to run the course every year, dozens of psychologists have been able to increase their knowledge base about adult ASD so they could better serve these patients. I also thank Tony Brown and Pat Abbott at the Autism Diagnostic Research Centre for inviting me on more than one occasion to offer lectures and workshops to cognitive-behavioral therapy clinicians in the United Kingdom. These opportunities to meet with clinicians practicing in different countries have enriched my understanding of the needs of adults with ASD.

The colleagues who have been the most directly supportive of this book are those who helped with the manuscript preparation. While all of these people fit into one or more of the networks mentioned above, I list them here to highlight their generosity with their time to give me detailed comments on drafts of this book. They are Candice Baugh, Kathryn Cody, Ruth DeRosa, Brenna Maddox, Rebecca Sachs, and Pat Schissel. Matthew Lerner kindly allowed me to recruit from his Social Competence and Treatment Lab at Stony Brook for research assistants, where I found Elliott Keenan, Fatema Noor, Hayley Rein, Amanda Stoerback, and Lauren Wagler, who helped with critical research and administrative tasks while I prepared my first draft.

I read Tony Attwood's first book about Asperger syndrome 20 years ago, and saw him do a lecture not long afterward. I was awestruck because he described in such a comprehensive yet accessible way what I had been observing in some of my patients. Because I have admired his work ever since, it was a great honor for me to have him take the time to read and then support this book by writing the thoughtful Foreword.

I will forever be grateful to Jacqueline Persons, the series editor for the first edition of this book. She took a chance on what, at the time, was a seemingly obscure topic in the world of cognitive-behavioral therapy. If not for her progressive thinking and compassion for these adult patients, there would be no editions of this book in existence. Similarly, I need to thank my dear friend Ann Kring for suggesting that I organize my thoughts and to make an initial proposal of the concept to Jacqueline.

The editorial support I got from The Guilford Press was invaluable, and I want to thank Jim Nageotte and Jane Keislar for their patience and support throughout. Both were willing to help at a moment's notice, no matter how big or small my question was.

Paul Gordon and Laura Specht Patchkofsky were also extremely helpful during the various phases of production. Last, but not least, I thank Kitty Moore. Though she was not involved in this second edition, her faith in and cheerful support of the first edition gave me a level of confidence that I carried forward into this more recent work.

Thanks to all of my friends, many of whom have already been mentioned as colleagues. Most especially I am grateful to my steadfast "dinner group": Mary Brady, Arnetta McKenna, Eddie Velazquez, Pam Wolff, and Kathleen Ziccardi.

I thank my husband, Lider, for tolerating my bouts of absence from family life while writing and, as always, for making sure I eat and cheering me on. My son Gabriel, who came into my life since the first edition, was always available to remind me not to take things too seriously. I am proud of my older son, Sean, who now works for a developmental disabilities service agency, and I have enjoyed the many interesting collegial discussions we have had about the field. My father, Raymond Gaus, after several years of listening to me talk about my work, proudly labeled himself an "Aspergian." As a professional, I must say he does not meet criteria for the diagnosis, but having lived with him, I cannot say he is very far away from it either. My mother, June Gaus, who also follows my work, has been married to him for almost 60 years and does not deny his claim. Because he is one of the most loving people I have ever known, I must credit him for giving me insight into the capacity for caring and empathy that does indeed exist in people with "Aspergian" traits, whether they are diagnosable or not. I also need to thank my mother for picking him out of the crowd all those years ago.

Contents

Introduction   1

    The Book's Intended Audience 2
    Terminology 3
    Mental Health Needs of Adults with ASD   4
    Removing Barriers and Bridging Gaps 5
    Origins of My Ideas   6
    A Philosophy of Change 11

1. Defining Autism Spectrum Disorder   13
    in Cognitively Able Adults (Asperger Syndrome)

    What Is AS and Why Is the Term Still Used? 13
    How Does ASD Present in Adulthood?   18
    Understanding the Symptom Picture in Adults with ASD   33
    Strengths and Assets   43
    Chapter Summary and Conclusions 45

2. Conceptualization of Mental Health Problems   46
    in Cognitively Able Adults with Autism Spectrum Disorder
    (Asperger Syndrome)

    General Conceptual Model 47
    Core Cognitive Dysfunction in ASD   50
    Cognitive Dysfunction and Risk for Mental Health Problems 71
    CBT for Adults with ASD   77
    Chapter Summary and Conclusions   78

3. The Initial Assessment   79

    Intake Issues 79
    Diagnosis and Definition of Target Problems   91
    Chapter Summary and Conclusions 112

4. Individualized Case Formulation and Treatment Plan   115

   Case Formulation   115
   Treatment Plan   128
   Chapter Summary and Conclusions   139

5. Psychoeducation and Orientation to Treatment   140

   Psychoeducation   140
   Orientation to Treatment   145
   Chapter Summary and Conclusions   153

6. Intervention: Increasing Skills to Address   154
   the Core Problems of Autism Spectrum Disorder

   Review of Nomothetic Formulation   154
   "Habilitation" for Core Problems   155
   Increasing Social Skills   157
   Increasing Coping Skills   174
   Chapter Summary and Conclusions   182

7. Intervention: Addressing Comorbid Mental Health Problems   183

   Introducing the Cognitive Model to the Patient   184
   Identifying and Responding to Dysfunctional
        Automatic Thoughts   190
   Recognizing and Modifying Intermediate Beliefs   198
   Modifying Schemas   206
   Chapter Summary and Conclusions   213

8. Intervention: Addressing Emotion Regulation Problems   214
   Using Mindfulness-Based Strategies

   ER and ASD   214
   Mindfulness-Based Interventions in CBT   216
   Improving Identification of One's Own Emotions   226
   Improving ER Skills   236
   Clarifying Values   243
   Chapter Summary and Conclusions   247

9. Adjunctive Therapies and Interdisciplinary Collaboration   248

   Guidelines for Referral and Collaboration with Other
        Service Providers   248
   Adjunctive Services and Their Roles   250
   Chapter Summary and Conclusions   257

10. Obstacles to Treatment and How to Address Them   258

   Social-Interaction Difficulties as Challenges
        in the Psychotherapy Session   258
   EF Problems Interfering with Homework Completion   261
   Low Motivation to Be in Treatment
        or Rejection of the Cognitive Model   262
   Family Issues That Interfere with Treatment   262

Trauma History or "Complex" PTSD   263
Substance Use   264
Isolation and Lack of Supports   264
Financial Problems   265
Untreated Health Problems   267
Polypharmacy: Multiple Psychiatric Medications
    without a Rationale   267
Lack of Cooperation from Other Providers   268
Chapter Summary and Conclusions   268

11. Ending Treatment and Looking Ahead   269
When the Goals of Treatment Are Met   269
When Treatment Is Interrupted before Goals Are Met   271
Looking Ahead for Adults with ASD   274
Concluding Comments   277

APPENDIX. Therapy Resources   279
Professional Overviews   279
Therapy Tools and Workbooks   279
Autobiographical and Self-Help Books by Authors
    on the Autism Spectrum   280
Websites of Education, Advocacy, and Support Organizations
    for AS and ASD   281

References   283

Index   302

Introduction

The first edition of this book was titled *Cognitive-Behavioral Therapy for Adult Asperger Syndrome* (Gaus, 2007). As readers may have noticed, this second edition carries a different title. This is largely because of the impact the publication of the fifth edition of the *Diagnostic and Statistical Manual of Mental Disorders* (DSM-5; American Psychiatric Association, 2013) has had on the research literature, not because I am writing about a different patient population. *Asperger syndrome* (AS) was a relatively new term to mental health professionals in the United States when this book was first published in 2007. Treatment providers were slowly coming around to the idea that autism spectrum disorders (ASD) can affect people who are verbal and have average or above intellectual functioning, as seen in AS. Now, 11 years later, this understanding is more widespread, but there remains a tremendous struggle in both the scientific and clinical communities to achieve consensus on how to define, classify, and label this phenomenon. The patients I described 11 years ago, who were diagnosed with AS at that time, would now be diagnosed with ASD instead, if DSM-5 criteria are used. They are the same people, struggling with the same problems in daily living, but the words we use to diagnose them are not.

My main objective in writing this and the previous edition of the book is to provide a guide for practitioners who are treating adults who have ASD, but do not have cognitive or language impairments. The ever-changing terminology has created a challenge for me and my colleagues. When these patients show up in our offices, week after week, with a willingness to work hard to improve their lives, looking to us to help them, the exact label that is attached to the phenomenon loses importance. Yet, our commitment to use evidence-based interventions requires us to stay tuned to the research literature, where the labels of phenomena have a significant impact on how we can interpret and apply the findings of studies. I have met this challenge by synthesizing the current literature that is relevant to treating these patients, while maintaining a person-centered approach to treatment planning. With that, cognitive-behavioral therapy (CBT) continues to offer the most promise for helping these individuals. The CBT literature is full of interventions shown to be effective for other clinical problems that are commonly comorbid with this syndrome (e.g., mood and anxiety disorders), have potential for addressing the core deficits in ASD itself, and have shown promise for youth with ASD. Despite its utility, CBT is not made available to adults with ASD as often as adults in the general population. The chapters ahead are designed to improve that.

This book offers an updated definition of AS (in the significantly changed terminology found in DSM-5) and how it manifests in adulthood (Chapter 1), an evidence-based rationale for applying CBT to the problems that affected patients encounter (Chapter 2), guidelines for assessing the complex presenting problems seen in this population (Chapter 3), a model for conceptualizing cases for individualized treatment plan design (Chapter 4), and psychoeducation and orientation to treatment (Chapter 5). Detailed instructions and case examples for using CBT to build needed skills (Chapter 6) and decrease symptoms of comorbid psychiatric disorders using traditional (Chapter 7) and mindfulness-based (Chapter 8) CBT approaches in adults with ASD are also provided. The necessity for interdisciplinary collaboration is addressed (Chapter 9), as well as strategies for handling obstacles in therapy (Chapter 10) and ending treatment (Chapter 11).

The Book's Intended Audience

The aim of this book is to help increase the number of therapists available to treat this underserved population. More than a decade after the first edition, I am happy to see that many of the barriers to appropriate therapy have been tackled with an increased willingness to bridge the gaps between separate fields of research and clinical practice (Cooper, Loades, & Russell, 2018; Maddox & Gaus, 2018). Nonetheless, I have continued to observe instances in which professionals in the "mainstream mental health community" do not consider themselves qualified or interested in serving people with developmental disorders. Therefore, they may not market their services or accept referrals from the adult ASD population. Likewise, professionals in the "autism spectrum community" are still focusing more on children and the behavioral interventions that are most fitting for the younger population. This leaves a large proverbial "crack" for adults with ASD to fall through, as they suffer from various problems in daily living and/or comorbid mental health disorders that warrant effective psychotherapy (Maddox & Gaus, 2018).

There are many skilled and experienced clinicians in both of these communities who, with a willingness to look outside their respective literatures, can use their existing talents to help adults with ASD. They include psychologists, social workers, psychiatrists, speech–language pathologists, and educators. I hope this new edition can serve as a resource to any of these professionals who come into contact with this population. For example, clinicians serving the general adult population in "mainstream" mental health settings are encountering ASD incidentally in patients who have sought help for a mood or anxiety disorder. This has become increasingly apparent to me over the last 11 years, as I have been invited more often to provide training workshops to groups of psychotherapists who do not identify themselves as ASD specialists, but are eager to learn about ASD because they already have patients on their caseloads with the diagnosis. These meetings have been most exciting for me, as I have been inspired by the compassion and dedication of so many therapists to learn about something new so that they can best serve their patients. Adding to the hopefulness I feel has been the wide range of locations in which I observed this interest, from therapists working in the most remote rural settings to the most densely populated cities across Sweden, the Netherlands, England, New York, Massachusetts, North Carolina, Tennessee, Iowa, Kansas, Minnesota, Utah, and California. Likewise, specialists in the field of childhood ASD are receiving an increasing number of requests to serve adults with this diagnosis. Most importantly, I wish to raise awareness and interest in graduate students and interns who are just entering their respective fields of research and practice because the quality of treatment available to the adults of the future is dependent on them.

Terminology

Chapter 1 details the changes in terminology that have taken place with the publication of DSM-5, but the subject is touched on briefly here for the purpose of establishing the language to be used throughout this book. DSM-5 does not include the term *Asperger's disorder* that was described in the previous edition (DSM-IV-TR; American Psychiatric Association, 2000). In that earlier version, it was included in a collection of disorders called "pervasive developmental disorders" (PDD), alongside but distinguished from the classic "autistic disorder." In the current version, the broad category label of PDD has been replaced with the term *autism spectrum disorder* (ASD), and the symptom presentation that made up an Asperger's disorder diagnosis is now subsumed under that, along with the classic autistic disorder presentation. Now a series of specifiers are to be used to differentiate a more severely affected individual from a less functionally impaired patient.

To illustrate, a person who would have been diagnosed with Asperger's disorder in DSM-IV-TR would now be diagnosed in DSM-5 with:

- 299.00 autism spectrum disorder
  - *requiring support with social communication (Level 1)*
  - *requiring support with restricted repetitive behaviors (Level 1)*
  - *without accompanying intellectual impairment*
  - *without accompanying language impairment*

As can be seen, the proper use of the recording procedures outlined in DSM-5 results in a very wordy set of phrases, instead of the two-word term offered by DSM-IV-TR. It would be quite cumbersome to repeat that phrase every time I make references to this population of people throughout this book. In an attempt to resolve this, I turned to the research literature to see how investigators are describing subjects who have ASD, but do not have intellectual or language impairments; how are they communicating about their research with subjects who have the symptom profile we once called "Asperger syndrome"? What I found there did not help! One consistency is, in more recent peer-reviewed journal articles about this population, the word *Asperger* does not appear in any titles. However, the language researchers use to differentiate their subjects from those with a more impaired "classic" autism profile is not consistent. In a sampling of peer-reviewed articles published between 2013 and 2017, the variety of terms used by authors includes:

- *ASD without intellectual disability*
- *Cognitively able subjects with ASD*
- *Cognitively high-functioning subjects with ASD*
- *High-functioning ASD*
- *ASD with normative cognitive ability*
- *Intellectually able subjects with ASD*
- *ASD with no intellectual impairment*

Without consensus in the scientific community, I was left to choose a phrase that will succinctly capture the population of people who are the focus of this book.

As a side note, I am uncomfortable with the term *high functioning* when talking about people on the autism spectrum with any level of impairment. I find it misleading because, although these individuals have higher intellectual and verbal abilities than people who are considered "low functioning," they are not *functioning* at the level of their *potential*. As an ironic example, many of these adults are unusually adept at using their sophisticated verbal skills to describe their sense of frustration at failing to turn their talents into a meaningful career or occupation. I prefer the term *cognitively able*, first used by Ami Klin and his colleagues (e.g., Klin, Jones, Schultz, Volkmar, & Cohen, 2002b), or Lynda Geller's (2003) "with independence potential."

For practical purposes in this book, the reader should assume I am including all patients on the autism spectrum who are "cognitively able," have "independence potential," or, to be consistent with DSM-5, are without significant intellectual or language impairment, when using ASD. When summarizing research articles, I use ASD without intellectual disability (ID) to be consistent with the language of investigators. Finally, when I refer to people who are not on the autism spectrum, I use the term *typical* or from the *general population*. It is worth noting that in the autism community, some people use the term *neurotypical* (NT) to distinguish people without from those with ASD.

Mental Health Needs of Adults with ASD

Adult patients typically come to a therapist for help with social problems that they are attributing to ASD and/or for help with secondary psychiatric disorders, most commonly anxiety or mood symptoms. The mental health problems seen in these individuals are often related to their attempts to fit in with society. Contrary to the popular belief that people with ASD are aloof and disinterested in others, these individuals are desperate to have friends and lovers. Chronic stress comes with their dramatically uneven profile of strengths and deficits. Generally bright and often successful with academic pursuits, they fail in the interpersonal domain of functioning. They lack the ability to interface successfully with other people because, as Gray (1995, 1998, 2015) describes it, they lack "social understanding." This deficit underlies mistakes (e.g., missing cues, making inappropriate comments, crossing boundaries) that lead others to see them as rude, bizarre, or threatening. Their tendency to focus intensely on one interest area can take on an obsessional quality because they may be unable to discuss anything outside of that topic (e.g., computers, coin collecting, aviation). Many also have difficulty with judgment and problem solving, which in lay terms would be called "common sense." These deficits affect both social and occupational arenas because their behavior interferes with healthy social and sexual relationships and causes them to be unemployed or working at jobs far below their academic and intellectual level. The resulting isolation and sense of failure leave them tremendously vulnerable to anxiety and mood disorders.

I conceptualize all of these problems as stemming from a basic *information-processing disorder,* and I present research that supports that idea in Chapter 2. People with ASD have an idiosyncratic way of processing both social and nonsocial information that has been present since birth or early childhood. Their unique perception has adversely affected their development and social experiences, resulting in negative consequences. It causes them to exhibit behavior that is unappealing to others and contributes to the recurrent rejection and ridicule they encounter. It also leads to impairment in nonsocial areas of functioning, such as organization and self-direction, which increases the level of stress in daily living.

Intervention can have the most dramatic impact when it comes early in life, but many of today's cognitively able adults with ASD were not identified as being on the autism spectrum when they were children, so they did not have the opportunity for early specialized intervention. However, I do not believe these individuals have "missed the boat" for the chance to make improvements in areas of functioning with which they are struggling. Considering a lifespan developmental perspective, it is widely accepted that learning and growth do not stop at age 18 or 21 for typical people, so there is no reason to believe it would cease for adults with ASD. That a new skill learned at any age can affect development in a positive way from that point on is an assumption that I make throughout this book.

A psychotherapist can help these adults by teaching them to (1) recognize and modify automatic maladaptive thoughts, (2) recognize and regulate emotional experiences, (3) more accurately "read" the behavior of others to better understand social interactions, and (4) modify their own behavior in response. This new learning helps the individual with ASD improve social functioning, increase coping/stress management skills, and prevent or reduce symptoms of anxiety and depression.

Removing Barriers and Bridging Gaps

A theme that runs through this book is *integration.* Since the publication of the first edition, in which I had no references that directly supported the use of CBT for adults with AS, there has only been a handful of studies done that directly assessed the efficacy of CBT to treat mental health problems of this population. Thankfully, we can bolster the rationale for its use if we consider multiple literature sources, such as theory and research on:

- Information-processing dysfunction in ASD
- Social cognition in typical people
- The risk factors and effects of stress in typical people
- Cognitive dysfunction in typical people with anxiety or depression
- Emotion regulation impairment as a transdiagnostic mental health problem
- The efficacy of CBT for typical people experiencing anxiety and mood disorders
- The efficacy of CBT for youth with ASD

If we combine what we know from these separate areas, we do have enough evidence to offer CBT to adults with ASD. I provide a review of these data in Chapter 2, where I highlight the findings that have practical implications for adults with ASD and refer the reader to the primary sources and more detailed literature reviews.

Origins of My Ideas

I have worked almost exclusively with more cognitively able adults on the autism spectrum for the past 20 years. When I became interested in this population, there was no intervention literature about these adults upon which I could draw. So, the biggest challenge I faced was the need, mentioned above, to integrate information from a variety of disparate sources. My current conceptualization of the clinical problems characterizing adults with ASD resulted from a process of linking separate literatures and clinical experiences, which began 35 years ago and many years before I met my first patient with AS. I share this background here as a foundation for the treatment approach I describe in the chapters ahead.

Early Misgivings and Misconceptions

During the summer after my high school graduation, I had my first encounter with the autism spectrum. I worked as a teacher's aide in a special education school where one of the students was diagnosed with autistic disorder. This 6-year-old girl was nonverbal, screamed frequently, and did not seem to enjoy any of the classroom activities. As an inexperienced teenager, I grew fearful of her because at least once a day, she would succeed in pulling my hair *very hard,* despite my efforts to prevent her from doing it. I finished out that summer figuring I would never see another person with autism again, and that was fine with me.

I had another encounter several years later when working on my undergraduate honors thesis at Hofstra University with Junko-Tanaka Matsumi as my faculty advisor. Titled "Cross-Situational Assessment of the Behavioral Repertoire of an Autistic Child," it would also be my first conference presentation (Gaus & Tanaka-Matsumi, 1987). As a budding behaviorist, I was excited about the idea of applying scientific principles to the study of aberrant behavior, and my thesis was predicated on a school-based naturalistic observation of a 7-year-old boy diagnosed with autistic disorder. He was nonverbal, had severe ID, was socially withdrawn, and exhibited high rates of self-stimulatory behavior; my project focused on measuring the frequency of each of these behaviors across different settings. I had not forgotten about the discomfort I had felt with the girl who pulled my hair a few years before, and although I would not have admitted it at the time, my work was driven by a desire to understand behavior that seemed so bizarre that it repelled me. I wish I could say my interest in autism flourished from that point, but it did not. My thesis had brought me some satisfaction in that I could better explain and predict my subject's behavior by the end of the study, but I was not particularly drawn to the population. Shamefully, my limited experience with only two cases of autism had left me with the vague and misinformed concept that working with autism meant working with children and that all these children were nonverbal. Even worse, because of my naive and simplistic perspective, I had failed to understand these two young people and their daily struggles.

Although my thesis did not direct me to further autism-related work, it did bring me the good fortune of Dr. Tanaka-Matsumi's mentorship. She sparked my love of empiricism and a desire to become a scientist–practitioner, which landed me in the clinical psychology doctoral program at Stony Brook University, State University of New York. There I was immersed in a stimulating environment where the many facets of clinical psychology were introduced by faculty members who were leaders in their fields. It was a privilege to learn about behavioral parenting intervention from Susan O'Leary, marital discord and therapy from Daniel O'Leary, CBT and psychotherapy integration from Marvin Goldfried, problem-solving therapy from Thomas D'Zurilla, fundamental and applied behavioral principles from Edward (Ted) Carr, adult psychopathology from John Neale, and child psychopathology from Alan O. Ross.

Outside of some brief mention of autism and ID in the psychopathology courses, developmental disorders (DD) were not a focus during my training. Peers who worked in Ted Carr's research group had the most exposure to those clinical populations because their subjects were children with DD. However, my clinical practicum experiences were shaping my preference for work with adult patients and for psychotherapy as an intervention modality over classroom or parent interventions. In addition, my research was targeting an adult population, as I had joined the research group of Alan O. Ross. Despite his long history as a child psychologist with an interest in child abuse, at the time I came to Stony Brook he was working on research questions about adults; his investigations were aimed toward the identification of factors that could cause an adult to, as he put it, "snap" and injure a child. My objective was to develop and validate a behavioral measure of frustration tolerance, which would be used to study high-risk response styles in adults. A long series of experiments with undergraduate subjects resulted in a reliable instrument and a completed dissertation, but I graduated before it was ever used on clinical populations. Nevertheless, the work raised my curiosity about a wide variety of adult problems, including anger, aggression, and anxiety.

My predoctoral internship in a veterans affairs (VA) hospital, where I worked mostly with combat-related posttraumatic stress disorder (PTSD) and substance abuse, solidified my interest in CBT and adult psychopathology. It was also during that year that I made the decision to pursue a career as a clinician, not a researcher. When I finished the internship, autism was further from my mind than ever before and *Asperger syndrome* was a term I would not hear for several years. But I was about to enter a field that would gradually lead me to the work I describe in this book, a field that would force me repeatedly to adjust my thinking because it exposed me to phenomena that were inconsistent with my previous conceptions (or misconceptions). Each discovery would cause me to adopt a new idea and to slightly shift the direction of my practice. Many of the basic assumptions underpinning this book were formed this way, and the experiences that spawned them are presented below in the order in which they occurred.

Discovery 1: Children with DD Become Adults with DD

After I completed my degree at Stony Brook, I needed to work in a clinical setting where I could get the supervision required to qualify for a state license to practice. I would have loved to work in the VA where I had interned, but they were not hiring at the time I needed a job. So, I took a position at a large and well-established DD service agency in New York City, which provides programs for people with ID, autism, and other DD.

I was hired by the adult residential department to design behavioral intervention plans in a group home for people diagnosed with ID and/or autistic disorder and "severe challenging behavior." It did not seem as interesting to me as the VA, but I did need the supervision and, quite frankly, I also needed to make some money! With my solid behavioral training, research background in frustration/aggression, and clinical interest in adult populations, I was confident that I could do the job. I agreed to the standard agency requirement of an 18-month commitment.

As I worked in the group home, I found it intriguing to see how DD manifested in adulthood. I previously had held the belief that DD were childhood disorders. I quickly learned that, although these problems have their *onset* at birth or in early childhood, affected individuals are impaired by their symptoms throughout their lives. My fascination was overshadowed, however, by the frequent and severe aggressive behavior demonstrated by these adults, which made my job quite unpleasant. In fact, when a male resident pulled my hair during my first week (a mild behavior in this setting), I thought back to my experience with the girl in summer school 10 years before and asked myself, "For this I got a PhD?" In some ways, it was worse than the earlier experience, despite the fact that I was older and trying to be more objective. When a grown man pulled my hair, it felt much more like an assault than when a 6-year-old girl had done it. I nonetheless resolved to stick it out until I fulfilled my commitment, at which point, I promised myself, I could resign to do something else. I could use the clinical hours toward the eligibility requirements for state licensure, so my time would not be wasted. I was not willing to cut my hair, so I would simply have to be more clever about keeping it out of harm's way.

Discovery 2: Adults with DD Have Similar Mental Health Problems as Typical Adults

The majority of the individuals I served in residential services would not fit the profile of the patients I describe in this book; almost all residents had ID and fewer than half of those had an ASD. However, most of them had comorbid psychiatric disorders that had never been properly diagnosed, and this omission raised my curiosity. Thus, although I had not received any specialized training in DD before this job, in some ways my "mainstream mental health" background was a better preparation for the issues I was encountering. This is one of the reasons I remained at the agency for 13 years!

The intrigue was found in my observation that most staff in that service delivery system did not recognize the presence of mental health problems in adults with DD. The field was dominated at the time by a view that problem behavior in people with DD is the result of their learning history and could be reduced or eliminated by teaching and reinforcing an alternative adaptive behavior. I agreed with that view (and still do), but I did not believe it applied to *all* the problems a person with a DD could have. This one-dimensional approach failed to take into account the possibility that a mood disorder, for example, could affect an adult with intellectual impairments. I was repeatedly asking colleagues the question "If psychiatric disorders strike a proportion of the *nondisabled* adult population, why *wouldn't* these phenomena be present in a certain proportion of the population of adults *with* DD?"

I searched for resources and found that, although they were a small minority, other professionals in the DD field were asking the same question, including members of the interdisciplinary organization called the National Association for the Dually Diagnosed

(NADD), devoted to providing treatment guidelines (e.g., Fletcher & Dosen, 1993; Gardner & Sovner, 1994; Matson & Barrett, 1993; Nezu, Nezu, & Gill-Weiss, 1992), and the editors of a special section in the *Journal of Consulting and Clinical Psychology*, devoted to the topic of mental illness in persons with ID (1994, Vol. 62, No. 1). Most of these guidelines included the behavioral approaches that were traditionally applied to this population (assessment and manipulation of environmental antecedents and consequences of aberrant behavior) but also promoted more multidimensional or "biopsychosocial" case formulation models.

I was lucky to have supportive and forward-thinking administrators working with me on my cases in the residential facility. Together we recognized that some of the more complex behavior problems were multidetermined and would need a multifaceted treatment plan that included *medical, psychosocial,* and *environmental* interventions. The *individualized treatment planning* approach that is described in this book has its roots in the work we did in the group home setting. We recognized that each component, whether behavioral, cognitive, or pharmacological, is necessary but not sufficient to ameliorate complex problems in adults with multiple disorders.

Discovery 3: People with DD Can Benefit from Psychotherapy

As soon as I became a state-licensed psychologist, I started a private practice and soon after began working in an outpatient clinic for people with DD. Again, I was challenged to try something for which I had never received formal training, and I found it necessary to integrate ideas from separate literatures and experiences. My doctoral training had given me a solid foundation in CBT, but not in applying it to people with DD. My experience at the agency up to that point had not involved psychotherapy but did teach me to understand the various forms of cognitive dysfunction present in people with DD. When I tied these two concepts together by offering *cognitive*-behavioral therapy to people with known *cognitive* dysfunction, it seemed so fitting to me, yet I was surprised when I could not find very much written about it. In fact, the idea of offering any type of psychotherapy to people with DD was foreign to many professionals in the field at that time. The range of psychological services traditionally sought for this population was limited to environmental or staff/parent training interventions and was based on a purely behavioral orientation. Thankfully, publications began to appear that addressed this new trend of offering "talk therapies" to people with DD (Nezu & Nezu, 1994; Strohmer & Prout, 1994), including one that focused on CBT exclusively (Kroese, Dagnan, & Loumidis, 1997). With those publications and my work at the agency came an ever-widening circle of colleagues who were doing similar work with whom I could exchange ideas.

Discovery 4: Symptoms of Autism Can Present in People Who Have Strong Cognitive and Verbal Abilities

It was in my private practice that I met Joe, my first patient with AS. Meeting him led to one of my most important revelations and brings me to the subject of this book. The initial phone call came from Joe's brother, who said, "I want you to see my brother, who I think has Asperger syndrome." I responded, "What's that?" I thought he had said, "assburger syndrome." He told me that it was "high-functioning autism," so I scheduled an appointment, satisfied that the presenting issue was probably somehow related to my

DD specialty. As soon as I got off the phone, I grabbed my then-new copy of DSM-IV (American Psychiatric Association, 1994) and went to the section on PDD. Sure enough, there it was: Asperger's disorder. I was a little embarrassed that I had not encountered this term on my own (this was early 1995), as the DSM had been sitting on my desk for months at this point. But I got over it quickly as I became enthralled by the research I did on this phenomenon.

I was even more intrigued when I met Joe, whose case is detailed in Chapter 1. This 55-year-old man had a master's degree from an Ivy League institution and had worked and lived independently for years, but demonstrated odd social behavior and struggled with simple problem solving in daily living. It was during his assessment that I experienced my fourth important revelation. I realized that it was possible for a person to have the social difficulties and behavioral eccentricities of autism (as I had always defined it), but also have average to superior intelligence and sophisticated verbal abilities. I also assumed that Joe could not be the only person like this, and that others with similar problems may also have reason to seek help from mental health professionals. I shifted the focus of my practice at that point toward the understanding of these often misunderstood individuals.

Discovery 5: Some Things Are Better Left Unchanged, or Don't Throw the Baby Out with the Bathwater

Since I entered the "autism spectrum community" I have come to enjoy the fact that I am indeed part of a community. This field is unique in that there is much productive interaction outside the clinical setting among professionals, individuals on the spectrum, family members of those on the spectrum, support networks, and advocacy groups. This involvement enriches my understanding of this population, keeps me constantly informed, and has brought me some wonderful friends.

With this has come the unpleasant realization that, compared to other fields, there seems to be so much controversy, emotion-laden debate, and division within the community surrounding ASD. There is ongoing controversy about defining autism as an epidemic and to what extent environmental events are causal. There is disagreement about the utility of alternative medicine and holistic approaches to treat autism. There are arguments about separating "high-functioning" from "low-functioning" people on the spectrum, in terms of definition and eligibility for resources and services. Related to that was a struggle over use of the word *cure* when research funding and treatments are being sought; families of severely affected children cited the pain, suffering, and debilitation they witnessed in their loved ones as a reason to seek a cure, when cognitively able adults argued that being on the autism spectrum has brought them unique qualities and talents, and the idea of a cure was offensive to them because it would mean a sacrifice of their individuality. Some resolution has been found in the call for autism *acceptance* and the growing popularity of the term *neurodiversity,* which acknowledges the need for society to embrace people with all types of neurobehavioral profiles, but unrest continues. A recent example is seen as people grapple with the elimination of the term *Asperger's* from DSM nomenclature. Many adults, who had finally found a home in the world of support/advocacy networks based on that term, became terrified they would be thrown back out into the cold world where they were sorely misunderstood.

As a clinical psychologist, I remain apolitical in this community. I may have many tasks and roles, but I have only one objective, which I have held since the earliest days of my doctoral training: *to help patients reduce their psychological distress by using scientifically based interventions.* I would apply that principle in my work with any patient, regardless of the form or severity of distress presented. While working with adults with ASD, there is a particularly delicate balance between the need to target aspects of their functioning that interfere with a sense of well-being and the need to preserve those parts of themselves that constitute unique strengths and assets. As I work to maintain that balance with each of my patients, my goals are based on my long-standing clinical objective, not politics.

When treating mental health problems in any population, such as depression or anxiety, the ultimate wish of the therapist and patient is to *eliminate* the problem or drive it into total remission—the disorder is considered to be completely undesirable. However, I find it difficult to view ASD in this same way because I do not believe the associated phenomena can be totally eliminated in an adult patient, nor do I believe that should be the goal of treatment. A major assumption behind the material I present in this book is that *ASD is driven by an idiosyncratic information-processing system* that leads to numerous negative consequences for the affected individual. The related problems are what bring patients into treatment and indeed must be addressed using the strategies I describe in this book. With that, I also assume that the idiosyncratic information-processing systems associated with ASD are not *universally* faulty. Unconventional ways of looking at the world can be assets to adults with ASD and the people around them. For many, their unique thinking styles have led them to invent effective strategies for coping and adapting to a world that seems strange to them. I agree with Tony Attwood, clinical psychologist and author of this book's foreword, when he tells each of his AS patients that "he or she is not mad, bad, or defective, but has a different way of thinking" (2007, p. 332). This way of thinking, along with a unique interaction style, is intertwined with the individual's personality. It is part of the essence of each individual and has led to the talents, unique abilities, and appealing qualities of the person. To eliminate the ASD would be to eliminate the patient!

A Philosophy of Change

As a result of meeting so many adults with ASD, I have developed a philosophy of change for my work with them. I maintain a strength-based, lifespan developmental perspective as I collaborate with patients to help them *alleviate the distress* that they describe. As with any typical patient in CBT for an anxiety or mood disorder, the therapist's job is to teach the patient to identify and modify the cognitive activity that is causing problems in living, not to change the individual's entire personality. For adults with ASD, this means to:

- Teach new cognitive and behavioral skills that were never learned.
- Teach compensatory strategies for deficits that cannot be changed.
- Facilitate self-acceptance.
- Teach strategies to decrease or prevent symptoms of comorbid mental health problems, such as anxiety disorders and depression.

The Global and Regional Asperger Syndrome Partnership (GRASP) is a support, education, and advocacy network for people with AS. When the founder, Michael John Carley, launched the organization, he defined the mission with a statement that is still relevant and in which therapists can find words of wisdom:

> We will work . . . to teach ourselves, through education and understanding, to maximize the talents brought on by our condition; to harness the unique capabilities and celebrate the accomplishments inherent in our community . . . [and] to minimize the damage brought on by our condition; to reduce the harm caused when our behavior diverges from non-autistic norms. (GRASP, 2003)

When people with ASD find ways to manage their stress, form satisfying relationships, and achieve occupational goals, they continue to have unique ways of processing information. At that point, their uniqueness is something to celebrate. By providing psychotherapy to these individuals, we have the privilege of sharing in that celebration.

CHAPTER 1

Defining Autism Spectrum Disorder in Cognitively Able Adults (Asperger Syndrome)

This chapter introduces the most recent definition and diagnostic criteria for autism spectrum disorder (ASD) and provides the historical context for the *Asperger syndrome* (AS) term that is still used by some. That is followed by a description of how ASD manifests in adulthood and why affected individuals may seek out a psychotherapist. The factors adding to the complexity of the symptom picture in adult ASD are outlined, including differential diagnosis and common myths. To round out the picture of adult ASD, the chapter ends with a discussion of the strengths often seen in these adults and how they may serve to make them particularly responsive to cognitive-behavioral therapy (CBT).

What Is AS and Why Is the Term Still Used?

AS was first recognized in the United States in 1994 when it was introduced as one of the pervasive developmental disorders (PDD) in the fourth edition of the *Diagnostic and Statistical Manual of Mental Disorders* (DSM-IV; American Psychiatric Association, 1994), shortly after it was introduced in the *International Classification of Diseases* (ICD-10; World Health Organization, 1992). Termed *Asperger's disorder* in that volume of DSM (*Asperger syndrome* in ICD), the general features are very similar to the symptoms seen in the longer-known autistic disorder—that is, "impairment in social interaction" and "restricted repetitive patterns of behavior, interests and activities" (p. 77). In contrast to traditional or "classic" definitions of autistic disorder, however, there are no clinically significant delays in cognitive development, language, development of age-appropriate self-help skills, adaptive behavior, or curiosity about the environment. In other words, people with AS are verbal and do not have comorbid intellectual disability (ID), as do many individuals with autism.

Although the concept of AS was new to mental health practitioners in the United States when DSM-IV was published in 1994, it was 50 years old in Europe. Hans Asperger, an Austrian pediatrician, first described a set of features common among a group of his patients in 1944. His German-language manuscript received little attention until 1981, when Lorna Wing connected his descriptions to the cases she was seeing in the United Kingdom (Attwood, 1998; Wing, 1981, 2000). Internationally, there are differing perspectives on the specific criteria to be used when making the diagnosis, but most authors agree that it is on a spectrum with autistic disorder and that it involves severe problems in social perception and behavior that appears in people whose intellectual and language functioning is relatively intact (Attwood, 1998, 2007; Ghaziuddin, 2005; Klin, Volkmar, & Sparrow, 2000; McPartland, Klin, & Volkmar, 2014; Wing, 2000).

Current North American Criteria: DSM-5 and ICD-10

The criticisms of current classification systems for ASD are many and the debates among researchers in the autism field have only intensified since the first edition of this book was published 11 years ago. The most recent controversy, for example, has surrounded the significant changes reflected in the publication of DSM-5 (American Psychiatric Association, 2013); only 19 years after being introduced to the DSM system, the category termed *Asperger's disorder* was removed as a more dimensional system for describing behavioral symptoms and impairment severity was introduced. A single category of autism spectrum disorder is used, with several specifiers allowing the diagnostician to indicate the presence of certain features and to rate severity. The practical implications of this change on any individual vary greatly, depending on the role one plays in the autism community. So, the impact is quite different for each of these players: practitioner, researcher, parent of school-age child, early intervention specialist, special education teacher, young adult with ASD, middle-age adult with ASD, and so on. Because this book is meant to be a clinical manual for practitioners interested in treating cognitively able adults with ASD (AS) and similar conditions, a comprehensive review of the controversies would be outside its scope (for more extensive discussion, see McPartland et al., 2014; Ozonoff, 2012). This section outlines the current diagnostic criteria and highlights the issues that would be relevant to clinical work with adult patients.

Most clinicians serving adults are required to use either DSM-5 or ICD-10 when assigning a diagnosis to a patient. Which system one chooses would depend on the individual circumstances of a case, including the requirements of any third-party payer for the services. For example, many health insurance companies, as well as U.S. government-funded health plans (Medicare, Medicaid) require a clinician to code the treating diagnoses using ICD-10 in order to pay for therapy. On the other hand, adults who are applying for Social Security disability benefits or state-funded vocational assistance may ask a therapist to fill out government forms requiring a DSM diagnosis, though I have observed that such forms have not been updated for DSM-5 (at the time of this writing, many of these forms still ask for DSM-IV classification). Because both systems are in use, clinicians may find themselves referring to the same patient as having ASD or AS interchangeably, depending on the documentation requirements of the service delivery system within which the therapy is being provided. For that reason, a summary of each is presented here.

An abbreviated summary of DSM-5 criteria for ASD is shown in Table 1.1. The reader can refer to DSM-5 (American Psychiatric Association, 2013) for an in-depth description of the symptoms and associated features. Similarly, the diagnostic criteria summary of AS from ICD-10 is presented in Table 1.2, and the reader can find a more detailed description in the primary source (World Health Organization, 1992). Chapter 3 covers the specific assessment approaches that are currently used as best practices for diagnosing ASD in adulthood.

A few points worth noting here in comparing the two systems. First, the two core symptom categories are the same in both systems; affected individuals have *impairments in social communication/social reciprocity,* as well as *restricted, repetitive patterns of behavior and interests.* Second, the two systems differ in that DSM-5 criteria are dimensional while ICD-10 (which is very similar to DSM-IV-TR; American Psychiatric Association, 2000) criteria are categorical. Different manifestations of ASD would be described by *varying severity levels on a scale* in each of the two core symptom areas in DSM-5 (all subjects have the same label, but differ by numbers 1, 2, or 3 assigned on the level of severity scale, with 1 representing mildest and 3 the most severe). Conversely, in the ICD-10 system, different symptom presentations are described by *varying labels* (e.g., subjects would have different labels: autistic disorder vs. AS vs. pervasive developmental disorder not otherwise specified [PDD-NOS]). DSM-5 does require some categorical information in that the clinician is directed to specify the presence or absence of intellectual impairment, as well as the presence or absence of language impairment. However, some flexibility has been built in that it is helpful for clinicians who are diagnosing adults, as the DSM-5 system does allow for a symptom to be counted, whether it appears currently or *by history.* The acknowledgment that symptom presentation may fluctuate across the lifespan is also noted in the third criterion, which describes how some behaviors may be prominent at some points and masked by various factors at other points in a person's life. This is particularly important for clinicians who are working with people who have been alive for several decades!

The remainder of this section is used to comment on two other general issues that can arise with adult patients because of these ever-shifting diagnostic terms. The first is that there have been significant and frequent changes in how ASD has been defined within the lifetimes of adult patients—more so for older adults. Because of this, clinicians commonly see adults who have had *long histories of misdiagnosis* or confusing labels that often did not quite fit the problems they were experiencing. In both the DSM and ICD systems used before the early 1990s, clinicians had only *two* categories to choose from for patients presenting with autism symptoms: autistic disorder and PDD-NOS—as already mentioned, AS did not exist. Then, when AS was introduced, it was presented as one of five PDDs; the umbrella expanded and more verbal and cognitively able people were identified. Now, with the new DSM system, clinicians have *one* category, but more flexibility in applying it, as there is a more dimensional system of symptom identification. The sort of "flip-flopping" of terms over the last 30 years has adversely affected the quality of treatment for adult patients, and clinicians need to be sensitive to the stress this has caused for many.

The second issue relates to concerns that both patients and professionals have about people with AS potentially *losing their identity or being denied access to services* because the AS category does not appear in DSM-5. These are valid concerns and have been the subject of many sessions with my patients as well as conversations with my colleagues.

TABLE 1.1. DSM-5 Criteria for ASD

A. Persistent deficits in social communication and social interaction across multiple contexts, as manifested by the following, currently or by history (examples are illustrative, not exhaustive; see text):

1. Deficits in social–emotional reciprocity, ranging, for example, from abnormal social approach and failure of normal back-and-forth conversation; to reduced sharing of interests, emotions, or affect; to failure to initiate or respond to social interactions.

2. Deficits in nonverbal communicative behaviors used for social interaction, ranging, for example, from poorly integrated verbal and nonverbal communication; to abnormalities in eye contact and body language or deficits in understanding and use of gestures; to a total lack of facial expressions and nonverbal communication.

3. Deficits in developing, maintaining, and understanding relationships, ranging, for example, from difficulties adjusting behavior to suit various social contexts; to difficulties in sharing imaginative play or in making friends; to absence of interest in peers.

   Specify current severity:

   Severity is based on social communication impairments and restricted repetitive patterns of behavior (see Table 2 [on page 52 of DSM-5]).

B. Restricted, repetitive patterns of behavior, interests, or activities, as manifested by at least two of the following, currently or by history (examples are illustrative, not exhaustive; see text):

1. Stereotyped or repetitive motor movements, use of objects, or speech (e.g., simple motor stereotypies, lining up toys or flipping objects, echolalia, idiosyncratic phrases).

2. Insistence on sameness, inflexible adherence to routines, or ritualized patterns of verbal or nonverbal behavior (e.g., extreme distress at small changes, difficulties with transitions, rigid thinking patterns, greeting rituals, need to take same route or eat same food every day).

3. Highly restricted, fixated interests that are abnormal in intensity or focus (e.g., strong attachment to or preoccupation with unusual objects, excessively circumscribed or perseverative interests).

4. Hyper- or hyporeactivity to sensory input or unusual interest in sensory aspects of the environment (e.g., apparent indifference to pain/temperature, adverse response to specific sounds or textures, excessive smelling or touching of objects, visual fascination with lights or movement).

   Specify current severity:

   Severity is based on social communication impairments and restricted, repetitive patterns of behavior (see Table 2 [on page 52 of DSM-5]).

C. Symptoms must be present in the early developmental period (but may not become fully manifest until social demands exceed limited capacities, or may be masked by learned strategies in later life).

D. Symptoms cause clinically significant impairment in social, occupational, or other important areas of current functioning.

E. These disturbances are not better explained by intellectual disability (intellectual developmental disorder) or global developmental delay. Intellectual disability and autism spectrum disorder frequently co-occur; to make comorbid diagnoses of autism spectrum disorder and intellectual disability, social communication should be below that expected for general developmental level.

Note. Reprinted with permission from the *Diagnostic and Statistical Manual of Mental Disorders, Fifth Edition.* Copyright © 2013 the American Psychiatric Association. All rights reserved.

TABLE 1.2. Summary of ICD-10 Criteria for Asperger's Syndrome

1. *Lack of clinically significant delay in language or cognitive development; self-help skills and adaptive behavior during first 3 years appear normal.*

2. *Abnormalities in reciprocal social interaction*—at least one of the following:
   - Inadequate use of eye-to-eye gaze, facial expression, body posture, and gesture to regulate social interactions
   - Lack of peer relationships involving sharing of interests, activities, and emotions
   - Lack of social–emotional reciprocity (e.g., impaired response to the emotions of others; failure to modulate behavior according to context; weak integration of social, emotional, and communicative behaviors)

3. *Restricted, repetitive, stereotyped patterns of behavior, interests, or activities*—at least two of the following:
   - Restricted interests, abnormal in terms of intensity, content, circumscribed nature, or focus
   - Compulsive adherence to nonfunctional routines or rituals
   - Stereotyped or repetitive motor movements (e.g., hand or finger flapping, twisting, or whole-body movements)
   - Preoccupation with parts of objects or nonfunctional aspects of play materials
   - Distress appears with small changes in the environment

4. *Not attributable to other pervasive developmental disorders or mental disorders (e.g., schizotypal, schizophrenia, reactive and disinhibited attachment disorder, obsessional panic disorder, or obsessive–compulsive disorder).*

Note. Adapted with permission from *The ICD-10 Classification of Mental and Behavioural Disorders: Diagnostic Criteria for Research* (World Health Organization, 1993).

I am happy to share that I have been reassured by several factors in the 4 years that have passed since the publication of DSM-5 and the time of this writing. The first was already mentioned: AS still appears in ICD-10, a system that therapists are often called to use by third-party payers. Inspection of the criteria shows that the description is very similar to that of DSM-IV-defined AS. For situations where DSM-5 is required or chosen by a therapist, there is a note that appears in that volume that says, "Individuals with a well-established DMS-IV diagnosis of . . . Asperger's disorder . . . should be given the diagnosis of autism spectrum disorder" (American Psychiatric Association, 2013, p. 51). In other words, a provision is there to ensure that any previously diagnosed person will not be left without an ASD diagnosis, as some patients of mine had feared. My confidence that no legitimate case of AS will be excluded from the new ASD definition has some empirical support, as well. Wilson and colleagues (2013) used a sample of 150 adults in the United Kingdom who met ICD-10 criteria for an ASD and compared the diagnostic outcomes of each case using DSM-IV-TR and DSM-5. By taking full advantage of the flexibility that is offered in the DSM-5 description (symptoms can be observed currently or by history) and using the least stringent coding methods regarding symptoms that may have been present historically, 98% of the subjects who met ICD-10 criteria for AS also met DSM-5 criteria for ASD. Using a less stringent method is often necessary when diagnosing adults, as it is not always possible to get all the details of their early developmental histories.

As mentioned previously, the struggles we face in trying to standardize our language for describing the complexities of ASD are likely to continue for decades to come. In the meantime, readers are among a growing set of practitioners who are trying to help these adults every day as they appear in psychotherapy offices and clinics across the country. No matter which specific terms are used to define the social and behavioral problems seen in the adult patients described in this book, I encourage the use of an individualized approach to treatment plan design and intervention. I see no reason why we cannot continue to do that even though our past, present, and future classification systems are imperfect. Furthermore, while Asperger's disorder no longer appears in DSM, it cannot be erased from the collective consciousness of our community. In the United States, it has become a "household word" with which many people have become quite familiar, as there are numerous fictional characters that have appeared in countless television shows and movies since the first edition of this book. Patients who have come to identify strongly with the *Asperger* term can be assured that it will not disappear just because of DSM-5.

How Does ASD Present in Adulthood?

The purpose of this section is to familiarize readers with the various ways in which ASD may present in adults who are seeking help in treatment settings. The prevalence of such cases in the general population is useful to know so that clinicians have a sense of how frequently a person with this diagnosis may show up in practice settings where adults are served. Unfortunately, there is a paucity of data on the epidemiology of adult ASD. Prevalence studies are clouded by inconsistencies in how ASD is classified, and most large-scale studies are based on child samples. We can only make inferences about the U.S. population of adults with ASD by looking at child data on all the ASD and adult prevalence reports from outside the United States. The most recent estimate published by Christensen and colleagues (2016) in the United States for all ASD was 14.6 per 1,000 (1 in 68) children across a multisite study conducted in 2012. Of the ASD sample, 10% met criteria for AS (DSM-IV-TR) specifically, which converts to about 1.5 per 1,000 (1 in 680). When the absence of ID was used as the defining factor, 68% of the ASD sample were represented, which converts to 4 per 1,000 (1 in 250) children having an ASD without ID (IQ $\geq$ 70). In a child study conducted in Finland that focused on AS specifically (Mattila et al., 2007), the rates were estimated to be 2.9 per 1,000 (1 in 344) when ICD-10 criteria were used. For adult ASD, the only recent comprehensive study was conducted in the United Kingdom by Brugha and colleagues (2011) and estimated that in the populations of adults living in the community, approximately 9.8 per 1,000 meet criteria for an ASD in general, or about 1 in 102. Subtype data were not available for this sample. Because we know that children with ASD do not just "grow out of it," we can assume from these data, as variable as the estimated rates are, that there is a fair number of adults living in our communities with these issues who do not have ID, but do have enough daily problems to compel them to appear in therapist offices for help. (see Maddox & Gaus, 2018, for a more extensive discussion).

Gender/Sex

Our access to an accurate ratio of male-to-female cases is also limited because the classification problems mentioned above are compounded by questions about gender differences in symptom manifestation and identification biases (Koenig & Tsatsanis,

2005; Kreiser & White, 2014; Lai, Baron-Cohen, & Buxbaum, 2015; Wilson et al., 2016). Generally speaking, all epidemiological studies have shown a higher incidence of male cases of ASD compared to female cases. The specific ratios have varied greatly across studies, however, from as high as 16:1 to as low as 2:1 (as reviewed by Kreiser & White, 2014; Lai et al., 2015). Recent child studies conducted by Christensen and colleagues (2016) found an overall ratio of boys to girls to be 4.5:1 for all ASD. Most relevant to the subject of this book was a study conducted in the United Kingdom with adults not previously diagnosed with ASD—in the investigators' analysis of people who met criteria for ASD without co-occurring ID, the male-to-female ratio was found to be 3.4:1 (Wilson et al., 2016).

Many researchers are suggesting that the gender differences cited above do not reflect true prevalence and that the male-to-female ratios reported would not be as high if several problems were to be addressed (Kreiser & White, 2014; Lai et al., 2015; Wilson et al., 2016). The theoretical and practical explanations for exaggerated prevalence differences involve many factors, but all surround the idea that *truly affected females are underrepresented in study samples,* not that males are overrepresented. Highlighting the most recent literature on this, Kreiser and White (2014) review the biogenetic explanatory models that have been offered by autism researchers for the gender/sex differences observed in ASD, including the brain differences model (e.g., assuming differences in brain structure, brain circuitry, and hormones account for different prevalence rates), greater variability model (e.g., assuming males have a genetic vulnerability to develop ASD), and liability/threshold model (assuming females have built-in compensatory mechanisms that cause the threshold for visible impairment to be higher than in males). These authors go on to suggest that while biogenetic factors may account for some of the variance observed in the male-to-female prevalence rates, there are likely social and cultural factors that inflate the disparity between male and female incidence reports. The two main categories of factors are (1) biases in research methods and diagnostic criteria and (2) nonbiological influences (sociocultural, familial, intrapersonal) on the unique manifestation of symptoms in females that cause their presence to be missed or downplayed by others.

Biases in epidemiological research, for example, lie in the common method of using convenience samples—studying cases that have already appeared in clinical settings. Because boys with ASD are more likely to be referred for services than girls (due to more disruptive and aggressive manifestation of ASD symptoms), females are underrepresented in these studies. Moreover, while both genders are experiencing the same core problems, the different phenotypical expression has biased our diagnostic criteria; the way we define and describe the phenomenon has been more heavily influenced by male cases. In a reciprocal bias process, the samples that inform our diagnostic system design have been mostly male, so the male manifestation has shaped how we define the disorder in general, further causing the female variation to be left out of the diagnostic system, further causing females to be left out of research because they do not meet the criteria, further causing the ongoing development and modification of diagnostic criteria to be based on biased samples—and on and on.

Keiser and White (2014) provide a schema for understanding the way biogenetic factors of female ASD develop into a unique manifestation of symptoms because of a complex array of gender-specific behavioral norms/expectations inherent in sociocultural systems (from school, community, ethnic group), familial systems (from home), and intrapersonal systems (from the individual's motivational, emotional, cognitive processes during development of socialization behaviors). All of these factors interplay to lead females with ASD to be more likely to develop compensatory strategies that mask their deficits enough to "get by" in the eyes of others, but which are not conducive to healthy social or emotional development. It has been reported that these girls are more likely to develop passive personalities, struggle with more internalizing problems, and be more prone to comorbid depression.

For the present purposes, suffice it to say that clinicians who are treating adults may see one woman with ASD for every two to three men, keeping in mind that the ASD symptoms may look different and be compounded by comorbid conditions.

Race/Ethnicity

Epidemiological studies in children have consistently shown disparities in the prevalence rates of ASD between various racial and ethnic groups (Durkin et al., 2017). The general trend noted in both U.S. and European studies is that ASD rates are higher within white-majority groups and lower within ethnic-minority groups (Begeer, El Bouk, Boussaid, Terwogt, & Koot, 2009; Christensen et al., 2016). The most recent Christensen and colleagues (2016) multisite study of 8-year-old children showed that the rates of ASD were highest in non-Hispanic white children (15.5 per 1,000), a significant difference compared to non-Hispanic black children (13.2 per 1,000), Asian/ Pacific Islander children (11.3 per 1,000), and Hispanic children (10.1 per 1,000).

Research that will help us understand the causes of these differences and the true prevalence of ASD in ethnic minorities is only in its infancy. Durkin and colleagues (2017) explored the hypothesis that socioeconomic status (SES) accounts for these differences. Considering that people in higher-SES groups would have more access to information, resources, and quality medical care, a child with ASD is more likely to be identified and treated than a child who may be struggling with ASD within a lower-SES family and community. Durkin and colleagues found that when they statistically controlled the SES factors, disparities between ethnic groups still showed up, suggesting that it is not that simple. While SES undoubtedly has some influence, other factors that are being discussed and explored in the field are biased assessment instruments (Harrison, Long, Tommet, & Jones, 2017), protective factors associated with some ethnic communities (Palmer, Walker, Mandell, Bayles, & Miller, 2010; Ratto, Anthony, et al., 2016), culturally influenced variations in parental perception, and description of child behavior/symptoms (Ratto, Reznick, & Turner-Brown, 2016).

Though we have almost no research to rely on, clinicians treating adult patients from ethnic-minority groups should consider that these individuals may have had unique experiences with their ASD identification and diagnosis as compared to non-Hispanic white patients.

Age and Cohort Issues

Since the first introduction of AS into North American classification systems, the attention paid to it in research and practice has primarily focused on children. It is a developmental disorder (DD) involving problems that usually first appear in children, so it makes obvious sense to channel resources into understanding early developmental processes and to intervene in a proactive way early in life. However, people born before the mid-1970s who currently meet criteria for AS or ASD without ID were already adults before the syndrome was made known in 1994 to the mental health community in the United States. They are at a particular disadvantage because their problems were not diagnosed and treated properly when they were children, yet they need effective therapeutic supports as much as today's newly diagnosed youngsters. When these individuals were children, they presented differently from their counterparts with the more familiar or "classic" autistic disorder of the 1950s, 1960s, and 1970s, the latter being mostly nonverbal, unresponsive to other people, and having ID. The more cognitively able children with ASD had average to superior intelligence and advanced verbal skills, were often academically successful, and had intense interests in certain topics (e.g., astronomy, insects, trains). This presentation (sometimes referred to as the "little professor syndrome") may have been endearing to parents and some teachers, but these children were typically disliked by their peers. They were plagued by anxiety, subject to anger outbursts, and sometimes classified in the education system as "emotionally disturbed," but in those earlier decades less likely to have been identified as having a DD. In fact, their profiles did not clearly fit any diagnostic category during the 40-year span between the 1950s and 1990s in the U.S. classification system. They have therefore lived most of their lives with an array of problems but without a diagnosis, or worse, with the wrong diagnosis. They have missed out on the benefits that educational and therapeutic programs designed to meet their needs would have brought them, and therefore are at a greater risk for problems in adulthood.

As mentioned, research studies on adults have not been nearly as many as those on children. Looking at the numbers of studies done on ASD in general, Cottle, McMahon, and Farley (2016) illustrated how the trend of growth in research has increased dramatically over the past two decades, but the number of studies done on adult ASD has not grown at nearly the same rate. Worse yet, there has been almost no focus on cohort effects or the needs of people with ASD in mid to later life (Wright & Wadsworth, 2016). For example, older adults who rely heavily on their parents are facing major losses of support as their caregivers age and die. Others are themselves becoming caregivers as their parents lose independence and need more help from them.

As an informal observation, I have noticed over the past 10 years an increase of attention by advocacy and support communities on the needs of adults, which has been pleasing. At the same time, I have been disappointed that there has been a bias toward offering help and resources to *young* adults without much mention of the needs of people who are 30 years old and up. To make a point in a discussion published elsewhere (Gaus, 2016), I sampled my caseload by looking at all the clinical contacts I had with patients meeting criteria for AS or ASD without ID within a 2-year period. Of the 68 cases, the age range was 19–77 years. Less than half of these cases were young adults (29, or 43%, were under 30). Of the 39 cases (57% of my cases) that were 30 years old or more, 24 (35% of the whole ASD caseload) were 40 or older, and 15 of those (22% of the whole ASD caseload) were 50 or older. While this is only a rough sketch of how ages are represented in one clinician's caseload in a specific setting and geographical region, it illustrates the fact that adults of all ages can appear in clinicians' offices.

Different age groups may present with different types of problems, partly because of cohort effects (e.g., inadequate support and education for earlier-born cohorts, technology influences on later-born cohorts) and partly because the types of stressors patients contend with are different depending on life stage (e.g., pressures on a 24-year-old are different from those on a 50-year-old). The case examples in this book illustrate some of these issues. To conclude this section, clinicians serving the adult ASD population can expect to see a heterogeneous collection of problems given the wide age range across the adult lifespan.

Presenting Problems

Psychotherapy is becoming more widely perceived as a viable treatment modality for individuals with ASD (Attwood, 2007; Gaus, 2011; Jacobsen, 2003; Koenig & Levine, 2011; Volkmar, Klin, & McPartland, 2014). To illustrate the multitude of symptom profiles a therapist may encounter and the wide variety of reasons an adult may seek treatment, I describe several case examples of patients as they presented at their intakes in my practice. These individuals are introduced before the theoretical and empirically supported explanations for the adult ASD symptom picture are presented, as a way to simulate the order of events in a practical setting. After all, a therapist usually meets and talks with a person who has a name and face *before* conceptualizing the reasons behind his or her problems. These individuals were selected because their symptom presentations are heterogeneous, and their primary complaints are representative of the common difficulties a therapist will observe in this population. Each case description is followed by a brief discussion of how it illustrates a unique manifestation of ASD. Please keep in mind that a *full evaluation was necessary for each before confirmation of the diagnosis could be made*; the information contained in these summaries is insufficient to diagnose ASD with certainty. The purpose of this section is to familiarize the reader with some of the clues that can appear during an intake. Details on conducting a comprehensive assessment, obtaining a diagnosis, and providing treatment for individuals with ASD are provided later in the book. The descriptions begin with Joe, my very first encounter with AS.

Joe: Severe Regression in Functioning Triggered by Stressful Life Event

Joe is a 55-year-old single Latin American man who was referred to the therapist by his brother, who had become concerned about him because Joe had been suddenly evicted from his apartment. This turn of events raised questions about his mental status and ability to care for himself. His brother had recently read an article about AS and connected the description to Joe.

Joe has a master's degree in engineering and has worked in that field in one company for more than 25 years. He has lived alone in the same apartment in New York City for the past 18 years without incident. His eviction was a shock to his family because they had seen no warning signs. After checking into the reason for the eviction, his brother found out that Joe's apartment building had been sold to a new management company many months before. Because the change in management required Joe to write and send his rent check to a new place, he just stopped paying. Numerous notices and warnings that came in the mail were ignored by Joe, who simply stacked them neatly in a drawer.

His brother reported that Joe had always been a "loner," "a little odd," and "rigid." However, he was able to succeed in college and graduate school, get and keep a job, and live on his own without assistance. His siblings were in the habit of checking on him by phone on a weekly basis, although Joe never initiated contact with them. He never complained of any distress, there was no history of psychiatric illness, and no problems at work; he always received positive performance reviews from his supervisors. His family sometimes had minor concerns that his life was "boring" because he carried out exactly the same routine every day and had no friends or girlfriends. He did have a passionate interest in wild birds and spent his free time pursuing the subject by going to the library or watching documentaries on television. Because he never complained, the family assumed he was content.

At intake, Joe demonstrated flat affect, spoke in a monotone, and avoided eye contact. However, he articulately described feeling distraught about the incident, expressing shame and anger at himself for having handled the situation so poorly. He reported that he had felt very nervous by the change in building management companies, and this nervousness made him avoid writing the rent checks. When he began receiving the warning notices, he became so frightened that he did not know what to do and was afraid to tell his family about the problem. The worse the problem got, the more he avoided taking steps to address it.

Joe's intake description highlights some of the DSM-5 symptoms for ASD without ID (and ICD-10 symptoms for AS), presented earlier in the chapter. His "inflexible adherence to routines" could be seen in his total inability to shift his rent-paying routine and to practice adaptive problem solving when he received eviction warnings. Joe also demonstrated "restricted, fixated interests": his leisure activities focused solely on wild birds. In the social communication domain, he demonstrated a "deficit in developing, maintaining and understanding relationships" and "deficits in social–emotional reciprocity" in the way he interacted with his family as well as the therapist (American Psychiatric Association, 2013, p. 50).

Joe's case illustrates one common reason cognitively able adults with ASD are referred to psychotherapy: *a regression in functioning triggered by a stressful life event* or major change in circumstances. This also relates to issues commonly seen in *older adults*. Like Joe, many adults with ASD can achieve a high level of education and function adequately in a predictable, structured, and restricted set of circumstances. However, they may demonstrate *poor judgment* and *lack of problem-solving ability* when faced with an unexpected change. In lay terms, family members may complain that the individual seems to have "no common sense." A stressful shift in circumstances may occur in the individual's environment, as it did in Joe's case; other times a natural developmental change, such as the transition from adolescence to adulthood, can trigger the regression. The next case, Lorraine, is an example of this.

Lorraine: Frustration over Lack of Independence

Lorraine is a 22-year-old white Catholic woman who attends a community college on a part-time basis and lives with her mother, father, and one sister. She was diagnosed with PDD-NOS, as per DSM-III-R at the time (DSM-III-R; American Psychiatric Association, 1987), when she was in preschool, but a psychiatrist had more recently changed her diagnosis to AS (as per DSM-IV-TR). Lorraine was referred to therapy by her parents, who had growing concerns about her low frustration tolerance and anger outbursts. She agreed to meet the therapist because she wanted to learn to be more assertive and less dependent on her parents.

Lorraine's frustration had been increasing around her schoolwork. For all college classes she has taken to date, she has had to rely on a *scribe,* a person assigned to take notes in class and take dictation from her on written assignments. This special education accommodation was necessary because she had fine motor problems that significantly impaired her handwriting capacity. In recent months, her mother was acting as the scribe because her school had not been able to find one for her. This level of interaction was increasing the tension between them; Lorraine would often end study sessions by screaming, and during one episode she pinched her mother. She frequently stated that she was "tired of needing help" and concerned that the college credits earned thus far were not legitimate but really "belong to my mother."

Lorraine's parents reported that she had significant "autistic signs" since preschool, including unusual use of language, social detachment, severe tantrums, distress with changes, and hyperactivity. She steadily improved as she developed, and her parents attribute her success to the special education supports she received, such as intensive speech–language therapy. They have always considered her education a high priority, and they often had to legally challenge their school district for specialized services that were not readily offered to Lorraine. Her parents personally funded additional supports outside of school, most importantly by enrolling her in a therapeutic horseback riding program when she was 6 years old. Not only did this activity help her develop gross motor skills, ability to focus, and self-confidence, but she enjoyed it more than any other. As an adolescent, she began to ride in competitions, and at the time of intake, had been the sole owner of a horse for 3 years.

Lorraine's intake took place across two sessions. She came to the first with her parents and chose to have them remain with her for the entire session. Lorraine presented as a pretty woman who was well groomed and dressed neatly in an athletic outfit. She made eye contact when she shook the therapist's hand, but avoided it for the rest of the session, and her affect appeared consistently flat. Lorraine played a passive role as she looked to her parents to answer many of the therapist's questions. When she returned for a second interview by herself, her affect and expressions were as flat as before. She spoke very slowly with a low volume but clear articulation. She did not look at the therapist and there was a long delay between each question and her answer, but she appeared to carefully consider each one, and her answers were appropriately related. She reported that she felt appreciative of the support her parents had given her over the years but frustrated that she was still so reliant on them. She was in a 1-year-long relationship with a boyfriend (whom she described as "on the autism spectrum, too") and was enjoying the time spent with him outside of her parents' home. She wanted therapy to help her become more independent and more "in control" of her anger because her "yelling" was starting to bother her boyfriend. Throughout the session she looked down, as she sat with one foot on her knee and repeatedly ran her hand back and forth over the tread on the bottom of her sneaker. Twice during the interview, she directed the therapist's attention to the shoe and pointed out all of the special features in the design. She was slow to return to the topic when the therapist redirected her because she was intent on describing the sneaker, its unique qualities, and where it was manufactured. As she was exiting the office at the end of the session, she suddenly turned around and hugged the therapist, but with a flat facial expression and no eye contact.

Although Lorraine's parent-reported history indicated that she had more severe problems with social interaction and behavior as a child, she continued to demonstrate clinically significant symptoms of ASD (DSM-5 defined) as an adult. Some of the symptoms that were present in her current life, as per her and the parents' report, were observable during the intake sessions. Her poor eye contact and flat affect were examples of "deficits in nonverbal communicative behaviors used for social interaction." The delayed responses to the therapist's questions, difficulty returning to the topic when prompted, and the spontaneous hug (mood incongruent and socially out of context) were examples of "deficits in social–emotional reciprocity." Her intense focus on the details of her sneakers was an example of "preoccupation with unusual objects" as well as "unusual interest in sensory aspects of the environment" (American Psychiatric Association, 2013, p. 50). Poor handwriting skills represented motor coordination problems that are commonly associated features of ASD.

Many young adults with ASD share Lorraine's *frustration over lack of independence.* Their symptoms interfere with the ability to achieve occupational and financial independence, so they must rely on others to complete many activities of daily living. Young adulthood can be a particularly painful time for individuals with ASD and their families because the transition brings about changes that highlight the individual's disability. Typically developing people begin to take steps to leave the family home and pursue an occupation during the late teens and early 20s. Individuals with ASD who have had academic success in the structure of a high school environment, with or without special education supports, are often presumed to be ready for college or work at the same point as their typical peers. However, the changes in environment, schedule, and task demands that come with campus or work life often prove too drastic for individuals with ASD. When they find themselves struggling with tasks that they assumed would come easy, they and their families suffer confusion, disappointment, and frustration.

A different type of life-stage transition problem is illustrated in the next case. Carl is an older adult whose symptoms became most apparent only after the death of his mother.

Carl: Later-Life Diagnosis Prompted by Increased Support Needs

Carl is a 62-year-old single white man who lives alone in a house that he owns. He is not and never has been employed. He was referred to therapy by his psychiatrist following an incident in which he had threatened an in-home visiting nurse by pointing scissors at her. It was hoped that CBT may be helpful to address an increase in angry outbursts and other daily living problems.

Carl had been diagnosed with AS at age 59 (as per DSM-IV-TR) as part of an assessment of functioning completed for a guardianship evaluation. His IQ falls within the average range, though he has significant deficits in adaptive behavior, especially in the domains of health and safety, leisure, self-direction, and social functioning. He has cerebral palsy, which is secondary to congenital hydrocephalus. This causes him to walk with a significant limp, have a need to wear orthopedic shoes, and to have limited use of his right arm and hand. He also has diabetes, which is controlled by oral medication and diet.

Carl's mother had died about 12 years before. He has no family living nearby, but his cousin who lives in a different state is his legal guardian. She manages most of his affairs remotely by maintaining daily phone calls and making quarterly visits. He has a visiting nurse service, with one nurse making monthly visits, and daily assistance from a home health aide. Carl's cousin had applied for legal guardianship approximately 3 years prior, after Carl's dire circumstances were brought to her attention. She was contacted because she was Carl's only living relative when his house was about to be seized due to a large debt of back property taxes. She had not been involved in Carl's life because she lived so far away, but came for a visit when she learned of this urgent situation. What she found was that the house was in horrendous condition because Carl had been engaging in severe hoarding behaviors for close to 9 years, since his mother had passed away. He was not caring for the property or for himself, as he was also found to be in very poor health. At this point, it became clear that Carl's mother, who had cared for him his whole life, had been essential in compensating for his disabilities. When she died, no one knew that Carl had such deficits in independent living skills because he knew just enough to get by. Because he never had visitors, no one knew how poorly he was living. Carl was fortunate to have his cousin because she got right to work on helping him to stay in his house and improve his lifestyle. She and her husband took on the task of getting the house cleaned, obtaining guardianship, and bringing in the visiting nurse service to help him with his daily needs. Significant improvements were made in his life in a relatively short period of time. At the time of intake, he had already been enrolled in state-funded case management services for developmentally disabled adults and had been assigned a case manager (a.k.a., service coordinator). In addition, his case had ongoing monitoring of a surrogate court because he was not his own guardian, but was living on his own.

In the initial interview, Carl was pleasant and used humor to engage with the therapist. His jokes involved a lot of puns and plays on words. He elaborated on his lifelong hobby, which is learning about the work of the famous jeweler Fabergé. It was obvious that he had an elaborate knowledge base about the artist's life and pieces. He reported that his biggest problem was the nurse who visited him every month. He said she was pushy and nosy and he wished she would stop coming. He seemed to have a positive relationship with his cousin and the home health aide. He moved very slowly and at times appeared to be in pain (winced when he moved his leg), though he denied having any physical discomfort. He was very interested in the therapist's resident cat and dog, and told several stories about pets he had owned throughout his life. He repeated each story more than once and was not responsive to the therapist's nonverbal as well as verbal redirection attempts. At times he would say, "I know I told this story already . . . ," but would continue to tell it again with the exact same phrases and jokes as the previous time. Carl's cousin was able to send ahead summaries of his history, and also to be interviewed as part of the intake. Her most immediate concerns were around the increase in frequency of angry outbursts, overspending/compulsive purchasing of lottery tickets, and ongoing procrastination on self-care and housekeeping tasks.

Carl's symptoms and behavior during the initial interview illustrate several DSM-5-defined criteria for ASD without ID (or ICD-10-defined AS). Across his life, he failed to make his own friends or progress in "developing, maintaining, and understanding relationships." His perseverative storytelling style demonstrated both "deficits in social–emotional reciprocity" and "deficits in nonverbal communicative behaviors." His lifelong focus on Fabergé illustrates "highly restricted, fixated interests." In addition, Carl's compulsive lottery-ticket purchases would need to be explored further as a possible ASD symptom (e.g., ritualized patterns of behavior) and his denial of pain, despite wincing during the interview (also requiring further assessment), may be a symptom of hyporeactivity to sensory input as "apparent indifference to pain" (American Psychiatric Association, 2013, p. 50).

Carl's case illustrates several common problems faced by adults with ASD in *later life*. His access to professional supports was deferred for many years, as his mother ensured that his needs were met, which allowed him to live through most of his adult life in the community where he grew up. It was not until she was gone that his independent living skill deficits became problematic for him, but not immediately enough to prevent a decline in the condition of his home and personal health. Similar to Joe's case that was presented earlier, a fiscal crisis brought the aid of a family member and ultimately, professionals. Late diagnosis was a central part of Carl's story, as it is in the next case of Rachel.

Rachel: Late Diagnosis After a Long History of Misdiagnoses

Rachel is a 36-year-old single white woman who has a BA in English literature, is unemployed, and lives with her mother. She was referred to therapy as a result of a comprehensive psychological evaluation during which she was diagnosed for the first time with AS (as per DSM-IV-TR). The evaluation was completed at an autism specialty center only 3 weeks before intake, and she was looking for CBT in order to understand and come to terms with her new diagnosis.

Rachel reported a strong sense of relief at her diagnosis, as she had a long history of other diagnoses, none of which led to any effective treatment (e.g., obsessive–compulsive disorder [OCD], bipolar disorder, social phobia, schizophrenia). Her own research had led to the identification of AS and she self-referred to the diagnostic evaluation. Along with relief and a sense of vindication for her long-held belief that she had been mislabeled by educators and clinicians, she was also struggling with anger and sadness over not getting proper help much earlier in her life. Confusion over setting life goals and communicating her wishes to her mother were the most immediate stressors she wanted to address in therapy.

Information about Rachel's history came from her, her mother, and the report that generated from her recent evaluation. She had lifelong problems with anxiety, social relationships, behavioral rigidity, and sensory sensitivity, evidenced as early as 2 years of age. Verbal behavior fluctuated between being overly talkative to being almost nonverbal. She became highly upset when routines would change and would cling desperately to her own established schedules and rituals. Though she performed well in many academic subjects, she was very anxious about going to school and even went through a period of school refusal during middle school. Labeled by various family members as "difficult," "attention seeking," and "a drama queen," Rachel reported feeling misunderstood by most people. She had no siblings and her parents divorced when she was still a child. She stayed with her mother, who has always been a strong source of support. She was successful and reported feeling happy at times during college, once she found a niche with a major she liked and professors she trusted. The years after graduating were marked by frequent job changes, living situations, unstable relationships, and multiple major depressive episodes. Finally, when she was in her early 30s, Rachel moved back in with her mother and withdrew from all activities outside the home. It was during that period that she was researching possible causes for her sensory sensitivity to certain smells and stumbled on a description of AS.

Rachel came to the intake interview dressed in dark-colored, loose-fitting sweats. She sat in a slouched position and made only fleeting eye contact. Though she initially appeared sullen, her speech was rapid and energized, at times even pressured. Her animated verbal behavior was not matched by any nonverbal signs; her lack of gestures or body movements seemed incongruent with her speech. Her answers to questions were on-topic and relevant, but highly detailed. Her mother joined part of the session. Rachel did use more eye contact and nonverbal communication with her. While the two agreed that they argue quite often about Rachel's current lifestyle and seeming lack of goals, they appeared to have a close and caring relationship.

Rachel's evaluation took place when DSM-IV-TR was still in use and she clearly met criteria for AS. If we use DSM-5 terminology, she meets criteria for ASD without ID. Examples of how her symptoms were shown through her history, as well as in the interview, include deficits in social communication, such as "reduced sharing of interests," "poorly integrated verbal and nonverbal communication," and problems with "developing, maintaining, and understanding relationships." In the restricted and repetitive patterns of behavior domain, she showed "inflexible adherence to routine" in childhood as well as adulthood. Finally, one of her most prominent sets of daily living problems surround "hypersensitivity to sensory input," particularly tactile (driving her clothing choices), olfactory, and auditory (American Psychiatric Association, 2013, p. 50).

Rachel's case of *late diagnosis after a long history of misdiagnoses* is a perfect illustration of the consequences faced by bright and verbal girls whose ASD was not identified properly in childhood. This is an example of a *female with true ASD* who is left out of the research on clinic samples, as I discussed in an earlier section of this chapter. While Rachel's determination to find the right help for herself is a sign of one of her many strengths, she suffered unnecessarily for many years. The lack of guidance she received caused a long delay in mapping out a viable career path for herself, as she felt for many years that her talents and abilities were being underutilized. Rachel's job instability and significant *underemployment* is one of the most pervasive problems faced by adults with ASD. The next case, Rose, is another illustration of this problem.

Rose: Frustration over Occupational Problems

Rose is a 41-year-old single Irish American Catholic woman who was referred to therapy by her case manager because of a recent increase in angry outbursts and anxiety. Rose also has a long history of socially inappropriate behavior that has interfered with her occupational functioning. She lives with five other people in a group home for adults with developmental disabilities. The most recent psychological evaluation completed for Rose listed her diagnosis as PDD-NOS (as per DSM-IV-TR). She is unemployed and attends a full-time prevocational training program.

Rose's expressions of anger, which involve frequent episodes of screaming and occasionally include physical aggression toward others (shoving, punching), began approximately 6 months ago, soon after she was asked to resign from her job. She was employed in the clothing fitting room of a department store for 1 year. Her work was overseen by a job coach who periodically visited the store, interfaced with the employer, and provided her with guidance and feedback. Her performance was hindered by a number of repetitive behaviors about which her employer expressed concern. She tended to leave her work area without permission, walk around the store conversing with coworkers and customers, often using intrusive methods to initiate conversations (e.g., loudly interrupting, asking personal questions). Despite the support and direction provided by her job coach around these issues, she continued to demonstrate the interfering behaviors, and the employer asked her to resign. This was the second retail job she had held within the past 5 years; she had previously been asked to resign after 2 years in another department store for similar reasons. Because of this pattern, she was not set up with another job. Instead, Rose was referred to a prevocational day program, with the goal of teaching her social skills and strategies for impulse control. She has been attending regularly for the past 6 months, but expresses great dissatisfaction with the program and wishes to return to work.

Rose's mother reported that Rose had developmental problems since infancy, including swallowing problems, difficulty reciprocating affection, delayed language development, problems developing peer relationships, and difficulty with changes in routines or schedules. She was diagnosed with "minimal brain damage" by a neurologist and later classified with "mental retardation" by her school district because she was placed in special education when she entered kindergarten. Her education through 12th grade was marked by numerous changes in school and classroom settings because she did not appear to "fit in" anywhere. For example, she functioned at a higher intellectual level than her peers when placed in classes for students with ID, and she would become easily bored by the work. When placed in classes for "emotionally disturbed" students, she was given academic work more suited to her cognitive ability, but her lack of social skills contributed to poor relationships with peers and she was constantly "picked on." After graduating from high school, she continued to live with her parents and attended various vocational training programs, succeeding occasionally at temporary or seasonal retail jobs. She had numerous psychological evaluations throughout adulthood, all of which reported Rose's Full Scale IQ to be in the borderline range of intellectual functioning, with a significant difference (> 20 points) between Verbal (low-average range) and Performance (mild ID range) IQ scores. When she was 27, it was finally suggested by one psychologist that her symptoms and social history were consistent with an ASD and she was diagnosed with PDD-NOS. She moved into her current group home residence when she was 33.

There were two intake sessions for Rose—the first she attended alone and the second with her mother, who came to provide historical information. Rose appeared as a heavyset woman, neatly dressed in a color-coordinated casual outfit and well groomed. She was very talkative from the outset, making good eye contact and enthusiastically answering the therapist's questions and comments. She demonstrated a lack of awareness of social boundaries, however, as she walked over to the therapist's desk on her way in and tried to read some of the documents on it. She also interrupted the therapist frequently as the interview progressed, although she would stop herself, put her hand over her mouth, and say, "Oh. Sorry. I can't help it sometimes!" She was very articulate as she described her problems and goals for therapy. At times, she would make an odd hand gesture to emphasize a point; she would raise one hand and splay her fingers stiffly and wave the hand back and forth in that position. She reported that she "hated" the day program she was attending because it is for "lower-functioning" people—she whispered when she said, "I'm sorry, but it is for people who are retarded. I am not retarded." She also demonstrated some insight in that she voluntarily reported problems controlling her anger, that she was "too hyper," "stressed out," and wanted to learn how to focus better on her work.

Because Rose's developmental history was marked by some language and cognitive delays, she did not meet DSM-IV-TR for AS, but her profile is consistent with ASD as described in DSM-5. Like the previous four cases, Rose's independence potential is much higher than her current level of functioning in daily living. Her presentation at intake included several difficulties with social interaction, including "deficits in nonverbal communicative behaviors used for social interaction" (failure to read nonverbal cues and boundaries communicated by others), lack of "social–emotional reciprocity" (poor turn taking in conversation), and "stereotyped or repetitive motor mannerisms" (odd hand gestures; American Psychiatric Association, 2013, p. 50).

Rose's impairment in social interaction had manifested most dramatically in her work life—*occupational problems* are typical for adults with ASD. Many of her intellectual abilities were significantly more advanced than her social skill level, leading to unsuccessful experiences in almost any vocational setting she entered. Like many adult patients, her social behavior interfered with her performance whenever she was given a chance to work at a job that was suitable for her cognitive ability. On the other hand, when placed in a training program on par with her social functioning level, she quickly became bored and frustrated because the tasks were not intellectually challenging enough. As part of a vicious cycle, her social functioning regressed further because she expressed her anger in disruptive ways due to poor impulse control and difficulty with emotion regulation (ER).

The following description of Seth is also marked by vocational underachievement due to deficits in social functioning and extreme stress reactions.

Seth: Occupational Problems and Maladaptive Stress Responses

Seth is a 44-year-old single Jewish unemployed man who was referred by his vocational counselor to address problems with interpersonal behavior. Seth lives with a roommate in an apartment about 15 miles outside New York City and receives weekly visits from a staff member of an assisted living program for adults with developmental disabilities. He is pursuing an associate's degree and takes one course per semester. He is financially supported by Social Security disability benefits.

Seth's vocational counselor had been working with him for several months as part of a supportive employment program for people with disabilities. The counselor reported that Seth's options for job placement were limited by his poor interaction skills and high anxiety. Seth talked incessantly, asked intrusive questions, and became overwhelmed by minor demands (e.g., could not manage more than one college course at a time, despite the fact he was not working). The staff from both his employment and residential programs reported that Seth was developmentally disabled, but they were unsure of his diagnosis because he did not appear to have ID.

Seth had social and emotional problems from early childhood. His developmental milestones were achieved on time and he appeared to be intellectually above average in many areas. However, he always preferred to play alone and engaged in behaviors that annoyed other children. As a consequence, he had no friends. He was identified as "emotionally disturbed" by his school and by the time he reached high school, he was placed in a special vocational program for students with learning and behavioral problems, where he remained until he turned 21. There he developed an interest in computers, which was encouraged by his teachers. In his early 20s, he was able to apply the skills he had learned when he was hired by a large aerospace company as a computer operator. His job involved data entry; he worked there full time for 12 years, while living with his parents and taking courses toward his associate's degree on a part-time basis. Long shifts and interpersonal difficulties caused Seth to feel pressured constantly on the job. In his last year there, at the age of 35, he had begun to engage in self-injurious behavior (scratching and picking the skin on his hands and forearms). He performed the behavior in private, but the scabs and skin marks, along with other odd behaviors at work, drew the attention of coworkers. Eventually, a counselor with the employee assistance program at the company urged him to go into the hospital. He voluntarily entered a private psychiatric hospital, where he stayed for 2 months. He was given the diagnosis of psychotic disorder-NOS. After discharge, he returned to work for several months, but he continued to have difficulty coping, so he left the position and went on long-term disability. Seth remained at home, continuing his coursework for 7 years, until he moved into the apartment where he was living at the time of intake.

There were three intake sessions, two with Seth alone and one during which his parents joined him. Seth came to the sessions neatly dressed and groomed. He was slightly overweight, with thinning gray hair. He avoided eye contact but spoke freely. He had excellent articulation, to the point of sounding pedantic, and he spoke in a monotone. He appeared enthusiastic about the interview and seemed to enjoy sharing information about his life with the therapist. Several times when he smiled, he flapped his hands at the same time. His focus on details made transitions from one topic to the next slow because he would not shift until he had exhausted all of the information on a subject. For all sessions, he had some difficulty terminating the discussion when the time was up, and he appeared to ignore both the verbal and nonverbal cues the therapist was giving him to indicate that it was time to stop.

Seth's historical and current behavior was marked by several symptoms of DSM-5-defined ASD. His childhood years were characterized by "deficits in developing, maintaining, and understanding relationships," which had continued into adulthood and manifested as poor relationships with his coworkers. During the interview, he demonstrated signs of other interactional difficulties, such as "abnormalities in eye contact and body language," and poor demonstration of "social–emotional reciprocity" in conversation when he failed to respond to the therapist's cues to switch topics or end the session. Throughout his life, he had demonstrated "inflexible adherence to routines" and became highly stressed when routines were unpredictable. Indeed, unpredictability seemed to constitute a common precipitating factor for his self-injurious behavior in childhood as well as adulthood. He also demonstrated "repetitive motor mannerisms" (American Psychiatric Association, 2013, p. 50) during the interview when he flapped his hands.

Like many adults with ASD, Seth was *unemployed*, despite his experience and talent in working with computers. Although he was taking college courses, he was making relatively slow progress toward a higher education, considering his intellectual abilities.

It is common for adults like Seth to have a low frustration tolerance and *maladaptive reactions to stress*. Sometimes the behavioral manifestations of these maladaptations can lead others to see these individuals as bizarre or dangerous, such as what occurred in response to the self-injury in Seth's case.

Frequently, extreme responses to stress lead to the development of comorbid psychiatric disorders, as illustrated by the case of Bob.

Bob: Severe Anxiety and Depressive Symptoms

Bob is a 29-year-old single Jewish man. He holds a bachelor's degree in communication arts but is unemployed, lives with his parents, collects Social Security disability benefits, and attends a part-time psychiatric day treatment program. Bob also has diabetes. He was referred to treatment by an evaluating psychologist in October 2001 to address acute symptoms of anxiety and depression triggered by the World Trade Center disaster the month before.

Bob's parents reported that his current episode of severe anxiety and depression began a few days after 9/11. Bob was at home on Long Island, about 10 miles outside of New York City, when his mother phoned him and told him about the attack. He then watched the news coverage on TV throughout most of the day. He began questioning his family members repeatedly about the event, how it could have happened, and whether it would happen again. He reported that he could not sleep soundly and would lie in bed thinking about it over and over again. When he questioned family members about it, their answers would temporarily alleviate his anxiety, but then he would feel compelled to start questioning them again shortly thereafter. These episodes happened 10–20 times a day and were straining his relationships with his family members. His parents also reported frequent angry outbursts, which included verbal aggression toward them.

Bob has a long history of learning, social, and emotional problems. In elementary and middle school, he received special education services because of learning disabilities. He had problems making friends in all grades and had been to see mental health professionals on and off. His parents could not recall any diagnosis, but he was said to exhibit "behavior problems" and social difficulties. They reported that he became extremely upset whenever there were unexpected changes in routine, appeared "bothered" by wearing certain types of clothing (e.g., would "act itchy"), had some facial tics, and appeared indifferent to his peers. In high school, he no longer received special services, but his social adjustment continued to be poor. He went away to college but believes his parents forced him to do so. Socially he improved slightly while at college, and he was able to make some friends on campus. Although he kept in touch with them after graduation, he described them as "mentally impaired." When Bob was 21 he was diagnosed with diabetes, which was a shock to him and his parents. When he was 26, he experienced a severe decompensation marked by symptoms of anxiety (obsessions and compulsive behavior) and depression, triggered by a major social disappointment (a former high school female peer rejected him). A psychiatrist at the time diagnosed him with major depressive disorder and OCD. He has been treated by a psychiatrist since that time.

Bob and his parents came to the intake together. During the interview, he made no eye contact and displayed psychomotor retardation, sitting in a slumped posture and looking steadily toward the floor. However, he appeared to attend to the interview, in that he responded to each question and interchange—albeit in a very negative and defensive fashion, with a constant scowl on his face and expressions of anger and hostility toward the therapist and his parents throughout the session.

Bob was manifesting many acute mood and anxiety symptoms at the time of intake, leading to differential diagnosis challenges when considering the presence of ASD. Some of the clues for DSM-5-defined ASD that were present in the above description, however, include his historical failure in developing, maintaining, and understanding relationships and his rigid "adherence to routines." The "abnormalities in eye contact" (American Psychiatric Association, 2013, p. 50) demonstrated during the intake could easily have been attributed to his depression, but his parents reported that he had poor eye contact during social interactions ever since he was a very young child.

Bob's case illustrates a common phenomenon seen in adults with ASD: The inability to cope with stress and change contributes to the development of *comorbid mental illness*. Like many patients with ASD, Bob suffered from comorbid anxiety symptoms. He met criteria for OCD and a mood disorder (major depressive disorder). Because his case is the most complex of the examples given, we revisit it the most throughout the book. His detailed case formulation and individualized treatment plan are presented in Chapter 4.

These seven cases constitute a heterogeneous sample of adult patients in terms of age, gender, level of intellectual functioning, level of independence, academic achievement, and severity of symptoms. Their presenting problems varied, as they came into therapy asking for help with ASD specifically and/or because of some other mental health issue, such as depression, anxiety, or anger. Certain features tie them together: They all have some type of impairment in social functioning that was evident early in life, and they all demonstrate behavioral eccentricities that would be considered, in DSM-5 terminology, "restricted, repetitive patterns of behavior, interests, or activities" (American Psychiatric Association, 2013, p. 50). For all seven cases, their symptoms have the consequences of *isolation and poor social support systems*, a *sense of failure* in attaining interpersonal or occupational goals, *chronic stress* in daily living, and a *lack of coping abilities* resulting in *maladaptive responses* to stress.

Understanding the Symptom Picture in Adults with ASD

As these cases illustrate, the symptom picture is complex for more cognitively able adults with ASD. Their problems can be difficult to conceptualize and accurately diagnose because they are long-standing and driven by multiple causes. The rest of this chapter attempts to provide a clearer understanding of the origins of complaints and behaviors typically seen in adult patients at intake. To achieve greater clarity, it is not only important to understand what ASD *is*, but also to understand what it *is not*. The next two sections address the latter point by discussing areas of possible confusion and misconception that involve differential diagnosis and common myths. A general conceptualization of the problems faced by adults with ASD when they seek psychotherapy follows in Chapter 2, including core problems and comorbid conditions.

Differential Diagnostic Issues

The symptoms of adult ASD manifest in a wide variety of ways, as illustrated, so there may be a lack of clarity in mental health practitioners about how to diagnose the syndrome, particularly in adults. At times, symptoms mimic other disorders, including anxiety and mood disorders; at other times, adults with ASD experience true symptoms of comorbid disorders while also meeting full criteria for ASD. First, I focus on differentiating ASD from other conditions. Comorbidity issues are covered in Chapter 3. The disorders that can have similar features, and therefore can easily be confused with ASD, are social (pragmatic) communication disorder (SCD), psychotic disorders, ADHD, anxiety and related disorders, mood disorders, and personality disorders (PD). As mentioned earlier, clinicians serving adults may be called upon to use DSM-5 or ICD-10, depending on the circumstances. Differential diagnosis issues are similar in both systems, but DSM-5 has some changes in how the broad diagnostic categories are organized and also some rule-out guidelines. The DSM-5 language is used, but ICD-10 is mentioned where differences are relevant to a clinician.

Social (Pragmatic) Communication Disorder

SCD was newly introduced in DSM-5. It did not exist in earlier versions of DSM. It is also not listed in ICD-10 or earlier versions. The category is meant to describe individuals who have significant *problems with social communication,* but who do not have restrictive and repetitive patterns of behavior as seen in people with ASD. This phenomenon has long been discussed in the speech–language pathology (SLP) literature, and the term *pragmatic* is one used in that field to describe the social use of language. So, a person could have well-developed language skills (e.g., articulation, vocabulary, sentence formation), but if that individual makes *poor use of language to modulate social interactions,* a speech–language pathologist would call it a problem of "poor pragmatic skills." The disorder has many overlapping features with ASD when it comes to social communication deficits. If a patient presents with social communication problems, both SCD and ASD would be considered. SCD would be assigned if the patient does not have marked problems in the restricted, repetitive patterns of behavior domain. This diagnostic category is so new that there have been many concerns raised about its validity and the reliability of instruments that are meant to assess for it (Brukner-Wertman, Laor, & Golan, 2016; Norbury, 2014; Reisinger, Cornish, & Fombonne, 2011; Simms & Jin, 2015). In a study by Wilson and colleagues (2013) in the United Kingdom comparing DSM-IV-TR, ICD-10, and DSM-5 in an adult clinic sample, it was found that a portion (19%) of the sample that met criteria for ASD using ICD-10 would have their diagnoses converted to SCD when DSM-5 was applied. This could be partly due to a portion of those cases having been PDD-NOS before and not quite fitting into a specific ASD or AS symptom profile. This could also be due to the possibility that restricted and repetitive behaviors shift and change across the lifespan and may not be present at the time of the clinical assessment of an adult, thereby being mistaken as being absent. Further research is needed in this area to fine-tune differential diagnosis techniques between ASD and SCD. For the present purposes, clinicians should be thorough in assessing the restricted and repetitive behavior domain of symptoms to be sure those symptoms have always been absent before assigning a diagnosis of SCD.

Psychotic Disorders

Some of the symptoms and associated features of ASD can be erroneously identified as psychosis (Van Schalkwyk, Peluso, Qayyum, McPartland, & Volkmar, 2015). Sometimes, adults with ASD may show an *intense preoccupation with a particular area of interest* and build an *elaborate internal life* around it (e.g., a specific video game series, comic book, or anime character). They may have problems organizing themselves and their environment (executive function deficits). Difficulties with *stereotyped motor mannerisms* and *rigid adherence to routines* or ideas may look like positive symptoms of *schizophrenia*. They may have a *suspicious and untrusting attitude* toward people that can be mistaken as paranoia but which has actually emerged in response to lifelong histories of being bullied, ridiculed, and rejected by others, as well as their processing deficits, which cause social misperceptions. Likewise, there is a *lack of spontaneous seeking to share enjoyment, lack of social reciprocity,* and *flat or inappropriate affect,* all mimicking negative symptoms. In addition, when facing extreme stress, individuals with ASD may show a marked deterioration in functioning that is not clearly linked to an episode of another psychiatric disorder.

Professionals working with individuals with ASD have nicknamed these incidents as "meltdowns," and they are often extreme anxiety reactions to "sensory overload." Dramatic, bizarre, and destructive behaviors may emerge during these episodes, such as sudden withdrawal ("shut down"), incoherent speech, screaming, destroying property, or self-injury (banging head on wall, punching, scratching, or cutting self). However, these signs of distress tend to disappear once the stressful factors are removed or resolved, and the individual can quickly return to his or her previous level of functioning. This "bounce-back" effect is not usually observed in persons experiencing a true psychotic episode. Other differentiation features are described by DSM-5, Ghaziuddin (2005), Crespi and Badcock (2008), and Solomon and colleagues (2011). Age of onset for ASD is early childhood, but usually late adolescence or later for schizophrenia. Hallucinations and delusions are absent in ASD. Social pragmatic language is more impaired in ASD. A careful interview is needed to differentiate delusions from the overvalued ideas and rich fantasy life that can be seen in ASD, and also from the literal ways these patients interpret the interviewers' questions (Chapter 3 covers this area in more detail).

Attention-Deficit/Hyperactivity Disorder

Problems with *attention* and *motor control* are commonly associated features of ASD. Some studies have shown high rates of overlap in the symptom pictures of ASD and attention-deficit/hyperactivity disorder (ADHD). Child studies have shown high rates of comorbidity in ADHD samples. For example, Gillberg and Gillberg (1989) found that 21% met criteria for AS and another 36% had some "autistic traits." Conversely, in a sample of clinic patients who met criteria for AS, 28% also met criteria for ADHD (Ghaziuddin, Weidmer-Mikhail, & Ghaziuddin, 1998). More recent epidemiological studies showed that about 30% of children with ASD across all subtypes had comorbid ADHD profiles (Simonoff et al., 2008) and similar rates were shown in one adult study (Lever & Geurts, 2016). Many adults with ASD with whom I have worked had previously been diagnosed with ADHD before it was determined that they instead or in addition had ASD.

In contrast to earlier editions, DSM-5 allows for a comorbid diagnosis of ADHD with ASD. ICD-10 does not, stating that the symptoms must "not meet criteria for pervasive developmental disorders." No matter which system the clinician is using, differential diagnosis issues must be addressed for both documentation and treatment planning purposes (Craig et al., 2015; Ghaziuddin, 2005; Taurines et al., 2012). Research in this area is in its infancy, but both brain imaging and social cognition measures have been able to identify some overlapping and distinguishing features when people with ASD alone, ADHD alone, and ASD + ADHD are compared (Buhler, Bachmann, Goyert, Heinsel-Gutenbrunner, & Kamp-Becker, 2011; Craig et al., 2015; Taurines et al., 2012). These findings suggest that people with ASD alone or ASD + ADHD compared to ADHD alone have fewer problems with inhibitory control, more deficits with social cognition (e.g., theory of mind [ToM]) abilities, more significant social communication deficits, and more impaired adaptive behavior. When using the individualized case conceptualization approach outlined in this book, it is important to focus on symptoms of inattention or impulsivity if they are present and to ensure that the best empirically supported therapies are included in the treatment plan for these types of problems.

Anxiety and Related Disorders

DSM-5 radically changed the way "anxiety disorders" are categorized. For example, OCD, traditionally considered one of the anxiety disorders, has been removed from that section and given its own category along with conceptually similar conditions, which is called "obsessive–compulsive disorders and related disorders." Posttraumatic and acute stress disorders have also been removed and put into a separate "trauma- and stressor-related disorders" section. I discuss these disorders together here because, despite the division into separate chapters, DSM-5 still acknowledges a close relationship among anxiety disorders, obsessive–compulsive and related disorders, and trauma- and stressor-related disorders (American Psychiatric Association, 2013, p. 265). In addition, most research cited here was done using DSM-IV or ICD-10 categorization of anxiety disorders.

Every adult patient with ASD I have met has struggled with anxiety in one form or another. Studies (using DSM-IV-TR criteria) of people with ASD of all subtypes have shown reliably that clinical levels of anxiety are much more likely to be observed in that population as compared to same-age peers without ASD (Maisel et al., 2016). The incidence of comorbid DSM-IV-TR-defined anxiety disorders, combining all categories, has been reported to range from 31 to 59% in adult samples without ID (Hofvander et al., 2009; Joshi et al., 2013). Because the comorbidity rates are so high, differentiating ASD from some anxiety disorders is a complex task (Tsai, 2006). Chapter 3 elaborates more on the presentation of anxiety disorders as they appear with ASD in adult patients seeking treatment. Here the focus is on helping to differentiate between a patient with an anxiety disorder with *no ASD* and a patient who has an ASD (with or without a comorbid condition). The disorders that can most easily be confused with ASD are social anxiety disorder (SAD; aka, social phobia) and OCD.

SAD can be hard to differentiate from ASD, especially because it so often co-occurs with it (Bejerot, Eriksson, & Mörtberg, 2014; Rydén & Bejerot, 2008; White, Bray, & Ollendick, 2012). *Avoidance of social situations* is not necessarily seen in all cases of ASD. Some adults with ASD are quite gregarious and seek to engage people on a regular basis because they enjoy the company of others and seem oblivious to the consequences of their social mistakes. For those cases, SAD may not be as readily considered by a clinician. However, for those who do appear to be avoiding social interactions, the clinical presentation can in some cases mimic SAD, and in other cases, be a manifestation of a comorbid SAD. Swain, Scarpa, White, and Laugeson (2015) point out that low social motivation is not synonymous with social avoidance. In fact, high motivation could result in avoidance behavior because the fear of being judged is connected to the strong wish to succeed in social engagement.

One issue that can be confusing to the clinician is in the phrasing of the diagnostic criteria for SAD in DSM-5. Criterion E states, "The fear or anxiety is out of proportion to the actual threat posed by the social situation and to the sociocultural context" (American Psychiatric Association, 2013, p. 203). Similarly, in ICD-10-defined social phobia, Criterion C states that " . . . the individual recognizes that these (fears) are excessive or unreasonable" (World Health Organization, 1992, p. 93). If these criteria are taken literally, many of the adults I have treated with ASD who do exhibit the other symptoms of SAD would not meet full criteria. This is because some measure of fear about social encounters is arguably *in proportion* to the actual threat and *not excessive or unreasonable*. Any adult who meets criteria for ASD, by definition, has deficits in the skills necessary to have successful social interactions. It is not excessive or unreasonable for someone to fear social situations if the individual is not skilled enough to handle them. Most of the adults who present for therapy with this problem are painfully aware of their lack of skill and have learned avoidance as an adaptive strategy on the one hand, but on the other, the avoidance behavior ends up perpetuating the anxiety, which then contributes to the misunderstanding of social cues and other social cognition deficits that are central to ASD (White et al., 2013). Thus, the anxiety does reach the clinical levels necessary to meet criteria for SAD.

Thanks largely to White and colleagues, SAD is one of the anxiety disorders that has received the most research attention in relation to ASD, including as it occurs in adults (Maddox & White, 2015; Swain et al., 2015; White et al., 2012). They have provided substantial evidence that SAD and ASD are two distinctive, but commonly co-occurring disorders. The bidirectional relationship between them, described by White and colleagues (2013), results in the development of a vicious cycle of sorts that can be observed in adult patients. These studies offer some guidance for clinicians toward differential diagnosis among SAD alone, ASD alone, and ASD with SAD. In sum, people who have SAD alone will show a marked fear of, distress in, and active avoidance of social situations because of serious concerns about being negatively judged and evaluated. They may act in ways that lead to humiliation, but do not have marked social skill deficits, as do people with ASD.

People with SAD alone may have an earlier onset of social anxiety symptoms (elementary school), as opposed to cases of SAD where ASD is also present—those individuals may report a later onset (adolescence). People with ASD alone will demonstrate the social communication skill deficits and restricted, repetitive patterns of behavior that are central to the disorder, but do not demonstrate the fear of social situations, concern about negative evaluation or judgment, distress when exposed to social situations, and resultant avoidance of the feared social scenarios. For example, a person with ASD alone may have a low frequency of social engagement because he or she is not interested in people (low social motivation), not because he or she is fearful of them. Finally, people with both ASD and SAD exhibit more social impairment and skill deficits than people with SAD alone; they demonstrate social awkwardness that is not seen in SAD alone. In addition, people with both disorders may have insight into the role that their social skill deficits play in their social anxiety.

OCD can also be confused with ASD by clinicians. Symptoms under "restricted, repetitive, and stereotyped patterns of behavior" (American Psychiatric Association, 2013, p. 50), at least superficially, look like symptoms of OCD. The *intense focus on an interest area* can take on an obsessional quality, for instance. The *overreliance on nonfunctional routines and rituals*, as well as *repetitive motor mannerisms*, can appear to be compulsions. Some studies have suggested that there are some overlapping features seen in both OCD and ASD, such as attention-switching problems (Anholt et al., 2010; Kaur et al., 2016). Nevertheless, there is also enough evidence to suggest that these are two distinct disorders than can each occur alone in an individual, or can be comorbid.

Studies have shown that about 20% of patients seeking treatment for OCD have traits of ASD that were comorbid but distinguishable from the OCD (Bejerot, Nylander, & Lindstrom, 2001; Kaur et al., 2016). In a sample of adults with ASD and no ID seeking treatment for ASD-related problems, 24% met criteria for OCD, either currently or by history (Joshi et al., 2013).

While both conditions involve repetitive thoughts and actions, some investigators have compared the types of obsessive–compulsive symptoms reported by adults with OCD alone to adults who have ASD alone and those who have ASD + OCD. In one case-controlled study, the investigators administered the Yale–Brown Obsessive Compulsive Scale (Y-BOCS) to clinical samples of adults with ASD alone and those with OCD alone (McDougle et al., 1995). Although repetitive thoughts and behaviors were reported by all patients, qualitative differences in the content of obsessive thoughts and types of behaviors were reported between the two groups. For example, patients with OCD reported more thoughts with aggressive, contamination, sexual, religious, symmetry, and somatic content than patients with autism. However, patients with ASD alone reported more compulsions around repetitive ordering, hoarding, telling/asking, touching, tapping, rubbing, and self-damaging/self-mutilation than patients with OCD, who reported more cleaning, checking, and counting compulsions. In another study using the Y-BOCS (Russell, Mataix-Cols, Anson, & Murphy, 2005), comparisons were made between OCD alone and ASD with OCD (and without ID). In this sample, somatic obsession and repeating and checking rituals were significantly more frequent in the OCD alone group. Sexual obsessions were the only symptoms that were reported at a higher rate by ASD patients.

More research is needed in this area, but we have enough data to warrant efforts by clinicians to differentiate OCD from ASD in their patients, while also considering that the two distinct disorders can co-occur. Ghaziuddin (2005) suggests that in patients with OCD, the obsessions and compulsions are "ego dystonic"—that is, perceived as intrusive and unwanted by the sufferer. The compulsions serve the function of neutralizing the obsessions and alleviate negative affect in the short run (until the cycle starts again). The ritualistic behaviors that are core to ASD do not serve that neutralizing function seen in OCD, do not seem to cause distress, and the preoccupation with a narrow interest can actually be a source of pleasure for these individuals. For some, these interests develop into functional talents that can fuel a successful career or be an important source of life enrichment. If obsessional interests and ritualistic behavior are present along with the social communication deficits described for ASD, and the symptoms have been present since early childhood, then they are likely to be part of that syndrome. The topic of comorbidity is addressed in later sections, but for the purposes of this discussion, an additional diagnosis of OCD can be made when the preoccupations and ritualistic behavior represent a marked departure from the individual's baseline level of functioning, and are causing marked distress. Bob's case illustrates this phenomenon.

Mood Disorders

As with anxiety disorders, there is a high incidence of mood disorders comorbid with ASD. For example, in a study of psychiatric problems in adults with ASD, 65% met criteria for some kind of DSM-IV-TR-defined mood disorder (Hofvander et al., 2009). The rates of major depressive disorder have been reported to be from 33 to 77% in adult ASD samples (Joshi et al., 2013; Lever & Geurts, 2016) and from 7 to 25% for bipolar disorders (Joshi et al., 2013; Skokauskas & Frodl, 2015). One study of adult clinic outpatients seeking treatment for mood disorders in Japan showed significantly higher rates of ASD symptoms compared to the general population sample (Matsuo et al., 2015). Hence, this topic is addressed frequently throughout this book. It is difficult to ascertain whether some features seen in patients where ASD is suspected are part of the autism spectrum, part of a mood disorder, or both (Matson & Williams, 2014). At times the presence of a known developmental disability can obscure a clinician's view, and a mood disorder can be missed. This phenomenon has been called "diagnostic overshadowing" (Reiss & Szyszko, 1983, p. 396) in the literature on ID. With higher-IQ adults, where an ASD is less obvious, the overshadowing can happen in the opposite way: A person who presents for treatment of a depressive episode may have an underlying ASD that is unmasked only after the depression is successfully treated (Ghaziuddin, 2005). The typical overlapping features are discussed here with general guidelines for differentiating the source of the problem.

The impairments in social interaction that are hallmark features of ASD can make an individual appear *aloof* or *socially withdrawn*. Paired with the tendency of some individuals with ASD to demonstrate *flat affect*, these patients can appear similar to the way a person experiencing a *major depressive episode* may exhibit loss of interest in pleasurable activities. The preoccupation or *intense focus on one interest area* often presents as talking incessantly about a topic, and the individual has difficulty conversing about anything else. This symptom can be mistaken as the pressured speech seen during a *hypomanic* or *manic episode* of a *bipolar mood disorder*. Difficulty in *regulating emotion,* which is an associated feature of ASD, can manifest as *irritability, explosive outbursts,* or *lability*—and all can be symptoms of depressive or bipolar mood disorders. Finally, it has been documented that people with ASD are vulnerable to *disordered sleep* (Limoges, Mottron, Bolduc, Berthiaume, & Godbout, 2005; Matson, Ancona, & Wilkins, 2008; Richdale & Prior, 1995; Richdale & Schreck, 2009; Tani et al., 2004), which can also be a symptom of either a depressive or manic episode of a mood disorder. More research is needed to help differentiate between disordered sleep as part of the ASD phenotype and disordered sleep that is part of a separate, but at times comorbid, mood disorder. In the meantime, it is another factor that can make differential diagnosis challenging for the practitioner.

When considering mood disorders versus ASD during the diagnostic process, the clinician must consider developmental history and course of symptom development—guidelines that were mentioned previously for psychotic and anxiety disorders. If the social withdrawal, intense interest in one topic, irritability/anger outbursts, or disordered sleep have been present since early childhood and have appeared as stable problems accompanying the social skill deficits described earlier, then they are likely to be connected with ASD. However, if these problems present suddenly or involve a worsening of preexisting problems, they are more likely due to a mood disorder, with or without comorbid ASD.

Personality Disorders

Adults with ASD who have previously sought mental health treatment commonly have received a diagnosis of a PD at some point in the past. I have most often encountered the diagnoses of *schizoid personality disorder, schizotypal personality disorder,* and *borderline personality disorder* (especially in females) in patient histories. Studies in Europe of adults with ASD have found comorbid rates of PD to be as high as 62% in one sample (Hofvander et al., 2009) and 48% in another sample (Lugnegård, Hällerback, & Gillberg, 2011). For practical purposes one could argue that ASD *is* a PD, even though it is not classified as such in DSM or ICD. In fact, Wolff (1998) points out that Hans Asperger himself described the condition as a "lifelong, genetically based, personality disorder" (p. 127). Table 1.3 lists the general diagnostic criteria for PD from DSM-5. Every patient I have treated with ASD has met all four criteria. However, we must carefully consider the DSM statement that the "pattern is not better accounted for as a manifestation or consequence of another mental disorder" (American Psychiatric Association, 2013, p. 647). In fact, the criteria for both schizoid personality disorder and schizotypal

---

TABLE 1.3. DSM-5 Diagnostic Criteria for General PD

A. An enduring pattern of inner experience and behavior that deviates markedly from the expectations of the individual's culture. This pattern is manifested in two (or more) of the following areas:

　　1. Cognition (i.e., ways of perceiving and interpreting self, other people, and events).
　　2. Affectivity (i.e., the range, intensity, lability, and appropriateness of emotional response).
　　3. Interpersonal functioning.
　　4. Impulse control.

B. The enduring pattern is inflexible and pervasive across a broad range of personal and social situations.

C. The enduring pattern leads to clinically significant distress or impairment in social, occupational, or other important areas of functioning.

D. The pattern is stable and of long duration, and its onset can be traced back at least to adolescence or early adulthood.

E. The enduring pattern is not better explained as a manifestation or consequence of another mental disorder.

F. The enduring pattern is not attributable to the physiological effects of a substance (e.g., a drug of abuse, a medication) or another medical condition (e.g., head trauma).

Note. Reprinted with permission from the *Diagnostic and Statistical Manual of Mental Disorders, Fifth Edition.* Copyright © 2013 the American Psychiatric Association. All rights reserved.

personality disorder specify that ASD takes precedence if the criteria are met for one. The issue is complicated when assessing adults, however. For example, take a hypothetical "snapshot" of two 45-year-old men, one with schizotypal personality disorder and the other with ASD. Their presenting problems and current patterns of behavior could be identical. Both will have *odd beliefs and mannerisms,* both will have *few or no friendships,* and both will have *social anxiety.* So how can a clinician tell the difference? Unfortunately, there are little data to guide us on this issue (Ünver, Öner, & Yurtbaşi, 2015). Wolff (1998, 2000) offers a comprehensive discussion of this differential diagnosis question for children. In Wolff's (1998) estimation, schizoid and schizotypal personality disorders are highly overlapping conditions in the samples of children she has studied, and these problems "lie at one extreme end of the autistic spectrum, where it shades into normal personality variation" (p. 138).

Assessment is discussed in Chapter 3, but it should be mentioned here that I rely heavily on developmental histories when making a diagnosis. Even in older adults, gaining access to a family member who can give details about early childhood development is invaluable. ASD is the more appropriate diagnosis over schizotypal or schizoid personality if there is strong evidence for very early (preschool-age) problems with social development and restricted, repetitive patterns of behavior.

Common Myths

As a bridge between the differential diagnosis issues addressed above and the conceptualization of ASD that is coming next, I make a few more points about what ASD *is not.* As noted, the DSM-IV formulation (American Psychiatric Association, 1994) represented a radical change in the way ASDs were defined, by introducing AS and expanding our view to include individuals without ID or language impairment. Then the DSM-5 formulation (American Psychiatric Association, 2013) drastically changed things, yet again. Simply put, the diagnosis of ASD in adults who are verbal and have average or above-average intelligence is still easy to miss for many reasons. In addition to the differential diagnosis dilemmas already discussed, obstacles are created by a number of myths that many people, including professionals, continue to believe. Most are based on the old definition of "classic" autism that practitioners may have learned about in their training, or to which the public was exposed in the movie *Rain Man,* for instance. Table 1.4 lists some of the misconceptions that I have heard expressed as recently as the year of this writing. In the next section, following each myth is a related quote, paraphrased from what practitioners have said to me when trying to rule out ASD erroneously.

TABLE 1.4. Myths about ASD

- People with ASD are always aloof and uninterested in others.
- People with ASD have no relationships.
- People with ASD are usually male—it's a guy thing.
- People with ASD do not make any eye contact.
- People with ASD lack empathy for others.
- People with ASD are intellectual geniuses.

People with ASD Are Always Aloof and Uninterested in Others

"He can't have ASD because he is very talkative and engaging." By definition, people with ASD struggle with the complex skills required to interface successfully with others. However, many have a normal desire to interact with others, to belong to a social network, and to be liked. Some are so determined to talk to people that they will do so incessantly, despite signs that they are making social mistakes.

People with ASD Have No Relationships

"She can't have ASD; she is married." Some people have the basic skills to make a small number of friends and maintain those relationships in adulthood, even to the point of being married or in long-term romantic partnerships. They may complain that they do not feel confident or satisfied with these relationships, a report that is consistent with the ASD definition. However, a total absence of relationships is not necessary for the diagnosis of ASD.

People with ASD Are Usually Male—It's a Guy Thing

"She doesn't have ASD—isn't it a guy thing?" As discussed earlier, prevalence rates show a higher incidence in males, but the disparity between male and female rates may be inflated. Not only does it occur in females but the trend of late diagnosis in higher-IQ women is likely to be partially caused by myths and misconceptions that are held by laypeople and professionals alike.

People with ASD Do Not Make Any Eye Contact

"He can't have ASD. He made a lot of eye contact with me during the interview." Some people with ASD do exhibit complete avoidance of eye contact, especially when first meeting someone. Others cannot maintain eye contact and listen at the same time and must look away in order to process what is being said. However, many individuals do make eye contact consistently, even if there are some unique features. Just as described in DSM-IV-TR, the impairment is in "the use of eye-to-eye gaze . . . to regulate social interaction" (American Psychiatric Association, 2000, p. 84). Some people may show sporadic glances, whereas others may make *too much* eye contact to the point of staring. It is important to remember that the failure to utilize eye contact appropriately does not mean that eye contact is missing completely. Also, it is only one of the symptoms in a category and does not have to be present at all for the diagnosis to be made.

People with ASD Lack Empathy for Others

"She can't have ASD. She seems to really care about her ailing mother." People with ASD have difficulty with social reciprocity, as specified in the DSM criteria. This means they do not show "turn taking" in conversation and the spontaneous "give-and-take" of information and experiences that characterize socially satisfying interactions. They may also have difficulty with perspective taking—that is, imagining what another person might be thinking or feeling. In my clinical cases, I have found that these problems are often rooted in an impaired ability to show cognitive shifting. This issue is addressed in Chapter 2, where core deficits are described in more detail. What appears to be a lack of empathy may sometimes be a failure to "shift gears" at the rapid pace required by a social situation. With a history that is void of opportunities to practice reciprocal relating, a self-absorbed style may develop. Anecdotally speaking, when given the appropriate information and enough time to process it, patients with ASD can show as much empathy and concern for another person as the rest of the population. (Recent data supporting this clinical observation are presented in Chapters 2 and 6.)

People with ASD Are Intellectual Geniuses

"He can't have ASD. He does not have any kind of special talent or 'savant' qualities." It is true that people with ASD have scattered profiles of skills and deficits. There is great variability within each individual in terms of abilities versus disabilities. For example, a person with ASD may have superior mathematical abilities but extremely poor visual–motor coordination. However, there is also great variability across ASD patients. Some indeed have an area of superior ability that far exceeds the average person or their own ability in other areas. Others do not have such an exceptional talent, and it is not necessary for this to be present in order to make the diagnosis.

Strengths and Assets

Ironically, the characteristics that can put adults with ASD at odds with others or at risk for problems are the very same characteristics that contribute to their talents and abilities. When therapy goals are being set, it is important not only to identify the problems that are targeted for reduction but also to highlight the assets and coping strategies that the adult patient has already developed before coming into treatment. Although this chapter highlighted the vulnerabilities of these individuals, I have found that they are also incredibly resourceful and clever in designing strategies, often without any help, to negotiate their way through a world that is, to them, very confusing and threatening. The individualized treatment plan should always include interventions geared toward helping the patient recognize the things he or she *has already done to successfully adapt* and to build upon those self-taught skills. This approach is outlined further in a self-help book I wrote for adults (Gaus, 2011), which is largely based on a problem-solving approach driven by positive psychology concepts. Some of the common strengths are listed below. These are also the reasons I so thoroughly enjoy working with this population.

Creativity and "Unconventional" View of the World

Because these individuals have idiosyncratic perspectives, they often think of ideas that others would not. This resource can be useful in therapy during treatment planning problem solving.

Honesty

Due to a lack of understanding about "social boundaries," some individuals with ASD will not censor their thoughts when speaking. Although this absence of self-monitoring can get them into trouble socially, it can be useful in sessions because the therapist can often assess thoughts more readily than with patients who do not have ASD.

Sense of Humor

People with ASD often complain that they cannot understand humor and struggle to "get" what other people are laughing about. On the other hand, they will use humor effectively when they do "get it" and can be quite clever. Along with social skill building, these patients benefit from learning to utilize their humor to enhance their interactions with others.

Take Laura, for example, a woman who did not learn of her ASD diagnosis until she was in her mid-30s, but had always been aware of her difficulty understanding the nuances of social interactions. Even though she did not know why she was confused by the behavior of other people, sometimes she used cartoon drawing as a way of expressing the humor she saw in her struggle. Figure 1.1 is a cartoon she had drawn approximately 10 years before her diagnosis, after she learned what the term *brainstorming* meant. The cartoon depicts a typical meeting she would have to attend while working as a clerk in a large bureaucratic institution, a job that had been quite stressful for her. In it, she is making fun of her own overly literal interpretation of brainstorming by drawing actual brains whirling around the room, and her own need to protect herself from the apparent chaos, as suggested by the woman with the kerchief on her head who is trying to "keep her brain in her head." Not only was it helpful for her to laugh about

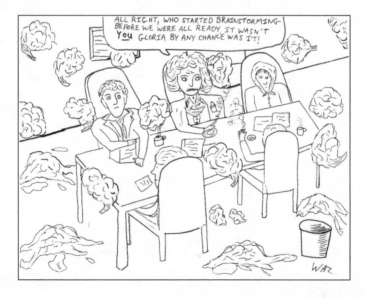

FIGURE 1.1. Cartoon by Laura, a person with AS for whom humor has served an adaptive function. Copyright © 1994 Laura Wysolmierski. Reprinted by permission.

this issue but she was also creating comedic common ground between herself and typical people. By illustrating how nonsensical some meetings can be, she connects with all of us who have been in similar situations at our jobs.

Responsiveness to Structure

Because the world can be confusing to individuals with ASD, they tend to adhere, sometimes rigidly, to any set of rules that does make sense to them. They rely on structured and predictable routines and are drawn to using logic to solve problems. For these reasons, many of these individuals find it easy to understand the cognitive model and the rationale behind the use of CBT.

Willingness to Observe and Evaluate Self

I admittedly work with a self-selected and motivated population of patients. With that, by the time the typical adult with ASD seeks outpatient treatment, he or she is acutely aware of "doing something wrong" in social situations. The patient is usually very open to feedback and willing to engage in self-observation exercises. Although some patients are not so compliant (discussed further in Chapter 10), on average these individuals make excellent candidates for CBT.

Chapter Summary and Conclusions

In this chapter, the reader was introduced to ASD and what it looks like in adult psychotherapy cases. The symptom complexity and areas of potential confusion were clarified through discussions of shifting classification systems, differential diagnosis, and common myths. Strengths and assets were also highlighted because therapists will find these characteristics crucial during the assessment and treatment planning phases of therapy. The next chapter presents the research evidence for core problems, a description of how they serve as risk factors for secondary emotional disorders, and a rationale for using CBT with these patients.

CHAPTER 2

Conceptualization of Mental Health Problems in Cognitively Able Adults with Autism Spectrum Disorder (Asperger Syndrome)

There is a growing body of evidence indicating that individuals with ASD, even those with average to superior intelligence, show cognitive dysfunction in several specific areas. In this chapter, I present those data and propose a general conceptual model that links basic research on core cognitive dysfunction to the clinical presentation of adults with ASD who seek treatment. The model is used to hypothesize how core information-processing differences are responsible for the struggles faced by individuals with ASD in their daily lives. These struggles, in turn, put them at risk for the development of a variety of mental health problems, and patients with ASD indeed often meet criteria for comorbid DSM-defined disorders. Finally, the cognitive dysfunction of ASD is considered within Beck's (1976) cognitive theory of emotional disturbance in typical people and serves as a rationale for using CBT to treat adults with ASD.

I recommend that therapists use an *evidence-based formulation-driven* model to understand and treat adult cases of ASD. As described by Haynes, Kaholokula, and Nelson (1999) and Persons, Davidson, and Tompkins (2000), clinicians need to refer to a general or *nomothetic* evidence base regarding the presenting problem (e.g., research literature on depression) and translate that information into an individualized or *idiographic* set of hypotheses that encompasses the unique factors affecting a particular patient. Weston, Hodgekins, and Langdon (2016) have recently called for that approach specifically for patients with ASD when CBT is being used. The general conceptual model presented in this chapter serves as a nomothetic model for understanding the presenting problems of adult cases of ASD, using the literature on cognitive dysfunction as the evidence base. Clinicians can use this foundation to generate an idiographic formulation of a specific case by assessing the unique way cognitive dysfunction and environmental factors interact in the life of an individual patient; strategies for conducting this type of assessment are then described in Chapters 3 and 4.

General Conceptual Model

ASD is a neurologically based set of information-processing problems. Affected individuals have unique ways of processing information from all sources, and these unique sources influence the way they learn about their world. This view is consistent with the theory of Klin and his colleagues, who propose that although ASD is a complex syndrome including an array of communication, learning, and behavioral symptoms, all of the problems can be traced to a "core social disorder" (Klin, Jones, Schultz, Volkmar, & Cohen, 2002a, p. 895). These authors contend that individuals with ASD have dysfunctional "enactive mind[s]" (Klin, Jones, Shultz, & Volkmar, 2005, p. 686) that produce a continuous interaction between idiosyncratic attention to social cues, erroneous interpretation of social information, and maladaptive behavioral responses—all which affect childhood development as well as current adult functioning. I find this process-oriented model useful when conceptualizing an individual adult psychotherapy case, as I consider the role of the core factors, or dysfunctional "enactive mind," in the development and maintenance of the presenting problems for which the patient is seeking help. Each patient presents very differently, and no two have the same profile of these deficits. Nevertheless, practitioners need to be familiar with all of these possible areas of dysfunction in order to formulate a comprehensive conceptualization and treatment plan.

Figure 2.1 illustrates my conceptualization of the problems commonly reported by adults with ASD in clinical settings. It is by no means a solid theory, but is based on evidence about cognitive dysfunction in ASD. The model is meant to provide a framework for the upcoming research review and a working understanding of the variables that may influence a person with ASD to seek psychotherapy. I hope that this model can guide clinicians to consider a wide range of factors during the individualized assessment and treatment planning process.

There is empirical support establishing that people with ASD process information in an idiosyncratic fashion. The types of information that people with ASD process erroneously can be classified into three major categories, and these appear at the top of Figure 2.1: *information about others, information about self,* and *nonsocial information.* These concepts are briefly introduced here, and supporting research is reviewed in the next section. *Processing of information about others,* or social cognition, is dysfunctional in people with ASD in that they demonstrate impairments in the ability to (1) formulate ideas about what other people are thinking or feeling ("theory of mind"), (2) use nonverbal cues to understand social interactions, and (3) make adaptive use of social language ("pragmatics"). *Processing of information about themselves* is dysfunctional in terms of the internal feedback loops involved in self-perception and self-regulation. People with ASD appear to have difficulty perceiving and regulating their own emotional experiences and have atypical sensation and motor experiences (hyper- or hyporeactivity to stimulation of any of the sensory systems). *Processing of nonsocial information* is dysfunctional in individuals with ASD who have problems managing input that is not necessarily related to other people. These problems include deficits in

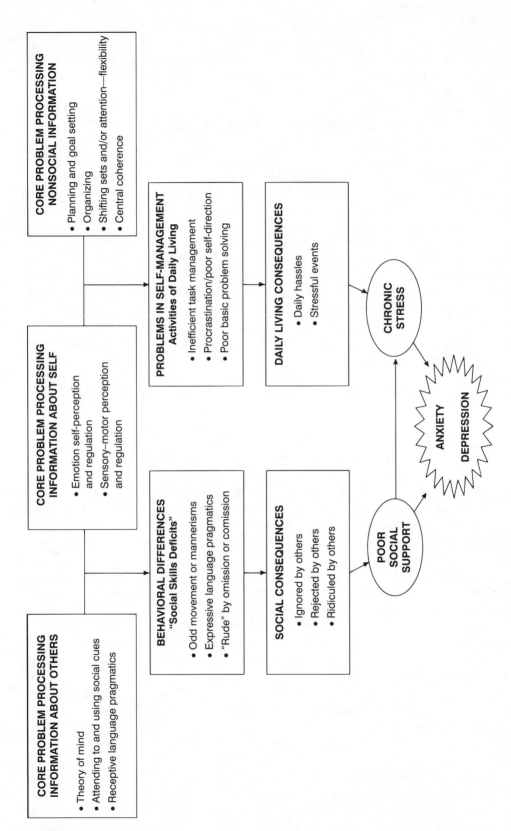

FIGURE 2.1. Core problems in ASD and pathways to mental health problems.

planning, organization, goal setting, and cognitive flexibility ("executive functions") as well as difficulty processing incoming pieces of information within a context ("gist" or "central coherence" or "seeing the big picture").

Dividing these information-processing issues into three separate categories is admittedly arbitrary, in that these phenomena probably occur in a dimensional way and interact with one another in a multidirectional fashion. Figure 2.2 represents the overlap that exists between the categories. Although researchers are still years away from establishing these connections or evidence for the direction of causality, a clinician can find these concepts helpful in understanding the history and development of a client's presenting problems.

Going back to Figure 2.1, the diagram illustrates how the core problems combine and lead to difficulties when these individuals interact with their environments. The *social skill deficits* noted in the midleft box are well documented in patients with ASD and are hypothesized to be the behavioral outcome of a combination of erroneous social inferences, self-perception problems, and a lack of typical social learning during critical periods of development. Because these individuals misperceive many social situations, they do not know how to respond to others or what others expect from them. Their *odd mannerisms, poor language pragmatics,* and *"rude" behavior* lead others to become frustrated or angry with them, resulting in negative *social consequences.* They experience being *ignored, rejected,* and *ridiculed,* without knowing why. The people in their lives who are more compassionate may try to tell them that their behavior is "inappropriate," but the people giving the feedback may not always understand *what* is different about the behavior or explain *why* it is different.

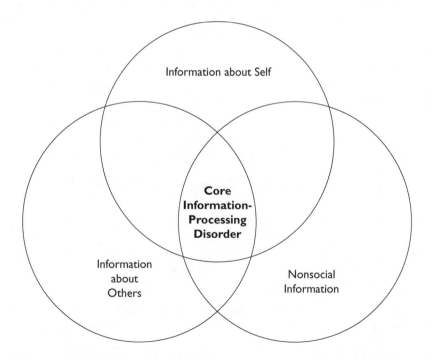

FIGURE 2.2. Interrelationship between core problems in ASD.

Difficulties in nonsocial domains appear as problems in *self-management* and *activities of daily living*, represented by the box on the midright side of the diagram. These difficulties are the behavioral outcomes of combined problems with executive function and self-perception. They appear as *inefficient task management, procrastination/poor self-direction,* and *poor basic problem solving.* It is common, but often surprising, to see a huge discrepancy between IQ and formal measures of adaptive behavior, such as the Vineland Adaptive Behavior Scales (e.g., Green, Gilchrist, Burton, & Cox, 2000). The folk stereotype of "the absentminded professor" is fitting in that the person may be brilliant but can barely take care of the tasks necessary for independent living. This leads to the *daily living consequences* of *frequent hassles,* as well as a preponderance of *stressful events.*

The model ends with the hypothesized outcomes of the repeated failures in the domains described above. The negative consequences of dysfunctional information processing and the resultant maladaptive behavior lead to *emotional distress,* as reported by adult patients seeking psychotherapy; the social consequences of ASD lead to *poor social support;* and the daily living consequences of ASD lead to *chronic stress.* Because poor social support and chronic stress are known risk factors for mental illness in the typical population (e.g., Cohen & Wills, 1985; Sarason & Sarason, 1985), they are hypothesized to increase the vulnerability in adults with ASD to develop comorbid conditions. As mentioned in Chapter 1, prevalence studies of psychiatric comorbidity in the adult population of people with ASD without ID have shown higher rates of *anxiety* and *depression* than in the general population (e.g., Hofvander et al., 2009; Joshi et al., 2012; Lever & Geurts, 2016). If we imagine the chronic stress to which people with ASD are subject, it is easy to assume that they would be at risk for many of the anxiety or mood disorders listed in DSM-5 (American Psychiatric Association, 2013). As a poignant illustration of this, Gillberg, Helles, Billstedt, and Gillberg (2016) reported that, in a sample of 50 men diagnosed with ASD without ID (which the authors termed *Asperger syndrome*) who had been followed in a Swedish prospective study since their diagnosis in childhood, 47 of them had at some point during the years since their first assessment met criteria for a comorbid psychiatric or neurodevelopmental diagnosis. In addition, if we conceptualize ASD as a neurodevelopmental disorder that causes dysfunctional learning experiences in the interpersonal domain, we could hypothesize a greater risk for personality disorders. These examples and others are discussed in more detail in Chapter 3, when assessment strategies and specific comorbid disorders are described.

Core Cognitive Dysfunction in ASD

This section presents the research findings that demonstrate the core cognitive dysfunction in ASD that was briefly introduced within the general conceptual model. Evidence that people with ASD have difficulty processing information about others, themselves, and in nonsocial domains is highlighted.

Dysfunctional Processing of Information about Others: Social Cognition

Perhaps the largest body of research regarding cognitive dysfunction in ASD is in the area of social cognition. As mentioned in Chapter 1, social cognition is the study of how people process social information. This field is not rooted in clinical psychology because historically the interest has focused on documenting how *healthy, typical* people understand others and themselves in the context of their social world. Research on attribution processes, social schema development, attention to social stimuli, person memory, and social inference are just some of the areas of basic social psychology that have cross-fertilized experimental cognitive science (Fiske & Taylor, 1984) to produce this literature over the past 60 years. Whereas social-cognitive science has provided information about how *typical people* generally process social information, clinical researchers have used those findings to begin investigating the role that *dysfunctional social cognition* may play in psychopathology. The following sections outline the research on social cognition and ASD; the subareas reviewed are *social inference* and *social language*.

Social Inference

Fiske and Taylor (1984) define *social inference* as a *process* by which typical people in social situations (1) decide what information to gather, (2) collect that information, (3) combine it in some form (interpret), and (4) make a judgment (about how to behave). The *product* is the outcome of the judgment made at the end of the process and leads to the action taken by the individual. In practical terms, when a person enters a social situation (any moment he or she must interface with one or more other human beings), that person must go through several cognitive steps in order to decide what to do or how to act. The decision is an *inference* because the person must "guess" what is going on to some extent; most situations a person encounters are not *identical* to any previous one in every regard, and in most situations, a person is not provided with any explicit instructions on what to think and do. However, most people guess correctly most of the time because they are using *educated* guesses. Their decisions are based on information they gather and analyze very quickly, while referring to their preexisting fund of knowledge about social rules and norms.

Using a simple example, a man on a business trip enters a crowded deli in an American city he has never before visited. Even though he is solely engaging in the task of grabbing a quick sandwich, he must go through a social inference process in order to successfully get his lunch. Using the steps outlined above, upon entering the store:

1. He must *decide what information to gather* ("I must find out where the line starts").
2. He must *collect the right information*, which requires him to know where to look ("I will look at the other customers and see where they are standing and which way they are facing"). To carry out this step, he must have the capacity to recognize other customers, differentiate them from employees, and see them as a group.
3. He must *interpret the information*. He has to assume the right meaning in what he observes. If he sees several customers standing one behind the other, all facing the same way, he must be able to recognize and label that group as "the line."
4. He must *make a judgment* about what he should *do* based on how he interpreted the information ("I think I should go and stand behind the last person in the line"). This judgment is based on the information at hand as well as his prior fund of knowledge about the social norms of his culture.
5. The *product* is the behavioral *outcome of the judgment* made at the end of the process. In this case, the outcome is seen when he acts on his judgment and stands in the correct place in the line.

Every step the man took in this example was based on his own information gathering and interpretation. Although he probably relied on some environmental cues (e.g., position of the deli counter, location of the cash register), it was necessary for him to be able to "read" the people in the store, as well, in order to have a successful outcome. He had never been in that deli before, yet he could make accurate guesses about the other people there, what they expected of him, and how he should behave. He made these accurate guesses without ever having met them and without speaking to anyone before deciding what he should do. It is also likely that he went through this process in a matter of seconds and without very much conscious thought.

People must make several hundred of these judgments every day. This example was a simple challenge because the man only needed to focus on *body language*. Most scenarios are far more complex and involve additional sources of social information, such as the *facial expression, voice tone,* and *social language* used by other people. There is evidence that people with ASD may have impairments in their ability to perform any or all of the steps of this social inference process. Theoretically, these deficits may be the reason for the maladaptive outcomes that are observed clinically in the social domain (Crooke, Winner, & Oswang, 2016; Winner, 2000, 2002), often called "social skill deficits" by clinicians and educators.

Let us consider a man with ASD in the deli scenario. This time, we start at Step 5, the behavioral outcome. The man with ASD enters the deli, proceeds to stand in front of the first person in the line, and begins to order his sandwich. When the employee ignores him because she is serving another customer, the man repeats his request in a louder voice. This behavior would be called, according to the social norms of his culture, "cutting the line," and would be considered rude. It would also be met by any number of unpleasant and hostile comments from other customers. By working through the steps of social inference, there are several points at which this man could have made an error, each resulting in the same unfortunate ending.

1. He may have made the wrong decision about *what information to gather.* He might have decided to look only for the location of the deli counter and not at the other customers.
2. He may have known what information to gather, but did not know *how to collect it.* He may have looked for other customers but did not know to look at their body language (standing position).
3. He may have gotten the first two steps right, but then did not *interpret the information* correctly. In other words, he may have seen the way they were standing but did not cluster them together as a group and/or did not recognize them as a "line."
4. He may have looked for, collected, and interpreted the information correctly, but made a poor *judgment* about what he should *do*—that is, he may have located the customer line and identified it as such, but he may not know the social rule about waiting at the back of a line or, more realistically, may not understand its importance. He may know the rule but think it does not apply to him if he is in a hurry, for instance.

When clinicians are working with adult patients with ASD, a common presenting problem is "lack of social skills." If social skill development becomes a therapy goal, it is important to consider that any number of these social inference errors may be present (Crooke et al., 2016; Winner, 2000, 2002). The research supporting this hypothesis is outlined below. Only studies that use adolescent or adult subjects are included in the discussion because they are most relevant to the clinical population that is the focus of this book.

SOCIAL PERCEPTION AND USE OF CUES

The first two steps of social inference, as defined above (*deciding what social information to gather* and *collecting it*) have been shown to be dysfunctional in persons with ASD. Klin and colleagues (2002a) and Klin, Jones, Schultz, Volkmar, and Cohen (2002b), through a series of seminal eye-tracking studies, asked how people with ASD without ID gather visual–social information. They designed a methodology that allowed them to observe the process by which subjects visually scan a naturalistic, dynamic social scenario. In one study (Klin et al., 2002b), they recruited 15 male adolescents with ASD without ID (whom they described as "cognitively able males with autism") and 15 matched controls. The social competence and severity of autism symptoms were measured. Using an eye-tracking device, the researchers were able to record the precise movements of subjects' eyes while they watched an emotionally charged set of movie scenes, depicting several adult characters in conversations that involved interpersonal conflict, tension, and strong negative emotions. The device then superimposed the actual pathways the eyes had followed directly onto the movie scene; the subjects had thereby left a set of digital "eye tracks" for the researchers to view. Tracking patterns were analyzed and significant group differences were observed in the time spent looking at four types of visual information in the movie scenes, on or around the main characters of the story: mouths, eyes, body, and objects (e.g., objects hanging on the walls of the movie set). The subjects with autism spent significantly more time looking at mouths, bodies, and objects, but significantly less time looking at the eye region than the control subjects. Interestingly, within the autistic group, the amount of time spent looking at eyes did not correlate with social adjustment. However, time spent looking at mouths predicted better adjustment and time looking at objects predicted poorer adjustment.

There have been many previous accounts of eye-gaze avoidance in this population, and, before this study, people tended to jump to the conclusion that individuals with ASD miss the social meaning of exchanges simply because they do not look at people's eyes. Based on this conclusion, the clinical solution would be to simply train them to make more eye contact. The data from Klin and colleagues (2002b), however, showed that social perception is not that simple in older teens and adults. In their study, the more socially competent subjects with ASD did not necessarily look at the eyes during the movie any longer than the more poorly adjusted subjects.

To further our understanding of eye-gaze patterns in adults with ASD, Kliemann, Dziobek, Hatri, Steimke, and Heekeren (2010) used eye-tracking technology to investigate whether people with ASD without ID are failing to orient toward eyes (not looking at all) or whether they are actively avoiding eye contact (looking away after seeing it). Orientation was defined by looking at the eyes, and avoidance was measured as frequency of looking away from the eyes once there had been a glance at the eyes. A group of 12 adults with ASD and matched typical controls were shown various faces expressing fearful, happy, and neutral emotion while their eye movements were tracked. Compared to controls, the subjects with ASD did look at the eyes (orient), but less frequently than typical controls. They also showed more frequent gaze shifts away from the eyes (avoidance). These preliminary data suggest that adults with ASD are not unaware of the eyes—they are not entirely missing them—but are looking at them and reflexively looking away.

Of course, these laboratory studies do not tell us how these adults may be using eye contact in real-life situations as opposed to watching images or what factors contribute to their relative social competence. They do, nevertheless, show evidence that these individuals are failing to look consistently at the one cue source (other peoples' eyes) on which typical people heavily rely during social exchanges.

MIND READING AND EMOTION RECOGNITION

The work of Baron-Cohen, Jolliffe, Mortimore, and Robertson (1997) suggests that even if adults with ASD are directed to look at other people's eyes, they are not very skilled at reading them. In other words, they show problems with the third step of social inference: *interpreting* the information gathered from other people. The ability to formulate ideas about the mental states of others, or ToM, is a crucial part of the social inference process. It is easy to imagine that any person who comes to the wrong conclusion about another person's thoughts, feelings, or intentions is apt to respond in a maladaptive way both emotionally and behaviorally. Baron-Cohen and his colleagues first raised the question over 30 years ago about the usefulness of ToM as a construct in explaining the social dysfunction of people with autism (Baron-Cohen, Leslie, & Frith, 1985). His group has investigated this question through dozens of studies in the years since then and has demonstrated repeatedly that people with ASD have some difficulty with intersubjectivity—that is, with formulating a ToM about others—and this deficit has come to be termed *mindblindness* (e.g., Baron-Cohen, 1995).

In one study, while developing a test called Reading the Mind in the Eyes, Baron-Cohen and colleagues (1997) showed a series of photographs to adults diagnosed with ASD without ID, as well as a sample of typical adults. These were photos of actors portraying different emotions and mental states. Some pictures showed the whole face, some the mouth region only, and some the eye region only. Subjects were asked to choose a mental state word from a pair of multiple-choice items that were presented with each photo. Compared to typical control subjects, those with ASD performed significantly more poorly when looking at all three types of pictures, but the effect was most pronounced when they looked at the eye region alone. It is as if they relied on aspects of the face *other than* the eyes to attribute mental states. Visual cues that may be found in people's eyes seem to be relatively useless to the person with ASD.

To find out whether these deficits in the ability to infer mental states is specific to visual information, Rutherford, Baron-Cohen, and Wheelwright (2002) presented to a group of adults with ASD without ID, as well as typical controls, an expanded version of the Reading the Mind in the Eyes test that included auditory information. In one part of the test, subjects were asked to listen to actors' voices portraying different emotions and mental states. The results showed that the subjects with ASD had significant deficits compared to typical controls in their ability to accurately infer the mental states conveyed by the actors from the vocalizations. This finding suggests that even nonvisual emotional information is not utilized effectively by people with ASD.

These research results lead to the question of whether these adults have a general deficit in recognizing and identifying faces *or* an impaired ability to read emotional information, regardless of its source. Hefter, Manoach, and Barton (2005) set out to answer this question by studying a group of 26 adults they defined as having social developmental disorders (SDD) of different types, including AS, ASD without ID, and *socioemotional processing disorder* (normal language and cognitive development with neurological evidence of right-hemispheric dysfunction). Through a series of tasks, they separately tested subjects' abilities to (1) identify faces, (2) recognize emotional expression from faces, and (3) recognize emotional expression from nonfacial cues (voice and body language). Diagnostic label did not predict ability on any particular test, and 10 of the 26 subjects performed within the normal range on face identification. The ability to recognize faces was not correlated with the ability to perceive facial expressions (emotions) or to perceive emotion in nonfacial cues. However, there was a correlation between the ability to read both facial and nonfacial emotional expressions.

In a similar study, a group of 23 adults with ASD (including some subjects with no ID and some with mild ID) and 23 age- and gender-matched controls were assessed using a variety of emotion recognition tasks across three modalities, which were facial expression, body movement, and vocal expression (Philip et al., 2010). In all tests, subjects were asked to identify the emotion portrayed in each of many types of stimuli. Four different facial expression tests presented photographs of faces with a variety of emotions and intensities. Body movement stimuli were movie clips of actors portraying emotion through their body movements, and subjects were asked to identify the emotion shown in each. Voice emotion stimuli were recordings of actors expressing emotion through their voice tone and again, subjects were asked to identify the emotions they heard in each recording. The ASD subjects showed significant impairments across all of the stimulus domains, and these effects were not accounted for by IQ or basic face-processing ability. These findings support the idea that adults with ASD show a deficit in processing nonverbal emotional information that is not related to the ability to recognize or identify faces. Even when they are directed to attend to faces, they fail to utilize cues about the mental states of others, whether that information comes from faces, voices, or body language.

In an effort to measure the neural processes that occur while subjects engage in the recognition tasks similar to the ones described above, researchers have recently been using electroencephalogram (EEG) technology that can measure a variety of processing phenomena in ASD. By attaching electrodes to the scalp and recording event-related potential (ERP), researchers are able to measure the latency between stimulus presentation during a recognition test and the precise moment the subject begins to process the stimulus (see Jeste & Nelson, 2009, for a review of these methods as used in autism research). In plain language, this technology allows us to capture the exact instant a stimulus (photo, video clip, audio clip) is "registered" by the subject's brain.

In a seminal study by Lerner, McPartland, and Morris (2013), 34 adolescents with ASD without ID were asked to do a series of emotion recognition tasks that involved both visual stimuli (faces varied by emotion displayed, age of actor, and intensity of emotion) and auditory stimuli (voice clips varied by emotion in the tone, age of speaker, and intensity of emotion). What made this study unique is that EEG technology was used to measure ERP activity *while* the subjects were doing these emotion recognition tasks. This allowed the researchers to look at correlations between task performance (emotion recognition ability) and *social information processing speed* as measured by the latency between stimulus presentation and ERP. Similar to findings in other studies, the sample as a whole demonstrated significant impairment in emotion recognition ability (albeit there was a lot of variability within the sample in terms of degree of deficit and on which tasks). More important was the finding that task performance was correlated with *processing speed*; the slower their processing speed, the poorer was their emotion recognition ability. This gives us a new understanding about the mechanisms of pathology that underlie the social cognition deficits that have been so well documented, pointing to the very earliest moments in a social interaction as being atypical for these individuals. More studies like this are needed in adults, but these data provide enough evidence for us to consider that a fraction of a second of delay in processing social information might well be enough to throw off the whole chain of events that are essential for successful social interactions.

One of the questions that can be raised about this line of research is that the subjects demonstrate these deficits under contrived, static, or artificial circumstances in the laboratory. Although the evidence is convincing for the presence of these deficits in this population, we still know very little about how these individuals perform in more naturalistic settings, with the exception of documented clinical observations.

In an effort to create a more naturalistic test of social cognition, Dziobek and colleagues (2006) designed the Movie for the Assessment of Social Cognition (MASC). The researchers hoped that the test would be useful in assessing these skills in subjects with ASD or schizophrenia. The test requires subjects to watch a 15-minute movie about four adults who get together for a dinner party. The video is paused 46 times and the subjects are asked to answer questions about the characters' feelings, thoughts, and intentions. The movie was based on the researchers' operational definition of social cognition and simulated the way it plays out in real life.

Dziobek and colleagues (2006) deliberately selected a group of highly intelligent and educated subjects with ASD to test the validity of the MASC in discriminating between them and typical control subjects. This method was employed in response to previous studies that had shown that some tests of social cognition fail to capture deficits in subjects with ASD who have high IQs (Happé, 1994; Ozonoff, Rogers, & Pennington, 1991). In the initial study, the ASD group had an average Full Scale IQ of 122 and education level of 16.7 years, and the controls were matched on age, gender, IQ, and education level. As predicted, the ASD subjects performed significantly more poorly than controls on the MASC, and more poorly than their own performance on the other tests of social cognition. This finding supports the presence of an impairment in the ability to infer the mental states of others—an impairment that appears to be most obvious in a naturalistic (complex and unstructured) social situation.

If a person cannot read cues about what another person is thinking or feeling, then certainly he or she cannot engage in the higher-order social inference process that we call *empathy*. This is a complex *cognitive-emotional* activity that allows people to be successful in relating to others and enjoy intimacy; indeed, it is "the 'glue' of the social world, drawing us to help others and stopping us from hurting others" (Baron-Cohen & Wheelwright, 2004, p. 163). Because it likely involves multiple processes, empathy is very hard to define and measure. Current researchers define it as a two-component process: the *cognitive* or "intellectual" understanding of another person's affective experience, as well as an *emotional* response to that experience (Baron-Cohen & Wheelwright, 2004; Rogers, Dziobek, Hassenstab, Wolf, & Convit, 2007).

For example, a woman learned that her coworker Jim had lost his mother unexpectedly. The cognitive component of her empathy would be stated as "I *believe* Jim is sad," whereas the emotional component would be stated as "I *feel sad* when I imagine what Jim is going through right now." According to the contemporary definition put forth above, both components must be present for full empathy to be experienced. The cognitive component is necessary but not sufficient; the assessment must be accurate as a prerequisite for the emotional experience to be fitting, but it is not sufficient without the latter.

One of the myths about people with ASD, as mentioned in Chapter 1, is that they lack empathy. I shared my anecdotal impression from clinical cases that they do indeed have the capacity for empathy, but may have some information-processing deficits that impede a full experience. Recent research on empathy and ASD has supported this notion. Baron-Cohen and Wheelwright (2004) did a critical review of existing measures of empathy and found that none of them measured the construct according to the current definition. Some were not pure enough in that they also captured other concepts. Other measures did not assess both the cognitive and emotional components of empathy. These authors designed a new measure, the Empathy Quotient (EQ), to overcome these flaws. It is a 60-item self-report device that asks subjects to rate (on a 4-point scale) the degree to which they agree or disagree with statements such as "I can easily tell if someone else wants to enter a conversation" and "I get upset if I see people suffering on news programs." They administered this test to 90 adults with ASD without ID and 90 age- and sex-matched controls. As predicted, the subjects with ASD scored significantly lower on the test than controls. However, as the authors pointed out, the test does not assess emotional empathy separate from cognitive empathy. They conducted clinical interviews with 50 of the clinical subjects after the test and asked them to generate possible reasons for their lower scores. The subjects described a difficulty with judging, explaining, anticipating, and interpreting other people's behavior (cognitive processes), but that they have no desire to hurt others. In fact, they reported, if it is pointed out to them that their behavior has been hurtful in some way, they will usually express remorse and desire to avoid such hurtful actions in the future.

Although these are anecdotal descriptions, they are consistent with my clinical cases; these individuals appear to make cognitive errors—that is, they fail to glean important information from other people—which then impedes their ability to experience the emotional component of empathy. If given the proper information, however, they will experience the feeling and show a desire to correct any errors they have made that may have offended others. They are failing to show an emotional response not because they are incapable, but because they never get that far. For example, how can a person experience an emotional reaction to the sadness of a friend if he or she does not even know that the friend is sad?

In an effort to isolate the different empathic components in adults with ASD, Rogers and colleagues (2007) sampled 21 adults with ASD without ID and 21 age-matched controls. They administered four tests of social cognition and one test of empathy, the Interpersonal Reactivity Index (IRI; Davis, 1980), which has four subscales representing subdomains of empathy. Two are assumed to measure the cognitive component of empathy: Perspective-Taking (tendency to spontaneously adopt the point of view of others) and Fantasy (tendency to identify with fictional characters). The other two are assumed to measure the emotional component of empathy: Empathic Concern (tendency to experience feelings of sympathy and compassion for unfortunate others) and Personal Distress (tendency to experience distress and discomfort in response to the extreme distress in others). Results showed significant group differences on the social cognition tests, with the subjects with ASD performing more poorly on all of those tasks. They also received significantly lower scores on the cognitive empathy subscales. However, the pattern of results was quite different on the emotional empathy subscales. On the Empathic Concern subtest, they performed similarly to the typical controls; there were no group differences on these scores. On the Personal Distress subtest, they scored significantly *higher* than the typical controls, suggesting that they become more upset than typical people when faced with the extreme distress of others. The authors are careful to point out that the Personal Distress subtest also taps into anxiety, and although the high scores could be a demonstration of empathy, they may also reflect the overall levels of generalized anxiety reported in the ASD population.

Dziobek and colleagues (2008) were able to demonstrate similar patterns of performance on another sample of subjects with ASD ($n = 17$) and typical controls ($n = 18$) by using a different empathy measure called the Multifaceted Empathy Test (MET). As with the IRI used in the previous study, the MET allows assessment of cognitive empathy and emotional empathy separately. Like the previous study, the subjects with ASD showed significantly more impairment in cognitive empathy, while they did not differ from the typical controls on the emotional empathy portion of the test. These findings are inconsistent with the popular belief that people with ASD are uncaring or lack empathy, but rather suggest that they may process the experiences of others in a unique way.

Social Language

This topic was included as a subsection of social cognition because language plays such an integral role in social understanding. Core problems in "social communication" are essential to the diagnosis of ASD in DSM-5, no matter the intellectual functioning level of the patient. When a clinician works with a patient, it is almost impossible to find the dividing line between dysfunctional cognition and dysfunctional understanding and use of social language. As mentioned in Chapter 1, people with ASD without ID tend to score within the normal range on standardized language tests (Landa, 2000; Paul, Landa, & Simmons, 2014), which means they do not have problems in the formal use of language, such as word or sentence production. On IQ tests, they often exhibit relative strengths on verbal subtests. However, as described in the SLP field, they have great difficulty understanding and using language in the flexible way necessary to meet social demands (Landa, 2000; Paul et al., 2014; Twachtman-Cullen, 1998). These deficits are in the *pragmatics* of communication—the social-cognition deficits outlined in the previous section are thought to play a major role in these language issues (Crooke et al., 2016; Landa, 2000; Twachtman-Cullen, 1998; Winner, 2000, 2002), and vice versa.

Interventions that are designed to directly target social language use are best implemented by speech–language pathologists, not by psychotherapists. Nevertheless, it is important for psychotherapists to be familiar with these deficits for several reasons. One is that psychotherapy is a highly verbal activity. Because patients with

ASD have a unique way of using language, a therapist must learn each patient's idiosyncrasies in this domain in order to effectively communicate with him or her. Individuals with ASD without ID often appear superficially to have great command of the language, but their formal verbal strengths tend to mask the deficits outlined here, which are subtler and may "fly under the radar." Another reason a therapist must be familiar with these factors is that they often play a contributing role in the presenting mental health problems for which the patient is seeking treatment. At times a referral to a speech–language pathologist is necessary once the assessment and initial case conceptualization are complete so that speech therapy can be integrated into the overall treatment plan.

The reader is referred to Twachtman-Cullen (1998) and Paul and colleagues (2014) for reviews of the deficits in language pragmatics found in ASD, and to Crooke and colleagues (2016) for the role social cognition plays in these problems. These speech–language pathologists have done an excellent job in describing these complex issues in a way that is easy for non-speech–language pathologists to understand. Some of these descriptions are briefly outlined below.

Twachtman-Cullen (1998) defines the "the communication system" on which human beings rely and suggests that there are three components. These distinct processes, which professionals often confuse, are:

1. *Speech*—the neuromuscular motor behavior that purveys verbal utterances; the mechanical transmission of the sounds.
2. *Language*—the code that is agreed upon by a group of people that specifies how concepts are represented by symbols (words) and includes rules for form (syntax/grammar) and content (semantics).
3. *Communication*—the use of speech and language for the purpose of exchanging messages between people.

People with ASD without ID do not have difficulty with speech or language but do struggle with communication, or *pragmatics*. A typically developing person learns the rules for tailoring language to fit social demands through childhood and adolescence, and these rules are dictated by the culture in which the individual is raised (Landa, 2000). However, people with ASD fail to learn these rules in the way their peers do, so by the time they are adults, they are struggling in the social domain, largely because of their problems with *communicative intentions, presupposition*, and *discourse management*. These three processes of pragmatic language use are described below. The overlap between this area of SLP and the social-cognition dysfunction outlined in the previous section is obvious in the following descriptions.

COMMUNICATIVE INTENTIONS

To be a successful communicator, one must be able to convey and read the intentions behind the words used in a sentence. People often say things that are not literal representations of what they mean. However, they still convey what they mean because the words they use are modulated through the social situation (context), intonation (voice pitch and loudness variation), facial expression, gestures, and environmental cues. People with ASD have difficulty using any or all of these tools to convey their intentions clearly to others. They also have difficulty perceiving intention from others that is conveyed in these ways.

For example, if your boss asks you to do a task that you do not want to do, you may say out loud to her, "Sure, I would be happy to do it." Your *intention* is to convey to her simply that you are *willing* to do it, not literally that you are happy about it. But the *social context* (you are responding to an authority figure) may have influenced your choice of words; you chose a phrase that, in your culture, is a polite way to agree to carry out a task. In a different social context, you may also choose those words but convey a different intention by using facial expression and intonation to modulate the message.

For example, you just finish telling your spouse that your day is overbooked and you are very pressed for time, and your spouse promptly asks you to stop at the dry cleaners to pick up some things on the way home. Because the request annoys you and you are not really willing to do it, you may say, "Sure, I would be happy to do it." In contrast to how you may have said this to your boss in the earlier example, you hiss the words through clenched teeth, and glare at your spouse while saying it. You are hoping your spouse picks up your intention through your intonation and facial expression.

People with ASD cannot easily flex their strategies for different contexts. They are overly reliant on the literal meaning of words people use and often suffer communication breakdown because of it. If the boss or the spouse in the above examples had ASD, that person may have taken the phrase to mean the exact same thing in both situations: that the speaker was literally going to feel happy while carrying out the requested task.

PRESUPPOSITION

A successful communicator can make a sound judgment about the knowledge, expectations, and beliefs that another person already has before formulating a message to deliver to that person. As described by Paul and colleagues (2014), the speaker takes into consideration how much preexisting information the listener shares with him or her when planning the content and form of the message to be communicated. These authors define presuppositional success as depending on an array of different abilities: A person must be able to regulate attention, have a fund of knowledge about social norms and rules, be flexible enough to consider different perspectives on the same situation, and have the language skills to phrase things in alternative ways. On a practical level, it involves knowing what the communication partner is expecting and being able to adjust language accordingly. In the previous example, when you decide to use a polite phrase when agreeing to do the task your boss requested, you were using your presuppositional ability. This ability allowed you to assume that you and your boss share the same expectations about each other's role; the boss's job includes assigning tasks, and your job includes complying with reasonable requests.

People with ASD show difficulties with adjusting language use in response to the ever-changing contexts within social situations. They do not know when and how to be formal or colloquial, when to elaborate on an idea or give a condensed version, how much background information to provide, how complex or simple the sentences used should be, and what topics are taboo in what situations—all because of a deficiency in the ability to presuppose the needs and expectations of the listener. These individuals also fail to provide signals that would allow others to make good presuppositions about them.

DISCOURSE MANAGEMENT

Last but not least, a successful communicator must be able to participate in an ongoing exchange of utterances that serves to build an agreed-upon hierarchy of topics and subtopics. The abilities that are involved in this process may be called "conversation skills" by a layperson. During successful discourse, people follow shared rules about topic management, conversational repair after a breakdown, and storytelling (narrative discourse). Although there has been no research on these processes in adults with ASD, Twachtman-Cullen (1998) presents Grice's (1975) four maxims (rules) for discourse and describes how they can be broken. All of these rule-breaking behaviors have been described previously in clinical cases of ASD and have also been observed in the patients I have treated.

1. *In regard to quantity, be informative without being verbose.* This rule is broken by someone who speaks "nonstop," without regard to cues the listener conveys indicating disinterest or desire to escape.
2. *In regard to quality, be truthful.* This rule is broken by someone who confabulates or fills in gaps with false information that he or she believes to be true.
3. *In regard to relevance, contribute only information that is pertinent to the topic and situation.* This rule is broken by someone who makes tangential comments.
4. *In regard to clarity, convey information that is clear and understandable to the listener.* This rule is broken by someone who initiates a conversation in the middle of a thought, without providing background information.

To summarize, evidence indicates that people with ASD, including those with average or above IQ, have problems with both social inference and social language. *Social inference* involves the ability to make accurate, educated guesses about what is required in a social situation, based on information from multiple sources. *Social language* refers to the understanding and use of language according to the current social context. These two processes are interrelated in the sense that a person cannot perform well in the social language domain if he or she has impaired social cognition, and vice versa. Many of the "social skill deficits" of ASD are driven by core problems in social cognition and social language.

Dysfunctional Processing of Information about Self

This section describes the various difficulties people with ASD demonstrate when processing information from and about the self. The decision to separate this area of dysfunction into a separate category from social cognition was somewhat arbitrary because, as I illustrate in Figure 2.2, all of the core deficits of ASD overlap and interrelate. This crude definition of categories is meant to illustrate that not only do people with ASD have difficulty "reading" others but they also have problems with the perception of information that is coming from internal sources, or *interoception*. For instance, Garfinkel and colleagues (2016) showed in a sample of adults with ASD compared to typical controls that the ASD subjects demonstrated lower interoceptive accuracy (measured by heartbeat detection tests) than typical controls and exaggerated interoceptive sensitivity to internal sensations, compared to typical control subjects. The difficulty in "reading" themselves is detrimental in social interactions, and it can also affect them when they are alone, so therefore is worthwhile exploring separately. Two major areas of functioning are affected by dysfunctional internal "feedback loops" of information: (1) the perception and regulation of arousal states, or *emotion*; and (2) the perception and regulation of *sensory–motor processing*.

Emotion Perception and Regulation

It is almost impossible to separate emotional from social experience. In fact, the dysfunction in the emotional life of people with ASD has been conceptualized and reported by researchers almost exclusively in a social context. Hobson (2005) discusses the major theme of emotion dysfunction in autism as "impairment in sharing subjective states and coordinating attitudes with other people" (p. 419). Marans, Rubin, and Laurent (2005), lending insight from the fields of SLP and occupational therapy, outline crucial considerations of ER factors when evaluating people with ASD. They attribute the poor social communication skills seen in this population partially to their poor ER skills. According to these authors, in order to attend to the most important aspects of a social situation, one must be able to maintain an "optimal state of arousal" or "steady internal state" (p. 980). Using Tronick's (1989) conceptualization of ER skill development in normal infancy, they divide the skill deficits seen in ASD into two categories: *mutual regulation* and *self-regulation*. The term *mutual regulation skills* refers to the ability to use others to regulate arousal states. These skills include abilities to:

- Understand and interpret the emotional state of the self and others.
- Interpret affective cues regarding the intention of others.
- Express emotions in a socially conventional manner as a means of seeking help from others.
- Respond to help that is offered by others.
- Maintain focus on social engagement.

Self-regulation skills involve abilities to:

- Recognize and interpret one's own physiological and emotional state.
- Be aware of one's own emotional reactivity and variable arousal in response to sensory sensitivities or social overstimulation.
- Attend to information in the social situation that is needed to solve problems.
- Grade reactions to coincide with the expectations of the current social situation.
- Use effective behavioral strategies that are socially acceptable to regulate experience.
- Use cognitive strategies to anticipate and cope with dysregulating events.

More recently, basic emotion research has focused on regulation processes and on examining, from a transdiagnostic perspective, how problems with emotion regulation (ER) may factor into psychopathology in general (see Kring & Sloan, 2010). Gross and Thompson (2007) have described a developmental model that suggests humans first develop ER skills and then learn to use them flexibly and in appropriate contexts. These skills and applications are *extrinsic* when they involve other people (similar to

Tronick's [1989] mutual regulation skills) and *intrinsic* when they involve the self (i.e., self-regulation skills). As we seek an understanding of their role in psychopathology, these authors suggest that we find ways to delineate problems with skills being deficient versus problems with intact skills being applied in inappropriate contexts. So, when a therapist is working with a patient it would be useful to answer the question "Has this person failed to develop ER skills, or does this person possess the skills, but is not applying them in an adaptive way?"

It is easy to make the connection between mutual regulation (extrinsic) skills and the deficits outlined in the earlier section on social cognition. To avoid redundancy, this section focuses less on the social aspect of emotional functioning and more on the internal and subjective experience of emotion, which is more closely tied to self-regulation (intrinsic) skills, as discussed by Marans and colleagues (2005) and Geller (2005). There are only a few studies that have explored the way people on the autism spectrum experience and respond to their own emotions, probably because these concepts are elusive and difficult to measure. The small body of research literature is reviewed here, however, with implications for conceptualizing adult psychotherapy cases. Two relevant areas of research focus to be summarized are alexithymia and emotion regulation.

ALEXITHYMIA

One of the prerequisite skills for modifying one's own arousal level is being able to recognize and label one's own emotional state. A deficit in the fund or accessibility of words to describe subjective mental states is called alexithymia by researchers of the general population and more recently identified as a phenomenon with considerable overlap with ASD (Fitzgerald & Bellgrove, 2006). Berthoz and Hill (2005) investigated the presence of alexithymia in a group of adults with ASD without ID. They administered two scales: the Toronto Alexithymia Scale (TAS-20) and the Bermond and Vorst Alexithymia Questionnaire—Form B (BVAQ-B). They also administered the Beck Depression Inventory (BDI) to all subjects. Results indicated that the subjects with ASD were more alexithymic than typical controls but also more depressed, as measured by the BDI. This finding leads to the question "How can a person report the presence of depressive symptoms if he or she is alexithymic or has difficulty identifying his or her own mental state?" Further analysis of these findings shows that alexithymia represents several types of disability that may not be equally prevalent in affected individuals. The TAS-20, which measures the more *cognitive aspects* of identifying one's own mental state, discriminated between the groups, but the BVAQ-B, thought to measure the more *emotional aspects* of alexithymia, did not. This finding suggests that self-evaluation deficits exist only for certain types of internal states.

The study by Rogers and colleagues (2007) presented earlier in the chapter is relevant to this discussion. To briefly review, Rogers and colleagues administered the IRI (Davis, 1980) to adults with ASD without ID and to a group of matched controls. The purpose of the study was to investigate the social concept of empathy. However, self-reporting of one's own emotional reactions was a critical method of responding to the items on the IRI. The pattern of results mirrors what was found in the alexithymia study. The subscales that measure the *cognitive* component of empathy—Perspective-Taking and Fantasy—seemed to reflect an underreactivity in ASD compared to typical people, whereas the subscales assumed to measure the *emotional* component of empathy—Empathic Concern and Personal Distress—reflected similar reactivity (empathic concern) or overreactivity (personal distress) compared to typical people.

Neither of these studies tells us how individuals with ASD actually experience their emotions, only how they *report* these experiences. Nevertheless, these studies provide preliminary information suggesting that people with ASD report *less* emotional arousal than typical people when test questions have cognitive elements, but *more* intense emotional experiences than typical people if questions are more purely directed toward emotion (e.g., BDI, and the Personal Distress subscale of the IRI).

More recent studies on alexithymia and ASD have examined whether the alexithymia is part of the core dysfunction in autism or is a separate but commonly occurring phenomenon in ASD. Bird, Press, and Richardson (2011) measured attention to faces during video clips using eye-fixation data in a sample of adults with ASD without ID. They also measured alexithymia and autism symptom severity and found that only alexithymia severity predicted eye fixation, not autism symptom severity. In another investigation, Cook, Brewer, Shah, and Bird (2013) assessed facial emotion recognition ability and alexithymia in a sample of adults with ASD without ID. Alexithymia was correlated with task performance, but autism severity was not. Finally, Shah, Hall, Catmur, and Bird (2016) examined the relationship among ASD symptoms, alexithymia, and measures of interoception. In a sample of adults with ASD without ID, they found that alexithymia was more closed associated with impaired introception than ASD symptoms. The authors of all three of these studies suggest that alexithymia is not a core feature of ASD, but a separate condition that co-occurs in a subgroup of people with ASD.

Obviously, many more controlled investigations are needed before conclusions can be drawn. However, these data give a practitioner some sense that people with ASD report on and perceive their emotions in ways that are different from typical people. These differences have important assessment considerations that are discussed in Chapter 3.

EMOTION REGULATION

Recent studies have demonstrated some unique factors in the intrinsic ER tendencies of people with ASD. Samson, Huber, and Gross (2012) examined aspects of ER in a sample of 27 adults with ASD without ID and an equal number of typical controls. They demonstrated significant differences on self-report measures of emotion experience (Positive and Negative Affect Schedule [PANAS]), emotion labeling (TAS-20), and ER (Emotion Regulation Questionnaire [ERQ]) in the ASD sample. The ASD subjects reported significantly more negative affect, but no less positive affect than the control subjects. Consistent with the alexithymia studies mentioned earlier, the ASD subjects reported significantly higher levels of alexithymia on the TAS-20. Most relevant here are the significant findings that ASD subjects reported on the ERQ: less use of cognitive reappraisal as an ER strategy, but more use of suppression as a strategy to regulate emotion. The authors suggest that this represents a less adaptive ER profile in the subjects with ASD.

In another study, Swain and colleagues (2015) examined the relationship between difficulties with ER and anxiety in a sample of 69 adults with ASD without ID. Measures of ASD symptoms severity (Social Responsiveness Scale [SRS]), social anxiety (Social Anxiety Scale [SAS]), and ER problems (Difficulties in Emotion Regulation Scale [DERS]) were administered. Multiple regression analysis showed that ER problems predicted social anxiety severity, based on self-report measures, especially the subdomains of nonacceptance of negative thoughts, impulse control difficulties, and limited access to regulation strategies.

While there is no doubt that ER problems are closely associated with ASD and the comorbid conditions commonly seen in affected adults, far more research is required to understand the mechanisms by which these phenomena are interrelated (Mazefsky et al., 2013). For example, Mazefsky and colleagues (2013) propose that ER problems are inherent in the core symptoms of ASD and therefore put individuals at risk for the development of behavioral (e.g., aggression, self-injury) and emotional (e.g., anxiety, depression) problems. White and colleagues (2014) provide a rich review of the research that supports this conceptual model, synthesizing disparate fields of study to make the argument that ER ability is inevitably compromised by the core processing deficits of ASD. Because ER problems are well documented as central to so many mental health problems in the general psychopathology literature, it is logical to consider that people with ASD would be vulnerable to the development of other mental health problems via their ER impairments.

In an attempt to more closely examine the relationship between ASD and some specific ER problems that are known to be associated with anxiety in non-ASD populations, Maisel and colleagues (2016) recruited 76 adults with ASD without ID and 75 typical controls. They measured three domains of emotion labeling/regulation that have already been documented in the etiology of anxiety disorders in the general population: intolerance of uncertainty (Intolerance of Uncertainty Scale–12 [IUS-12]); alexithymia (TAS-20); and emotional acceptance, defined as the ability to allow one's internal experiences to be as they are and not to push them away (Nonreactivity factor of the Five Facet Mindfulness Questionnaire [FFMQ-Nonreactivity]). They also measured the severity of ASD traits (Autism-Spectrum Quotient [AQ]), as well as three measures of anxiety (State–Trait Anxiety Inventory [STAI], Penn State Worry Questionnaire [PSW-Q], and Fear of Negative Evaluation Scale [FNE]). Structured equation modeling showed that ASD predicted ER impairment; the level of ASD directly predicted more intolerance of uncertainty, higher alexithymia scores, and lower emotional acceptance. In addition, the alexithymia and emotional acceptance scores mediated the relationship between autism severity and anxiety.

In sum, we have enough research evidence to consider that treatment-seeking adults with ASD are experiencing comorbid mental health problems, at least partially because of impaired emotion identification and regulation ability. While more studies are surely being done to bolster our understanding of the underlying mechanisms involved, the treatment implications of these findings are presented more in the chapters ahead.

Sensory–Motor Processing

As mentioned earlier, people with ASD appear to demonstrate dysfunctional processing of information about their own bodies, or interoception. This section focuses on how that affects the sensory and motor perception differences that are features of ASD. Ever since Kanner (1943) first described his cases of autism, it has been well documented that children with autism have atypical sensory–motor development (see Baranek, Parham, & Bodfish, 2005, for a review). These issues have been less well studied in adults with ASD. Anecdotally speaking, patients often report problems with one or more sensory systems in the form of hypersensitivity or hyposensitivity, and these problems can be a source of stress (Groden, Baron, & Groden, 2006).

SENSORY

Table 2.1 provides a summary of the sensory problems seen in ASD, adapted from Myles and colleagues (2005). Unlike previous editions, DSM-5 now includes "Hyper- or hyporeactivity to sensory input or unusual interest in sensory aspects of the environment (e.g., apparent indifference to pain/temperature, adverse response to specific sounds or textures, excessive smelling or touching of objects, visual fascination with lights or movement)" as a symptom of ASD (American Psychiatric Association, 2013, p. 50), whereas it was only mentioned as an associated feature of autistic disorder in DSM-IV-TR (American Psychiatric Association, 2000). Because these individuals are processing sensory information so differently from the typical person, they may have extreme reactions to situations that seem unremarkable to others. Some sounds that are universally aversive, such as fingernails being raked across a chalkboard, may not bother a person with ASD, but a sound that would be considered mundane by most people, such as someone chewing gum very quietly, may be considered highly aversive to him or her. These individuals may be prone to irritability when affected by particular stimuli. Often an unusual behavior may be the only way a person has been able to regulate or manage an overwhelming sensory experience (e.g., squinting, body rocking, restricted clothing choices).

Another coping strategy many individuals adopt is avoidance, which can be mistaken as oppositional behavior, stubbornness, or procrastination by loved ones and other supporters. Because they sometimes have difficulty reporting their internal states to others (i.e., due to alexithymia and social language deficits), they may not let others know what they are experiencing and what their reason is for avoiding a particular situation. For example, one man with ASD who had tactile sensitivities dreaded large family gatherings at his house (he was living with his parents). He actually enjoyed seeing his relatives and was not intimidated by the social demands. Rather, he was bothered by the fact that the house would be crowded, with a lot of movement and close physical contact with others (e.g., people literally bumping into him or brushing by him). His parents would get offended and tell him later that he was rude because he would withdraw to his bedroom within an hour after guests arrived.

An example of how a sensory issue arose in therapy is the case of a 52-year-old man who was seeking treatment for ASD-related problems and reported an extreme sensitivity to the sound of wind. He was often preoccupied with weather predictions, and the therapist initially thought that this symptom was part of a comorbid anxiety disorder. While the therapist was assessing the source of his anxiety, the man was finally able to describe how excruciating the sound of the wind was to him. The problem was exacerbated by the fact that his apartment had old windows that whistled on windy days, making it unbearable for him to be at home. This information was important for treatment planning. If the therapist had focused solely on his anxiety about the weather, it would have been insufficient to help this patient because he also needed

TABLE 2.1. Sensory System Problems in AS

System	Process	Location of receptor cells	Hypersensitivity problems	Hyposensitivity problems	Practical impact on the individual
Tactile	Touch	Skin	Light touch, deep pressure, fabric textures, clothing labels, clothing fasteners, temperature changes, low pain tolerance	Indifference to temperature extremes, high pain tolerance, sensation seeking (odd gestures or self-injury)	Physical discomfort when coming into contact with someone or something that might not bother a typical person. Will take drastic measures to avoid certain experiences, may ignore threats to health or safety, may experience social rejection because of odd, sensation-seeking behaviors.
Vestibular	Balance	Inner ear	Low tolerance to movement, difficulty changing speed and direction, gravitational insecurity	Difficulty staying still, sensation seeking (rocking, crashing into things)	Clumsiness, hyperactivity, and difficulty "shifting gears" make group games or sports an unpleasant experience, thereby reducing opportunities for positive social experiences.
Proprioceptive	Movement	Joints and muscles	Inaccurate perception of the position of body parts, lack of coordination	Difficulty inhibiting movement, odd gestures, tic-like mannerisms	Poor posture, difficulty carrying multiple objects, uneven gait, clumsiness. Poor coordination between visual and proprioceptive stimuli contributes to gross motor (e.g., sports) and fine motor (handwriting) problems. May exert too little or too much force when moving things or touching a person (e.g., during a handshake).
Visual	Sight	Retina	Low tolerance for certain lights or patterns	Poor depth perception, poor visual–motor coordination, poor visual tracking and convergence	May avoid certain lighting conditions (e.g., fluorescent) or patterns (e.g., looking at other people's eyes). Visual–motor problems (also mentioned above) affect enjoyment of physical activities.
Auditory	Hearing	Inner ear	Low tolerance for certain sounds, exaggerated startle responses to noise, difficulty filtering out background noise	Lack of response or indifference to auditory cues	May avoid circumstances that involve specific sounds (e.g., bells, buzzers, high-pitched sounds), may have difficulty engaging in conversation in noisy settings (e.g., parties). May miss important auditory cues that signal danger or that are crucial in social interaction.
Gustatory	Taste	Taste buds and lining of nose	Strong food aversions	Lack of interest in some foods	May rigidly stick to a very circumscribed diet. Although connected to the tactile problems described above, some food aversions seem to involve the texture of the food and not just the flavor.
Olfactory	Smell	Lining of nose	Strong aversions to some smells	Failure to notice strong smells.	May have difficulty in the workplace, for example, if others wear fragrances that are too strong for the individual or cleaning products are being used that are aversive.

Note. Adapted from Myles et al. (2005). Copyright © 2005 the Organization for Autism Research. Adapted by permission.

some problem-solving and environmental modification components in the treatment plan to help him minimize the impact of this noise intrusion.

MOTOR

Table 2.1 also makes reference to some of the motor problems observed in ASD. DSM-5 lists one motor symptom: "stereotyped or repetitive motor movements (e.g., simple motor stereotypies . . ."; American Psychiatric Association, 2013, p. 50), and also mentions associated motor features (odd gait, clumsiness). I have observed that repetitive motor mannerisms are not usually pronounced in adults with ASD. If they are present, they are usually observed only in short spurts while the person seems to be experiencing an intense emotion. For example, one patient of mine exhibits hand flapping and body rocking, but only while he is laughing; I never observed these behaviors at any other time. The same man engages in an unusual finger-splaying gesture while he is expressing frustration. He holds up both hands, spreads the fingers far apart, and moves them in a writhing fashion while he utters a sentence expressing his concern, such as "I am never going to get my computer fixed!" As soon as he stops speaking, his hands return to a normal position on his lap. Again, this gesture does not appear at any other time.

Other associated motor features include fine motor deficits (e.g., poor handwriting). As Baranek and colleagues (2005) point out in their review of these problems in children with autism, it is difficult to distinguish between voluntary and involuntary movement problems.

Affordance perception is the ability to calibrate motor actions with perceptual outcomes, or to be able to integrate motor planning with perceptual experiences of one's own movements. This type of perceptual–motor integration is necessary to be able to navigate the physical environment during everyday tasks (climbing stairs, going through a doorway, loading the dishwasher, etc.). Impairment in affordance perception has been demonstrated in adolescents and adults with ASD without ID (Linkenauger, Lerner, Ramenzoni, & Proffitt, 2012). The impairment is not with the ability to execute a movement, nor is it with the visual system per se, but rather with the brain's ability to *integrate* these processes in an adaptive way. Moreover, Linkenauger and colleagues (2012) found in their study that impaired affordance perception was associated with social communication skill deficits as measured by the Social Communication Questionnaire (SCQ). These authors suggest that the basic perceptual–motor deficits observed in people with ASD may play a role in their social impairment, as it could affect how they synchronize their own actions with the actions of others. This idea brings us back to the point made earlier in this chapter when describing Figure 2.2, the interrelationship between core problems in ASD: the perceptual–motor deficits noted here as a problem processing information about the self overlap with the problems processing information about others.

As a final point in this section, the motor idiosyncrasies observed in adults with ASD may also present clinicians with issues of differential diagnosis because problems with movement can be symptoms of several different conditions, including a wide variety of medical problems, neurological disorders, and other DSM-5-defined disorders, such as OCD, tic disorders, ADHD, and medication-induced movement disorders. At times, a psychotherapist may decide to send a patient to an occupational therapist for a thorough evaluation of sensory–motor problems and possible intervention.

Dysfunctional Processing of Information in Nonsocial Domains

This last section describes some of the problems people with ASD have in processing information that is not social in nature. Some types of information about nonsocial aspects of the environment are typically processed erroneously by people with ASD, and these deficits can affect their functioning in clinically significant ways. Although most of the evidence for these deficits is found in the neuropsychological literature, it is important for psychotherapists to be aware of them even if they have not received formal training in neuropsychology. For example, I am not a neuropsychologist and therefore not trained to remediate neuropsychological deficits—but I do need to understand how my patients process information at a basic level because it has implications for how I conceptualize their cognitive styles and related behaviors. In many cases, the nomothetic evidence base that is described below is sufficient for a therapist to generate hypotheses about an individual patient. In other cases, a practitioner may choose to refer a patient to a neuropsychologist for a comprehensive assessment battery in order to understand better the unique way that person is processing information.

Neuropsychological research in ASD has been challenged because the population of people meeting criteria is so heterogeneous. Inconsistencies in subject selection, group assignment in the literature, and changing nosological factors make it impossible, at this time, to describe a single neuropsychological profile or phenotype for ASD (Tsatsanis, 2005; Tsatsanis & Powell, 2014). Despite these constraints, the following section outlines some of the findings that are most relevant to a practitioner who is serving adult patients with ASD without ID.

Ozonoff, South, and Provencal (2005) and Tsatsanis and Powell (2014) provide reviews of the research that demonstrates that people with ASD without ID have some impaired abilities in flexibility, planning, goal-directed behavior, and use of working memory. These problems are not specific to ASD; they were first described as "executive functions" (EF) in patients with frontal lobe damage (Duncan, 1986) and later in patients with ADHD, OCD, schizophrenia, and various forms of dementia (as reviewed by Ozonoff & Griffith, 2000). Also relevant is the research showing a deficit in the ability to integrate stimulus details in order to make global meaning of the context in which the details appeared, or "central coherence" (Frith, 1989; Happé, 2005). Standard IQ tests are not sufficiently sensitive to capture many of these deficits, but neuropsychological tests can provide the type of information that is outlined below. Research most relevant to this book are the studies showing impairments in the categories of *flexibility, planning,* and *central coherence.*

Flexibility

The earliest studies of EF in autism were conducted using the Wisconsin Card Sorting Test (WCST), a neuropsychological test designed to measure cognitive flexibility by administering a series of card-sorting tasks. Compared to age-matched controls, adults with ASD without ID show a tendency to perseverate, or continue to sort cards using a previously learned set of rules, even when they are given feedback indicating that the rules are no longer correct (Rumsey, 1985). Such errors are significant even when the control subjects have other types of learning disabilities (e.g., dyslexia; Rumsey & Hamburger, 1990).

Although these studies, and others like them, have been offered as evidence of impaired set-shifting capacity in ASD without ID, the WCST is not a "clean" measure of that concept. In other words, performance on the test is also reliant on other EF operations, such as organization skills, working memory, inhibition, selective attention, and encoding of verbal feedback (Ozonoff et al., 2005). Even though all of these functions have been assumed to be impaired in ASD without ID, Ozonoff and colleagues (2005) have taken a component process analysis approach to tease out the specific areas of dysfunction in this population. For example, through a series of tests they designed, they were able to isolate flexibility operations from inhibition operations and provided evidence that people with ASD without ID can inhibit responses as well as controls, but show specific problems in set shifting (Ozonoff & McEvoy, 1994). Further testing of inhibition ability has shown that subjects with ASD without ID are *unimpaired* in this operation (Ambery, Russell, Perry, Morris, & Murphy, 2006; Hughes, Russell, & Robbins, 1994; Ozonoff & Strayer, 1997).

Studies that tested attention-shifting ability have demonstrated that adults with ASD without ID have difficulty making rapid alternations of attention between two different sensory modalities (Courchesne, Akshoomoff, & Ciesielski, 1990; Kleinhans, Akshoomoff, & Delis, 2005) and are slow to disengage from one visual cue in order to attend to another (Hill & Bird, 2006; Wainwright-Sharp & Bryson, 1993). Taken with the set-shifting problems described above, it is safe to conclude that people with ASD without ID have a variety of problems with cognitive flexibility, which may explain why they are so often referred to as "rigid" in clinical descriptions and by their loved ones.

Planning

The Tower of Hanoi is another neuropsychological test that has been used frequently in studies of EF in ASD without ID. This instrument, which is designed to test planning ability, requires the subject to solve a problem by identifying subgoals before acting to reach a target goal. In a meta-analysis of the EF literature in autism, where neuropsychological tests were used to discriminate between people with ASD and controls, the most powerful effect size was found for the Tower of Hanoi, compared to other tests (Pennington & Ozonoff, 1996).

Similar to the WCST, however, the Tower of Hanoi is not a *pure* measure. In addition to planning ability, it may tap the use of working memory, for example—that is, "the ability to maintain information in an active, online state to guide cognitive processing" (Baddeley, 1996, as cited by Ozonoff et al., 2005, p. 611). However, when more isolated tests of working memory are applied to people with ASD without ID, the results are mixed. For example, Bennetto, Pennington, and Rogers (1996) demonstrated a working memory deficit in people with high-functioning autism, but a study by Ozonoff and Strayer (2001) did not. However, a task analysis of the Tower of Hanoi test (Goel & Grafman, 1995) suggested that it specifically measures a subject's ability to resolve conflicts between the target goal and a subgoal. In other words, a move that may seem to be wrong in the immediate sense may actually be correct in relation to the greater goal. This finding raises confidence that the Tower of Hanoi test is indeed capturing planning deficits in people with ASD and is also conceptually linked to flexibility (Ozonoff et al., 2005). Hill and Bird (2006) demonstrated in a sample of adults with AS that there were very specific impairments affecting planning ability, which were response *initiation* and higher-level intentionality as seen in the difficulty engaging and disengaging flexibly in the service of a goal.

Central Coherence

Frith (1989) was the first to use the term *central coherence* to describe a typical person's tendency to process pieces of incoming information within a context and to try to find the "gist" of a collection of details, rather than focus intently on each detail by itself. Frith proposed that people with ASD have a weakness in this area, noting their tendency to demonstrate a detail-focused processing that is unable to extract "the big picture"; a focus and memory for the parts but not the whole. Happé's (2005) first review on this topic supported this notion, describing how, on tests of memory for words and sentences, people with ASD can recall individual words as well or better than typical controls. However, the recall of typical controls is aided when the words are presented in a sentence (context), but this effect is not seen in people with ASD (e.g., Tager-Flusber, 1991). On nonverbal visual tests, people with ASD excel at detecting details. On the Embedded Figures Test, for example, subjects with ASD outperform typical controls in finding a small shape within a larger design (Joliffe & Baron-Cohen, 1997; Shah & Frith, 1983), but show poor integration of object parts (Joliffe & Baron-Cohen, 2001).

Because the information-processing tendencies of people with ASD can account for their talents as well as their difficulties, Happé and Frith suggest that we consider the pattern of focusing on discrete details as a *cognitive style* rather than a deficit (Happé, 2005; Happé & Frith, 2006), citing several studies (e.g., Snowling & Frith, 1986) showing that some subjects with ASD *can* extract meaning and gist when given explicit instructions to do so, but will not do it spontaneously in open-ended tasks. Also, it is not clear whether this cognitive style is due to a specific tendency to reduce global processing, increase local processing, or both (Happé & Booth, 2008). The idea that this pattern is a *preference*—which means it can be an asset and is not necessarily an unchangeable deficit—is encouraging for clinicians who are working with adult patients on modifying their cognitions in specific situations.

In summary, neuropsychological studies of people with ASD without ID have demonstrated a general problem with processing that shows up even when these individuals are exposed to nonsocial information. Specifically, studies have repeatedly shown various difficulties with cognitive flexibility, planning, and a bias toward perceiving details and not the gist or "big picture" in a collection of related pieces of information.

Cognitive Dysfunction and Risk for Mental Health Problems

The core cognitive dysfunction described above causes individuals with ASD to engage in a multitude of maladaptive behaviors that lead to negative consequences for them, further compound their problems, and cause emotional distress. When one of these adults presents for psychotherapy, it is rare that he or she seeks help with an isolated core ASD problem, as illustrated by the seven cases described in Chapter 1. Usually the patient's ASD symptoms have become interwoven in a complex web of environmental stressors and comorbid mental health problems, and this web leads the therapist to a broader conceptualization of the individual's presenting problems. Another case is used to illustrate how this interweaving occurs for one individual, Pam, by referring to the terms used in the conceptual model in Figure 2.1.

Pam is a 46-year-old woman with ASD who works as an office clerk. Her core information-processing problems involve poor *task organization* and extreme *sensitivity to fluorescent lights*. She has a large fluorescent fixture hanging over her desk, which significantly affects her concentration and exacerbates her organizational problem. She also has a "social skills" problem with *pragmatic expressive language*, and she cannot formulate a phrase to request a change in her light fixture (although the reader can easily imagine how anxiety may also be playing a role, for the sake of this example, we explore only the factors listed). Because of these three deficits, Pam continued to work under the light (suffering in silence) and also continued to perform her job poorly. This undesirable situation then led to the *daily living consequence* of poor work productivity and the *social consequence* of her boss criticizing her.

As mentioned, each person with ASD does not struggle with all of the deficits outlined in the model. However, most adults with ASD, each with a unique profile, face enough of these issues in daily life to lead them into two of the biggest and most well-established risk factors for mental health problems (presented in the conceptual model depicted in Figure 2.1): *poor social support* and *chronic stress*, with the former contributing to the latter. Sarason and Sarason (1985) demonstrated that people who report higher levels of social support are less vulnerable to the effects of negative life events than those reporting low levels of social support. They also showed a positive correlation between self-report of social support and levels of social competence. In their study, people who reported less social support also demonstrated poorer social skills and were perceived by others as less interesting, less dependable, less friendly, and less considerate than people who had reported high levels of social support. Of course, these correlational data are plagued with "chicken or egg" questions. However, it is not necessary to prove the direction of causality between these variables in order to consider how people with ASD are at risk on all of the dimensions measured by Sarason and Sarason.

Cohen and Wills (1985) conducted a meta-analysis of studies that investigated the relationship among stress, social support, and well-being (physical and mental health). They concluded that there was sufficient evidence to support the hypothesis that perceived availability of interpersonal resources can act as a buffer against stressful events. The extent to which people are integrated into a social network is also associated with improved well-being, even in the absence of stressful life events. More recently, Pocnet and colleagues (2016) demonstrated in a large community sample of typical people that perceived social support (PSS) was positively linked to quality of life, regardless of the number of stressful life events reported.

If this research on stress in the typical population is considered when examining the lives of people with ASD, it is easy to imagine the risks they face. With the exception of Groden and colleagues (Groden et al., 2006; Groden, Cautela, Prince, & Berryman, 1994), researchers and clinicians have largely ignored the role of stress in the lives of people with ASD. There has been improvement within the last decade, after Baron, Groden, Groden, and Lipsitt (2006) edited a volume of relevant theory and research on stress and the autism spectrum. Attwood (2006), in that same volume, provides a clinical conceptualization of stress factors faced by children with ASD and later (Attwood, 2007) offered a description of stress factors in adults with ASD who are in college, on the job, or in a marriage. The need for more research on these issues has begun to be answered, as some investigators have looked at factors such as social support and stress in the lives of adults with ASD.

PSS has been shown to be significantly lower in adults with ASD without ID, as compared to typical controls and also compared to adults with other clinical problems, like ADHD (Alvarez-Fernandez et al., 2017). Self-report of the level of participation in society predicts self-report of life satisfaction (Schmidt et al., 2015), and PSS appears to buffer against anxiety development in first-year college students with ASD (Reid, Holt, Bowman, Espelage, & Green, 2016). Not surprisingly, adults with ASD without ID compared to typical controls report higher levels of perceived stress, stressful life events, and poorer ability to cope with stress in everyday life (Bishop-Fitzpatrick, Masefsky, Minshew, & Eack, 2015; Bishop-Fitzpatrick, Minshew, Mazefsky, & Eack, 2017; Bishop-Fitzpatrick, Smith DaWalt, Greenberg, & Mailick, 2017; Hirvikoski & Blomqvist, 2015), and these factors predict poorer social functioning (Bishop-Fitzpatrick et al., 2015; Bishop-Fitzpatrick, Mineshew, et al., 2017), as well as poorer self-reported quality of life (Bishop-Fitzpatrick, Smith DaWalt, et al., 2017).

In my practice, I have observed that the difficult life circumstances faced by adults with ASD bring various types of stressors. *Daily hassles* are prevalent because EF problems make self-management so difficult. Poor organization, for example, often leads to losing things (e.g., car keys, wallet, important papers). Poor planning makes it difficult to complete tasks or maintain a schedule. Sensory problems make what are normal environmental events for typical people (e.g., light, noise) stressful for adults with ASD. *Chronic stressors*, other than the loneliness and isolation mentioned above, are associated with unemployment or underemployment (i.e., working at a job that does not utilize talent, intellectual ability, or level of education) (Baldwin, Costley, & Warren, 2014; Holwerda, van der Klink, Groothoff, & Brouwer, 2012; Nord, Stancliffe, Nye-Lengerman, & Hewitt, 2016; Roux et al., 2013; Shattuck et al., 2012), including financial struggles and legal problems (Debbaudt, 2002; Lerner, Haque, Nothrup, Lawer, & Bursztajn, 2012).

Adding to the example of Pam, consider that she has a master's degree in English literature, has a Full Scale IQ of 135, and is forced to work as an office clerk, performing poorly, no less, because she cannot manage the multiple demands of being a university faculty member. Teaching was always her dream, and she is intellectually and academically qualified to do it—however, she experiences the chronic stressor of underemployment.

Sadly, these social support and stress risk factors are likely related to the high rates of comorbid mental illness discussed in other sections of this book, as well as the high suicide risk that has been found in multiple studies. Segers and Rawana (2014) provide a review of these findings. The authors remark about how recent most of the studies have been, with very little work represented before 2007. They reported on 10 studies and three case reports published between 2007 and 2013. In studies that looked at the occurrence of ASD in larger psychiatric samples of suicidal patients, 7.3–15% of those groups were people with a diagnosis of ASD, and the ASD-diagnosed patients were prone to use more aggressive and lethal means in their attempts than non-ASD patients. In samples of adults with ASD, 31% reported suicidal thoughts and 7.7% reported attempts. Incidence of completed suicide in adults with ASD was reported as 7.7%. Cassidy and colleagues (2014) investigated suicidal thoughts, plans, and attempts in a sample of adults with ASD. In their sample, 66% of the subjects reported having suicidal thoughts at some point during their lifetimes, and 35% had planned or attempted suicide.

Conceptualizing Problems of ASD within a Traditional CBT Framework

CBT refers to a set of strategies for dealing with mental health problems that has existed for over 50 years and has a huge empirical literature supporting its validity as a psychotherapy approach with typical patients. This large collection of therapeutic approaches is based on the assumption that cognitive activity affects emotions and behavior and that people can learn to monitor and alter that activity in order to bring about changes in mood and behavior.

Reviews by Butler, Chapman, Forman, and Beck (2006) and Hofmann, Asnaani, Vonk, Sawyer, and Fang (2012) provide meta-analytic support for the efficacy of CBT for a wide variety of mental health problems. Most relevant to the present discussion are the robust effects noted across outcome studies for CBT used with adults for unipolar depression, generalized anxiety disorder (GAD), panic disorder, agoraphobia, social phobia, or PTSD. Although adults with ASD were not included in any of the studies cited, they are at great risk for all of the mental health problems that have been treated successfully using CBT, and these comorbid disorders have been reported in clinical descriptions of ASD (e.g., Attwood, 1998, 2007; Ghaziuddin, 2005; Ghaziuddin & Zafar, 2008) and epidemiological studies (Hofvander et al., 2009; Joshi et al., 2012; Lever & Geurts, 2016). This reality warrants a closer look at the utility of CBT for these patients, which is facilitated in the chapters ahead. I believe that cognitively able people with ASD who seek treatment should be offered the same state-of-the-art interventions that are available to any typical person suffering from mood or anxiety disorders.

Beck's Cognitive Model

The foundation for CBT, the *cognitive model,* was introduced in the early 1960s, with slightly different versions being offered by Ellis (1962) and Beck (1963). Because Beck's model has served as the basis for many empirically validated adult psychotherapy protocols (Butler et al., 2006; Hofmann et al., 2012), it is used to guide the discussion of CBT throughout this book. Conceptualizing adult ASD cases in this fashion leads a practitioner to a wide variety of evidence-based interventions in the CBT literature.

Figure 2.3 depicts a visual representation of Beck's (1976) model for emotional disturbance, as illustrated by Persons and colleagues (2000). Beck proposed that people process information according to *schemas,* which are cognitive structures that guide and organize the perception of events and experiences. Schemas are based on core beliefs that are learned, beginning early in life, through interactions with the environment and the groups of people to which they belong (e.g., family, peers, culture, religious community). They influence the way a person thinks, feels, and behaves in response to the environment. An event will activate a related schema, which in turn triggers a cycle of cognitions influencing emotion/mood, which then influences behavior, which again influences cognitions, and so forth. This feedback cycle loops back and further influences the schema by reinforcing or modifying it. At times schemas cause a person to distort events and, in that sense, they can become maladaptive. Beck proposed that emotional problems or disorders are driven by a preponderance of such distortions.

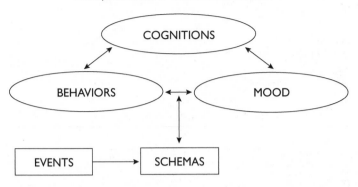

FIGURE 2.3. Beck's cognitive theory. From Persons, Davidson, and Tompkins (2000). Copyright © 2000 the American Psychological Association. Reprinted by permission.

Throughout life, schemas are continuously changing and evolving as new information is taken in, necessitating a modification of rules and beliefs. This process can also be maladaptive if a person fails to take in new information and "hangs on to" a previously functional schema that no longer fits with current life circumstances. Another problem can arise if there is a disproportionate amount of negative over positive beliefs about the self, others, the world, or the future. Such negative schemas may lead a person to focus selectively only on information that fits with those belief systems and ignore information that could possibly refute them.

Schemas and ASD

Considering the cognitive deficits that have been found in people with ASD, these individuals are at risk for developing a whole host of maladaptive schemas. The cognitive model assumes that fellow human beings are a great source of teaching, modeling, and reinforcing the beliefs that comprise schemas. However, social cognition deficits make it much harder for persons with ASD to infer and make use of information that comes from other people in a social context. They therefore miss out on a rich source of input for developing and evolving healthy schemas appropriately over time. Their cognitive inflexibility is also a risk factor in that they may hold on too strongly to a schema that is nonfunctional. Their frequent experiences of negative life events, such as social rejection and repeated employment failures, are likely to reinforce negative beliefs about self, others, the world, and the future.

Figure 2.4 is a duplicate of the core problems conceptual model shown earlier, with the added schema symbols, illustrating the points at which negative beliefs may develop or be reinforced. The struggles with *social skills* and *self-management* could easily give rise to *negative schemas about the self*. The *social consequences* of being *ignored, rejected,* or *ridiculed* typically foster the development of *negative schemas about others and the self.* The *daily living consequences* of *daily hassles* and *stressful events* may contribute to *negative beliefs about the world and the self.* Ultimately, all of the above can lead to negative ideas about what is to come—that is, to *negative schemas about the future.*

Figure 2.5 provides one more link between the problems inherent in ASD and the rationale for the use of CBT as an intervention to help people with ASD. The core problems of ASD are superimposed on Beck's (1976) cognitive model for emotional disorders,

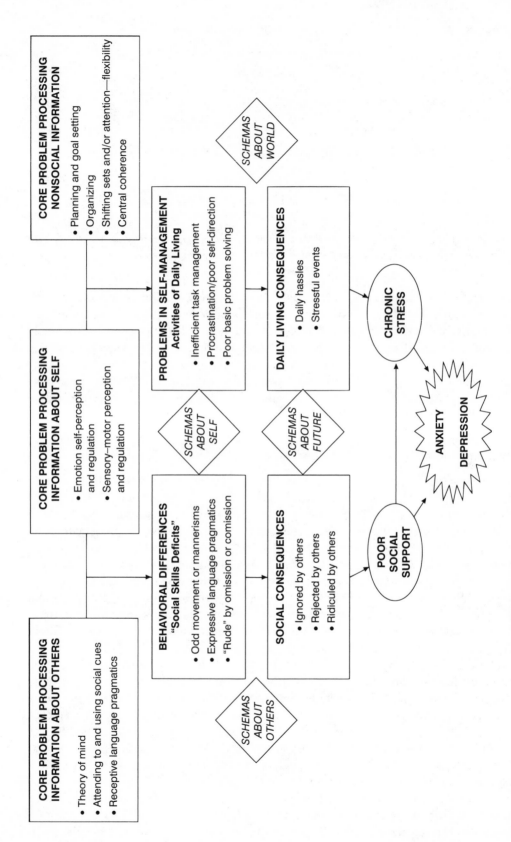

FIGURE 2.4. Vulnerability to maladaptive schema development in ASD.

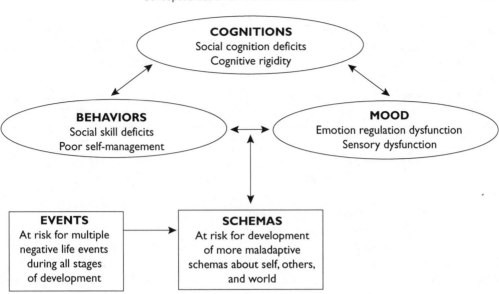

FIGURE 2.5. Core problems of ASD as vulnerabilities within Beck's cognitive theory. From Persons, Davidson, and Tompkins (2000). Copyright © 2000 the American Psychological Association. Adapted by permission.

showing how these factors increase vulnerability at each stage of the process, which is hypothesized to occur when negative schemas are activated by life events.

CBT for Adults with ASD

CBT, by definition, teaches people to monitor their own thoughts and perceptions with the hopes that they will become more aware of their interpretive errors. There is no reason to believe that people with ASD cannot learn to do this within a psychotherapy context. I presume that these adults can learn to reconceptualize social interactions and become better able to more accurately "read" the behavior of others. Once they understand others' motives and the rationale for the "codes of conduct" that exist in various social situations, they can more easily monitor their own behavior and adjust their responses to other people and situations. They can also be taught to recognize and modify the maladaptive patterns of information processing that contribute to their stress, anxiety, and depression.

Several authors have recommended the use of CBT for adult ASD (Attwood, 2004a, 2006, 2007; Attwood, Hénault, & Dubin, 2014; Cardaciotto & Herbert, 2004; Gaus, 2011, 2016; Hare & Paine, 1997; Kerns, Roux, Connell, & Shattuck, 2016; Powers & Loomis, 2014; Tsai, 2006), including one suggestion for the use of dialectical behavior therapy (DBT; Hartmann, Urbano, Manseer, & Okwara, 2012), but there are only a handful of empirical studies supporting its use with this population. A recent review of this literature by Spain, Sin, Chalder, Murphy, and Happé (2015) revealed six published studies where CBT was reported as a promising treatment approach for comorbid mood and anxiety problems in adults on the autism spectrum. Two were case studies (Cardaciotto

& Herbert, 2004; Hare & Paine, 1997), one was a quasi-experimental nonrandomized trial (Russell et al., 2013), two were randomized controlled trials (RCT; Russell, Mataix-Cols, Anson, & Murphy, 2009; Spek, van Ham, & Nyklíček, 2013), and one was a group-based case series (Weiss & Lunsky, 2010).

CBT with mindfulness components has been shown to be promising for adults with ASD (Conner & White, 2018; Sizoo & Kuiper, 2017; Spek, van Ham, & Nyklíček, 2013).

The potential for CBT approaches to be useful in adults with ASD is further supported if we look at the treatment studies showing the efficacy of CBT for adolescents with ASD without ID. RCT have shown CBT can reduce autism symptom severity (Wood et al., 2015), reduce some depressive symptoms (Santomauro, Sheffield, & Sofronoff, 2016), improve social functioning (Laugeson & Park, 2014; White et al., 2013), and that social functioning gains are maintained after treatment ends (Maddox, Miyazaki, & White, 2016). Meta-analysis of CBT treatment studies supports its efficacy for reducing comorbid anxiety symptoms in adolescents with ASD (Ung, Selles, Small, & Storch, 2015), as demonstrated, for example, in a study by Ehrenreich-May and colleagues (2014). Weston and colleagues (2016) provide a recent review and meta-analysis of 48 studies of the effectiveness of CBT for people with ASD (mostly children and adolescent subjects), showing some evidence that CBT can be used to target symptoms of affective disorders (anxiety and depression) as well as core symptoms of ASD.

We need more research before we can pinpoint which therapy components were the agents of change across all of these studies because the protocols were multifaceted. Nevertheless, these data provide important preliminary support for the rationale behind exploring the use of CBT for individuals with ASD. It is hoped that by providing a framework for conceptualizing adult cases of ASD and designing treatment plans that include empirically based CBT interventions, this book will encourage therapists and practicing scientists to work with, and study, this population further.

Chapter Summary and Conclusions

This chapter presented research findings supporting the existence of core dysfunction in people with ASD, in the form of problems processing *information about others* (ToM, use of social cues, language pragmatics), *information about the self* (perception and regulation of emotional and sensory–motor processes), and *nonsocial information* (planning, cognitive flexibility, and central coherence). A conceptual model was proposed that described how the core problems of ASD in adult patients serve as risk factors for the development of problems in living and comorbid mental health disorders. That conceptualization was then used to demonstrate how Beck's (1976) cognitive model for emotional disorders is a useful way to explain and address the anxiety and depression that are so often reported by patients with ASD. Finally, preliminary studies that support the use of CBT for patients with ASD were outlined. The next chapter discusses how the therapist can assess these problems in individual patients.

CHAPTER 3

The Initial Assessment

This chapter is meant to guide psychotherapists through the process of assessing an adult case where ASD is known or suspected. Cases such as these can appear in many forms and from a variety of referral sources (Maddox & Gaus, 2018). Typical scenarios include:

- A diagnostician who establishes ASD refers the patient for psychotherapy.
- A patient suspects ASD after being exposed to literature about it and refers self for treatment.
- A patient's child is diagnosed with ASD, leading to self-examination and consideration of diagnosis for self.
- A family member suspects ASD after being exposed to literature about it and refers a loved one for treatment.
- An inpatient psychiatry team suspects or establishes ASD for a patient who was hospitalized to treat a mental health crisis and refers for outpatient treatment upon discharge.
- A psychotherapist who is already treating an individual for a period of time realizes ASD may be present; that therapist may decide to continue working with a new conceptualization, or may refer out for a more specialized approach.

This chapter is divided into two major sections. The first addresses *intake issues,* including a more detailed presentation of the reasons adults with ASD seek treatment, and the special considerations involved in interviewing these patients. The second focuses on the information gathering that is necessary for *diagnosis and definition of target problems.* Guidelines are offered for establishing an ASD diagnosis, assessing comorbid conditions, highlighting patient strengths, and creating a problem list.

Intake Issues

Reasons for Seeking Treatment

Regardless of the referral source, patients with ASD come to psychotherapy with a wide variety of complaints about their life circumstances or sense of well-being. Three lists appear below. The first outlines the most common problems these patients report at intake and is framed in terms that represent *their* perspective. The second list presents the problems as described by referring family members, who may see the issues from a slightly different perspective. The third involves problems that are common in adults with ASD, but because of some of the embarrassment or shame that can accompany them, patients and families may not always report these right away.

Self-Reported Problems

LONELINESS

Most patients report some dissatisfaction with the number or quality of the relationships they have in their lives. Frustrated with the repeated failures they have experienced in the dating world, many of the single patients come to treatment hoping that the therapist will give them a shortcut to finding a romantic partner. These individuals have a healthy desire to be in a sexual relationship, if not a marriage. Some patients are also looking to increase the number of friendships in their lives.

DISCOMFORT IN SOCIAL SITUATIONS

Most patients are anxious in some or all types of social situations. They have all had a whole host of negative experiences with others, ranging from being ignored, at best, to being physically or sexually assaulted, at worst. A number of them have gained some insight into the role their own anxiety and/or lack of skill may be playing in the outcome of their social interactions. As a poignant example, a 25-year-old college student came to his intake session with a list of written questions he had prepared in advance. They were:

1. *What questions can I ask when I meet a person?*
2. *What are the questions I should not ask when I meet a person?*
3. *What are the topics that I cannot talk to a person about?*
4. *What are the things that I can do in a group conversation?*
5. *What are the things that I cannot do in a group conversation?*
6. *How many questions should I ask a person at a time?*
7. *When is it the wrong time to talk to a person?*
8. *What shouldn't I do in a conversation altogether?*
9. *What are some of the activities that I can do to meet some friends?*

DEPRESSION

Most patients report some level of sadness, "feeling down," or depression that they are experiencing at intake or have experienced in their prior histories. They also report a sense of helplessness about improving their lives and hopelessness about their futures. Some also report suicidal ideation.

INTERPERSONAL CONFLICTS/ANGER CONTROL PROBLEMS

In addition to the discomfort and anxiety that patients report, some complain of not being able to "get along" with others; they have repeated arguments and fights with other people. These are the individuals who are more outgoing and less avoidant, but more likely to display behavior deemed offensive or belligerent by the people in their lives. The conflicts may occur with family members, peers at college or work, bosses, or strangers in public places.

EMPLOYMENT DISSATISFACTION

Most adults with ASD report employment problems. A large portion of them are unemployed or employed part time while relying on Social Security disability benefits, despite the high level of education many of them have. Others are working full time, but their jobs do not relate to their talents, education, or interests. Still others have found success in careers that are related to their education and career choice, but the work setting is not well matched. Workplace problems result in stress because of task demands that exceed a patient's capacity to manage or difficulty understanding the social domains of the job (e.g., interfacing with coworkers, bosses, customers). There may be a sense of not being recognized for achievements or being passed over for promotion because the individual has difficulty understanding the subtle nuances of workplace culture and politics. In other cases, an individual may be pressured to take on job roles for which he or she is not socially equipped (e.g., management) because performance was excellent in a circumscribed set of responsibilities (e.g., computer programming).

FRUSTRATION WITH LIVING SITUATION

Many patients complain at intake about their living situations because they have not been able to achieve independence. Some are dependent on their family of origin or housing programs (e.g., group home, supportive apartment). The problem of sustaining employment has obvious financial implications that are exacerbated in large metropolitan areas, where even typical young people struggle to support themselves after graduating from college. The living arrangements of persons with ASD often involve an infringement on their rights to privacy and choice making. This is a powerful stressor contributing to the feelings of helplessness and hopelessness reported by these individuals.

SLEEP PROBLEMS

Sleep difficulties are very common among people with ASD and this is often reported at intake. In some cases, the complaint is poor sleep quality, in other cases an erratic sleep pattern, or sometimes a schedule that is out of sync with conventional sleep schedules.

Family-Reported Problems

ANGER OUTBURSTS

When family members are involved in the intake process, a common complaint surrounds patients' expressions of anger. They are described as having "meltdowns" that include explosive, unpredictable, or violent displays of rage entailing screaming, cursing, threatening others, stomping feet, destroying property (throwing and breaking items, punching holes in walls), self-injury (slapping or hitting self, banging head on hard surface), and, less frequently, physical aggression toward others (shoving, kicking, punching, choking). Parents who found a way to cope with these behaviors as their child was growing up may be finding the adult-sized version of a tantrum quite a bit more intimidating, frightening, and dangerous.

OBSESSIONS/INTENSE AND NARROW INTERESTS

Family members often express concern about the patient's "obsession" with a particular topic or activity (e.g., astronomy, sports, transit systems, aviation, cinema, meteorology). Although the activity itself is not maladaptive, there is a problem with the inordinate amount of *time* that the individual spends engaged in it, to the exclusion of other adaptive activities. Excessive computer use is the most common complaint; the person with ASD may be searching the Internet for items regarding his or her topic of interest, posting on social media sites, texting with others, or playing video games. Other time-consuming activities may involve watching TV programs or reading about a narrowly defined topic.

COMPULSIVE BEHAVIOR

The narrow interests discussed above often lead to repetitive, maladaptive behaviors that family members see as self-destructive. These individuals may make judgment errors about health, safety, or money because they are so immersed in their interest. One young man had spent thousands of dollars on mail-order dietary supplements because his interest was in nutrition and health. Not only was his mother concerned about the financial implications but she worried that he was taking too many of these vitamins and minerals without consideration for the health consequences. Another man had raised his mother's concern because he had become preoccupied with horse racing and was gambling his small income away at off-track betting facilities.

WITHDRAWAL/DEPRESSION

Family members are often concerned at intake about the individual's isolation and depressed mood. Sometimes a dramatic change in mood is what triggers a family member to refer a patient to therapy because it is usually accompanied by a change in the person's typical way of functioning (e.g., regression in self-care skills, less social engagement than usual).

LACK OF MOTIVATION/PROCRASTINATION

Perhaps the most frustrating issue for parents of adult children is the apparent lack of motivation to take responsibility for life decisions. The high level of intellectual functioning leads parents to say, "He should know better" or "She should be more interested in her budget." For example, the father of a young woman, a college senior at an Ivy League institution who had superior mathematical ability, was furious with her because, according to him, her procrastination had caused her to miss all of her graduate school application deadlines.

POOR HYGIENE/SELF-CARE AND ORGANIZATION SKILLS

Another source of frustration for family members is the patient's inability to take care of basic grooming and housekeeping responsibilities, or activities of daily living (ADL). The discrepancy between intellectual and adaptive functioning is puzzling to family members; it seems as though self-care should come more naturally. For example, it is easy to ask, "How can a person with an IQ in the superior range have difficulty brushing his or her teeth every day?" Even parents who have a good understanding of their adult child's disability become impatient over this issue if they are living together.

POOR SLEEP HABITS

Family members will often complain, even if the patient does not, about unusual sleep schedules—for example, "He is such a night owl," or erratic patterns of swinging from excessive sleeping to not enough sleeping.

LEGAL PROBLEMS

Sometimes a referral to treatment is triggered by an incident in which the patient gets "in trouble" with members of the community and/or the legal system. Unusual behaviors and poor social judgment often lead others to misconstrue the intentions of a person with ASD. For example, one 30-year-old man was arrested after being pulled over for a minor traffic violation. After a brief interchange, the police officer asked him to step out of his car while he did a complete search of the vehicle. The man with ASD became so anxious that he began pacing and muttering under his breath, causing the officer to become more suspicious of him and more confrontational. The muttering escalated to yelling and threatening of the police officer, and he was taken to the station for further questioning. Although he was eventually released, the experience led him to become fearful of police. His mother, who was not with him at the time, later assumed that his eye-gaze aversion and nervous tics had triggered the vehicle search, which marked the beginning of the unfortunate chain of events. Adults who have anger outbursts, as described in an earlier section, can also be vulnerable to getting into legal trouble. The adult version of aggression is termed *violence* by society and the criminal justice system, which puts some individuals at risk for being arrested and prosecuted (Debbaudt, 2002; Lerner, Haque, Nothrup, Lawer, & Bursztajn, 2012).

Other Problem Areas for Which People with ASD Are at Risk

The next three areas involve problems for which people with ASD are known to be at risk, but are also potential sources of shame and may not be reported during the intake process by the patient or the family.

SEXUAL PROBLEMS

Individuals on the autism spectrum are vulnerable to sexual problems because they are less likely than their peers to have had the educational or social experiences in adolescence through which typical people develop a healthy sense of sexual well-being

(Attwood, 2007; Attwood et al., 2014; Hénault, 2005; Koller, 2000; Nichols & Byers, 2016). This vulnerability can lead to a wide variety of clinical issues, with an equally varied set of interventions being warranted. Some common, though distinctive, presenting problems are lack of sexual information, preoccupation with sexual material, paraphilias, confusion about gender roles or sexual orientation, gender dysphoria, anxiety about interacting with potential dating partners, or aversion to touch. Patients and their families are often inhibited about these topics, and those with sexual problems usually do not initiate or engage in discussions about them until trust is built with the therapist. Nevertheless, it is important for the therapist to be attuned to these issues during intake and prepared to assess them further in later sessions, after rapport has been established.

SUBSTANCE ABUSE

Another issue that can be underlying presenting problems without being reported by the patients or their families is substance abuse. Alcohol and cannabis are the most common substances used (Sizoo, van den Brink, Gorissen van Eenige, & van der Gaag, 2009) by individuals with ASD. These substances may be overused because they can help relieve anxiety and stress (as a maladaptive coping strategy), and/or facilitate social interactions that would otherwise be strenuous.

SUICIDALITY

As mentioned in Chapter 2, suicidal thoughts, plans, and attempts are more prevalent in this population, and these phenomena are not always tied to a comorbid depression. While a therapist is more prone to assess for suicidal ideation in a depressed patient, for adults with ASD, a sensitivity to this risk should be there for all patients, regardless of presenting problem. Concerns about suicidality are sometimes reported at intake if present, but not always.

Interviewing Strategies

When a person with ASD comes for an intake, the goals are similar to the goals a therapist has for any new patient. Many of the points made in this section will seem like "common sense" to experienced clinicians and are not specific to this population. However, there are some special considerations and related modifications a therapist may need to make when interviewing a patient with ASD (Jacobsen, 2003). The goals at intake are to:

- Secure accurate information about current symptoms and history.
- Begin building a rapport with the patient.
- Begin learning the communication style of the patient.

Kingdon and Turkington (2005) offer useful guidelines for establishing a therapeutic relationship with adult patients who have schizophrenia. Although there are major differences between the needs of patients with ASD and those with schizophrenia, there are also some things they have in common. Both groups of patients are subject to problems with social cognition, idiosyncratic use of language, unusual beliefs, and trusting people. I share Kingdon and Turkington's commitment to maintaining flexibility in the use of CBT because of the perceptual problems with which these patients struggle. Kingdon and Turkington's concepts of *pacing, nonconfrontation,* using *"word-perfect" accuracy,* and *tactical withdrawal* are mentioned in the sections below, which outline basic guidelines for interviewing.

Pace Yourself

The first adjustment a therapist needs to make is to be willing to tolerate a slow rate of progress. Brenda Smith Myles has authored many psychoeducational materials for teachers and therapists to use with adolescents with ASD, and she has coined a term to help professionals set realistic expectations for progress with this population. She reminds service providers to work on "Asperger time," which means if you get "half as much done in twice as much time" than you would expect for any other patient, then you are successful (Myles et al., 2005, p. 13). Kingdon and Turkington (2005) also stress the importance of pacing so that the interaction does not overwhelm the patient. This means your initial interview may not be completed after only one session. You may need multiple meetings to gather all necessary information and to establish a working relationship with the patient.

When scheduling an initial session by telephone, I always tell new patients that there will be only one meeting, at the end of which we will make a mutual decision about meeting again. If at the end of the first session, the patient and therapist do agree to set up a second session, the therapist asks the patient if he or she is willing to meet three more times before deciding whether or not to embark on the therapy process, explaining that it typically takes a total of four sessions to decide what the treatment plan will look like. This approach serves two purposes. First, it truly does take that many sessions to get a solid understanding of the case, sometimes even longer. Second, pacing and structuring the intake in this way is also a rapport-building strategy. These patients often feel anxiety when entering a new relationship, and emphasizing their control over the process can minimize the pressure.

Learn to Speak the Patient's Language

People with ASD have verbal strengths and are usually quite articulate. However, they may use language in an unusual way and also may interpret what you say very literally. Therefore, a therapist must be cautious about his or her own use of language so as not to confuse or mislead the patient. Kingdon and Turkington (2005) discuss the importance of using *"word-perfect" accuracy* and honesty with patients who have psychosis. This means the therapist must be extra mindful of the words he or she is using, ensuring precision to the point of pedanticism. This degree of clarity is crucial for patients with ASD because they take words at face value. Our language is rich with idioms and phrases that do not really mean what they say, and we are not usually aware of our literal *inaccuracy.* Because these patients are so bright and articulate, even I, who supposedly know how important this is, still make mistakes in this regard. Take the following example from an interview I was conducting with a 38-year-old male patient with ASD and an average IQ.

THERAPIST: Comparing your life now to 10 years ago, it sounds like you have really grown.

PATIENT: (*Eyes widen, face flushes.*) No, I haven't. I have been the same height since I was 18 years old: 5 feet, 9½ inches!

Despite this man's intellectual functioning level, he took the word *grown* to mean that he had physically grown taller. A better way for the therapist to phrase this idea would have been:

"It sounds like you have achieved many of the things you wanted to over the last 10 years."

During the initial intake meetings, the therapist should take note of the words and phrases the patient uses to describe experiences, and should use those same words during further inquiry. Not only will the therapist sound clearer to the patient, he or she will also convey the desire to meet the individual on a common ground that has been partially designed by him or her. This is another way to give the patient control over the process and thereby reduce anxiety. Here is an example of the therapist using the patient's idiosyncratic phrase (italicized) to ask for more information.

PATIENT: I have things I have to do a certain way. I can't control it. Even if I want to change it really, really bad, I can't. I have *mental habits* that won't let me change.

THERAPIST: Which *mental habit* is bothering you the most lately?

PATIENT: Like starting my diet. I have a *mental habit* that says I can only start a diet on a Tuesday. I don't know why my mind thinks that because it doesn't make any sense. But I can't change it. I can't start on a Wednesday or a Thursday, even if I really, really want to.

THERAPIST: Do you have any other *mental habits* that are bothering you as much as the diet one?

At this stage of the interview it is more important to encourage the patient to continue sharing information with the therapist than for terminology to be technically correct. In a much later session, the therapist may choose to provide psychoeducation to the patient about "mental habits" and what they might be.

One final note about language: People with ASD sometimes have difficulty initiating a report of a distressing situation. Things that typical adult patients would spontaneously share with a therapist when seeking help are not reported by some patients with ASD, unless they are specifically asked about distressing situations. Their literal interpretation of social interactions leads some patients to believe that they should only answer questions the therapist asks. Also, they may not pick up on the general theme of a line of questioning or might fail to connect one topic to a *similar* one that might be relevant.

In the following example, the patient is describing a situation that was distressing to her, but the therapist needed to ask a very specific question before she could connect the situation to a possible pattern in her life. Typical adult patients who do not have ASD are able to make these connections more spontaneously.

PATIENT: The other day in class the professor was going on and on, and I couldn't follow him. I kept staring at the board and I kept watching him, but he might as well have been speaking Chinese. I wanted to run out of the room, but I was afraid it would be inappropriate.

THERAPIST: Have you ever had anything like that happen to you before?

PATIENT: Never.

THERAPIST: Have you ever tried to listen to a person who did not seem to make any sense? Or have you ever wanted to run out of a room when things were not making sense to you?

PATIENT: Oh, yeah. Last year at my father's retirement party, the speeches were like that. On and on and on and no sense. I get so freaked out when that happens because I'm the only one who can't understand it.

When the therapist asked the first follow-up question, the patient took it literally. She probably thought the therapist was asking if that exact situation had happened before with a professor in a classroom. When the therapist realized the question was not specific enough, she used elements of the scenario to help the patient generalize to other similar circumstances. Without the follow-up questions, the therapist was risking an oversight about possible anxiety symptoms. She also might have missed the preliminary information about dysfunctional automatic thoughts and schemas, which was revealed in the patient's last line, " . . . I'm the only one who can't understand it."

Convey Respect

It may seem obvious that the therapist should be respectful toward the patient. It is worth discussing briefly, however, because there are subtle ways that therapists can appear judgmental, usually if corrective feedback is given too early in the development of the relationship. Because these patients may display socially inappropriate behavior during the initial meetings, the therapist must be able to strike a balance between the *need to set appropriate boundaries* and parameters within the relationship, while also *giving the patient some latitude* in terms of his or her unusual mannerisms and unique style of communicating.

One strategy is to define as many boundaries as possible in advance. For example, it will alleviate some anxiety if the patient is given clear explanations of the therapist's "office rules." These are things that typical patients might be able to infer, but people with ASD need these explained to them with more specificity. Such rules include, but are not limited to, what door to use when coming into the office, where the bathroom is, where to sit while waiting, whether there is a sign-in procedure, whether or not to knock, when to make payments, and how long the session lasts. Giving these rules to the patient proactively minimizes the chances that he or she will make errors, which the therapist will need to "correct," thereby reducing unnecessary embarrassment for the patient. Even though these individuals have difficulty inferring the expectations others may have, they will usually comply once they know what they are.

In the same spirit, it is useful to give patients some warning that the session is nearing the end. Because of the problems with cognitive shifting, many people with ASD have difficulty stopping an interchange, even when there are clear signals that it is over. They may keep talking and stay seated, even after the therapist stands up and moves toward the door, for instance. To make ending seem less abrupt to patients, it is helpful to them to begin the wind-down process anywhere from 5 to 15 minutes earlier than the actual end. Here is an example:

> "We are 5 minutes from the end of the time, now. Let's start getting ready to bring it to a close."

One benefit of the boundaries *around* the session being clear to the patient is that the therapist can more easily be flexible *within* sessions in accepting some unusual behaviors. It is a priority to help the patient minimize anxiety in the initial sessions, as high arousal levels only hinder the process of the intake interview. Minimizing stress means that the therapist must allow the patient to use his or her own unusual or odd-looking methods of coping with anxiety. Kingdon and Turkington's (2005) guideline of being *nonconfrontational* applies here. The intake sessions are the wrong time for the therapist to teach social skills and give corrective feedback (unless the patient is doing something blatantly self-injurious or destructive to the therapist's property). So, for example, many patients do not make eye contact at first, and therapists *should not* prompt them to look at their eyes. Some patients may want to manipulate items in their hands or to "fiddle" with something while talking; this behavior is totally acceptable because it may actually help them to focus better on the interview. Some will even get out of their seats and walk around the room, inspecting the bookshelves or pictures on the walls. Again, this behavior should not be discouraged during initial sessions. Paradoxically, these actions help patients regulate their arousal and allow them to participate more fully in the interview, even though they would be deemed rude in a social situation.

As a therapist is getting to know a patient, he or she may unintentionally agitate the patient with a particular question or comment. Due to idiosyncratic perceptions and a history of negative experiences, a seemingly mundane question may suddenly trigger a panic-like or angry response. For example, one 22-year-old patient who appeared to be calm suddenly began to yell and slap his hand on the chair arm after I asked him how he liked to spend his leisure time. Kingdon and Turkington's (2005) *tactical withdrawal* is useful here. It is best to give up that line of questioning and move to something that is already known to be a safe topic.

To reiterate, it is counterproductive to insist that a patient comply with the therapist's agenda or strict code of conduct. The first reason is that the patient will experience the process as negative and will not trust the therapist; treatment is not likely to proceed past intake. The second reason is that the therapist will fail to get the information needed because the patient will be too aroused to concentrate on the task at hand. Therapists who find it difficult to refrain from commenting on socially inappropriate behavior can remind themselves that they will be addressing these issues as therapy goals at a later date.

Use Caution When Including Family Members

About half of the adult patients I see are fully independent in the therapy process; they schedule and attend their sessions by themselves, like typical adult patients. However, parents or siblings initiate the onset of treatment for the other half of the patients, making the initial phone calls to the therapist. It can be useful to include parents or siblings in the intake process because they can provide information about early childhood development and current functioning, both of which are particularly necessary to an accurate diagnosis. However, this is a practice that, if not done carefully, can jeopardize the dignity of patients as well as their trust of the therapist. Many of these patients assume a passive role when their family members are involved in their lives. They appear to let other people take care of the tasks of daily living for them, yet they often feel angry toward these helpers for infringing on their privacy and decision making. It is important for therapists to make it clear from the outset to everyone involved *who* the designated patient is, and how that person is in charge of what happens in the therapy process.

Preserving the adult patient's dignity starts at the point of the initial phone call. If someone other than the patient makes the contact, the therapist should encourage the caller to have the potential patient make the appointment. If the caller does not believe the patient will initiate this action, early assessment questions arise about the possible presence of:

- Low motivation for treatment
- High anxiety (avoidance of phone call)
- EF issues
- Depression
- Maladaptive dependence on family members

No matter which of these factors are contributing, the therapist should ask whether the patient can come to the phone at that moment, arrange to come to the phone at another time, or write the therapist an e-mail. A 5- to 10-minute conversation or brief e-mail dialogue with the patient is necessary in order to assess his or her own rationale for coming in, which may not be the same as the family member's motive. The following example illustrates the approach the therapist can take when the patient is ultimately available.

THERAPIST: Hello, _____, my name is _____. Your dad called me on your behalf to see if I could be of some assistance. Were you OK with that?

PATIENT: Yeah. He told me.

THERAPIST: What did he tell you about me?

PATIENT: Uh, you are a therapist of some sort.

THERAPIST: That's right. I am a [psychiatrist/psychologist/social worker]. Why did your dad think you might want to talk to a therapist?

PATIENT: He is worried because I don't go out that much.

THERAPIST: Is that something that you are concerned about?

PATIENT: It's not a big deal. It's always been like that. I'd rather stay home. My aunt is a nurse and she thinks I have something—Asperger's disorder. That's what got my dad into this. I say, it's always been like this, and it always will be like this. It's not a big deal. It's better when I stay home.

THERAPIST: Well, I do work a lot with adults who have Asperger's disorder. Maybe that's how your dad got my name. I don't know if that is what's going on for you, and I wouldn't know without meeting you. Let me just clarify something you just said. When I asked you if you were concerned about the same thing your dad is, you didn't really say yes or no. You explained that you believe things will stay the way they are, but I was not sure if you were content with that or not.

PATIENT: Well, I'm not happy about it, but I think we should just accept it. I looked up this Asperger thing online, and it does sound a little like me. But they said it is a lifelong thing. There is no cure. And I didn't know it the whole time, but I have lived with it for 25 years and I think I am doing OK. I just wish my father would let me be.

THERAPIST: Are you living with your dad?

PATIENT: Yes, unfortunately. That is part of the problem. He's always watching what I do. He should just worry about his own stuff and leave me alone.

THERAPIST: Well, it does sound like you have some things going on that are frustrating you, whether you have Asperger's or not. But it also sounds like you are trying to deal with things on your own and trying to gain some independence, you know, get some space between you and your dad. So, there are two things we could do. One is that we can skip making an appointment and you can explain to your dad that we talked just now, and that you have decided that you would prefer to continue coping with these issues on your own. I understand that your dad called me out of concern for you, but there really is no sense in meeting if you want to let things be for now. Or we could meet just once to talk about it some more, and then you and I, without your dad, could decide if I have anything to offer you to help in what you're dealing with right now.

PATIENT: I guess I could come in once. I wouldn't have to bring my dad?

THERAPIST: No. Not unless you need him to drive you. Even if you do, you would come into the session by yourself. Anybody who is with you would have to wait in the waiting room.

The extra time spent on the phone with a patient similar to this is a small investment to make. If an adult patient sees the therapist as an agent of the parent, especially when a desire for independence is an issue, as it was in this example, the therapist will have to work that much harder to establish trust and, in some cases, never will. The treatment will not be successful if the individual does not, on some level, believe he or she made the decision to come into therapy. Although in this example, the patient decided to come, the therapist would have been just as respectful of a different choice. In many of these types of conversations, the person chooses not to come in. Being allowed to exercise choice, in and of itself, can be therapeutic for some individuals, and sometimes such a person will call at a later date when he or she feels more interested or motivated to enter treatment.

Despite the above point, there are times when I do allow a parent to schedule the appointment for their adult son or daughter—for example, if the parent reports that the patient has expressed a willingness or desire to come to therapy but is so impaired by anxiety or related features that he or she is almost incapable of coming to the phone. In those cases, the individual is usually brought to the appointment by a family member. The case of Bob, introduced in Chapter 1, is one such example. The therapist should then use the greeting in the waiting room as the opportunity for the person to exercise some choice. The following illustrates this concept.

> "Hello, _____. I am _____. I know your mom made this appointment for you today, but it's up to you whether you would like her to come in with you right now. You can bring her with you into my office now, or we can ask her to wait out here and we can call her only if we think we need her for information or something like that. What would you like her to do?"

Even if the patient opts to bring the parent(s) in, the therapist still directs all questions toward the patient during the interview. If the patient is withdrawn and avoids engagement, the therapist must work hard *not* to let the conversation drift into one *about* the patient, as if he or she were not there.

Diagnosis and Definition of Target Problems

Establishing the Autism Spectrum Diagnosis

Sometimes a patient arrives with the formal diagnosis of ASD already having been made by a qualified mental health professional specializing in the assessment and diagnosis of ASD. In such cases, the therapist does not have to spend as much time interviewing the patient about history and symptoms of the ASD per se.

In the other referral scenarios outlined at the beginning of this chapter, more attention must be paid to this process. Patients who are seeking a diagnosis may have been introduced to information about ASD by the media, a family member, or another mental health professional. Other times a therapist who is already working with a patient for other reasons may realize that an ASD could be present.

The amount of time a therapist spends on this process depends on how the diagnostic information will be used by the patient. If the patient needs a detailed diagnostic report at the end of the assessment to use as part of an application to a program or service, for example, the assessment process will be more formal and may include more standardized testing. In those cases, a therapist may wish to refer to an experienced ASD diagnostician, before or during the initial stages of treatment. However, if the therapist and patient are only going to use the information to enrich the conceptualization of the presenting problems in order to design an effective treatment plan for the psychotherapy, the part of the assessment that focuses exclusively on ASD will be less formal and therefore less time-consuming.

As mentioned previously, diagnosing something that is essentially a developmental disorder is difficult when a person is well into adulthood because the symptom picture is influenced by so many factors. The following guidelines can help a clinician to access information about social functioning, past and present, as well as developmental history.

Interview the Individual

Ask the patient about memories of his or her own developmental history by inquiring about peer relationships, school experiences, and therapeutic services while growing up. Assess current social functioning by asking about the quantity *and* quality of relationships. For instance, when the patient reports on friends, ask for their first names to get a sense of how many there are. Then ask how often and through what means the patient socializes with those people. One young man said he had about 10 current friends, but further inquiry revealed that he had never met any of them in person, only through social media, and he did not have any other friends in his life at the time. Table 3.1 provides a list of questions to ask the patient during the interview.

Also pay attention to how the individual relates to you during the interview in terms of interaction skills. Table 3.2 offers guidelines for observing social behavior during the intake.

Interview Parents or Family Members

With the patient's permission, include people in the interview who knew the individual early in life. Ask about early development, social relationships, and behavior. In addition, supplement the information you obtained from the individual about special educational or therapeutic services by using the same questions with family members. Table 3.3 presents interview questions for family members.

TABLE 3.1. Interview Questions for the Patient during Initial Intake

Questions to ask the patient about developmental and social history

- Who were your friends?
- Were you satisfied with your friendships?
- Were you ever teased or picked on?
- What were your favorite activities/hobbies?
- What caused the most distress for you?
- How would you calm yourself down if you were upset?
- Were you in special education? If so, what for?
- Did you ever receive school-based or private psychotherapy? If so, what for?
- Did you ever receive school-based or private speech–language therapy? If so, what for?
- Did you ever receive school-based or private occupational therapy? If so, what for?
- Were you ever prescribed psychotropic medication? If so, what for?

Questions to ask the patient about current social functioning

- Who are your friends now? Can you tell me their first names?
- How often do you get to see your friends?
- What do you typically do for fun with your friends?
- Do you go out on dates? If so, how do you meet your partners?
- Do you have a boyfriend/girlfriend/romantic partner? If so, are you satisfied with the level of affection and physical intimacy in the relationship?
- If you are not currently dating, have you done so in the past or do you have plans to pursue it in the future? Why or why not?

TABLE 3.2. Observation Guidelines for Social Behavior during the Interview

- How does the patient use nonverbal cues to regulate the exchange (eye contact, gestures, body language)?
- How does the patient use language?
- Does he/she phrase things in unusual ways?
- Does he/she understand your questions the way you intend?
- Is he/she subject to tangential, circumstantial, or pressured speech?
- Is there a paucity of speech?
- How does he/she respond to transitions in the interview (e.g., change of subject, ending session)?
- Imagine yourself meeting the person in a social setting; would anything he/she does seem odd or eccentric?

Review Records

Ask the patient and/or family to provide copies of any reports of evaluations done on him or her, even if they are very old. These include report cards—teachers' narrative comments can provide clues about early social functioning. If the family did not keep records, they can sometimes be accessed from the school district. Although this was probably rare luck, I once had a 43-year-old man go back to his home district and get report cards from his elementary school years. The teacher remarks provided helpful evidence for the presence of ASD. Other useful documents include, but are not limited to, reports written by pediatricians, neurologists, psychiatrists, psychologists, social workers, speech–language therapists, and occupational therapists. For younger adults who received special education, access to their individualized education plan (IEP; a mandated statement of needs and goals that is provided by the school district) can be helpful.

TABLE 3.3. Interview Questions for Family Members during Initial Intake

- Did he/she have friends in the neighborhood, in preschool, in kindergarten?
- Did he/she have more or fewer friends at different stages (e.g., elementary school, junior high school, high school)?
- What caused him/her to become upset?
- What would calm him/her down after a distressing event?
- What were his/her strengths and talents?
- Did he/she have any significant fears, odd mannerisms, or rituals?
- Did his/her language development seem typical?
- Was his/her motor development typical?

Speak to Current Treating Professionals

In the first meeting, ask the patient for authorization to call any current or recent service providers who may be able to share insight into autism spectrum or mental health symptoms. These include, but are not limited to, psychiatrists, primary care physicians, case managers, or speech–language therapists. Other psychotherapists may also be involved for different reasons; some may have asked for a second opinion regarding ASD, whereas others may provide therapy in different modalities (group, family) or with different goals (supportive counseling).

Use Formal Testing Instruments, Screening Devices, and Symptom Checklists

A number of standardized instruments are available for use in diagnosing ASD. These devices vary greatly in terms of experience/training necessary to administer, age range of target subjects, functioning level of target subjects, and format/modality of administration. (See Campbell, James, & Vess, 2014, and Lord & Corsello, 2005, for more comprehensive reviews of available instruments.) As mentioned, the therapist will consider the possibility of referring the patient to an experienced ASD diagnostician in some cases. The most relevant instruments are listed below, with comments about the advantages and disadvantages of each. This information is also summarized in Table 3.4.

AUTISM DIAGNOSTIC INTERVIEW—REVISED

The Autism Diagnostic Interview—Revised (ADI-R; Rutter, LeCouteur, & Lord, 2003) is a structured interview meant to be carried out with the parent or other caregiver of the individual. It was designed to assess for autism in subjects of a wide range of ages and functioning levels. If used according to the guidelines, it is a reliable instrument to confirm or rule out an ASD, though a recent study of its use as a stand-alone instrument with adults has suggested that it could lead to overdiagnosis (Talari, Balaji, & Stansfield, 2017) and should be included as part of a battery of other instruments. Even a seasoned psychotherapist would need experience with ASD, as well as training and practice with the instrument before administering it. The interview will not be helpful to clinicians who, for example, are encountering their first cases of ASD and are searching for an instrument they can purchase and begin to use relatively quickly. However, it is worth the time investment for clinicians who intend to specialize in the formal diagnosis of ASD in adults.

AUTISM DIAGNOSTIC OBSERVATION SCHEDULE

The Autism Diagnostic Observation Schedule, Second Edition (ADOS-2; Lord et al., 2012) is a standardized protocol whereby a clinician observes and scores the social, communicative, and repetitive behaviors of the subject in a series of situations. It is applicable with people of all ages, but it may be less sensitive to symptoms in more cognitively able individuals. It is often described as a "gold standard" instrument for diagnosis of ASD because of its extensive empirical support for high reliability and validity ratings. Like the ADI-R, intensive training is required for the clinician to administer it competently.

TABLE 3.4. Assessment Instruments to Aid in the Diagnosis of ASD in Adults

Name of instrument	Author(s)	Age range	Format	Respondent for adult assessment	Level of training or expertise needed
Autism Diagnostic Interview—Revised (ADI-R)	Rutter, LeCouteur, & Lord (2003)	All	Structured interview	Other (caregiver or close companion)	High
Autism Diagnostic Observation Schedule–2 (ADOS-2)	Lord et al. (2012)	All	Behavioral observation	Self	High
Autism Mental Status Exam (AMSE)	Grodberg & Mount Sinai School of Medicine (2011)	All	Behavioral observation and interview	Self	Moderate
Autism Spectrum Quotient (AQ)	Baron-Cohen, Wheelwright, Skinner, Martin, & Clubley (2001)	Adults	Questionnaire	Self	Low
Empathy Quotient (EQ)	Baron-Cohen & Wheelwright (2004)	Adults	Questionnaire	Self	Low
Ritvo Autism and Asperger's Diagnostic Scale—Revised (RAAD-R)	Ritvo et al. (2011)	Adults	Questionnaire	Self	Low
Ritvo Autism and Asperger's Diagnostic Scale–14 Screen (RAADS–14 Screen)	Eriksson, Anderson, & Bejerot (2013)	Adults	Questionnaire	Self	Low
Social Responsiveness Scale, Second Edition (SRS-2)	Constantino & Gruber (2012)	All	Questionnaire	Self and other	Low

AUTISM MENTAL STATUS EXAM

The Autism Mental Status Exam (AMSE; Grodberg & Mount Sinai School of Medicine, 2011) is an observation tool that was designed to allow clinicians to observe and document social communication and behavior in the context of a general clinical exam, to serve as a screening device. It is an eight-item observational tool that guides the clinician to look for and score the presence and extent of autism symptoms, consistent with DSM-5 (American Psychiatric Association, 2013) by rating 0, 1, or 2 for each symptom. Validation studies have shown good prediction rates for classification on a gold standard instrument (ADOS) in children and adults of all functioning levels (Grodberg et al., 2014; Grodberg, Weinger, Kolevzon, Soorya, & Buxbaum, 2012). Like most of the tools described above, the AMSE should be used as a screening device when ASD is suspected, or to support diagnosis of ASD that is made during a more comprehensive evaluation that includes other diagnostic instruments. It gives the user objective ways to document the presence and severity of diagnostically significant behaviors, but warrants some practice with the nuances of judging the factors in a short period of time while ensuring fidelity to the instruction manual. The creators provide open access to the tool, but require the user to take a short online training session with posttests before downloading it.

AUTISM-SPECTRUM QUOTIENT

The Autism-Spectrum Quotient (AQ; Baron-Cohen, Wheelwright, Skinner, Martin, & Clubley, 2001) is a self-report questionnaire that is meant to be used only with individuals who have intellectual and verbal ability in the average or above-average range. Preliminary data support its discriminative validity in a clinic sample. It is only useful as a screening device and not as a definitive diagnostic tool. The test presents the subject with 50 questions, scored on a Likert scale, that assess five domains thought to be affected in people with ASD: social skill, attention switching, attention to detail, communication, and imagination.

EMPATHY QUOTIENT

The Empathy Quotient (EQ; Baron-Cohen & Wheelwright, 2004) assesses empathy and perspective-taking tendencies. It is a 60-item self-report instrument scored on a Likert scale. Because it only focuses on one feature of ASD, it is most useful if given as part of a battery of instruments, at the very least to complement the AQ described above, which was designed by the same group of researchers. Like the AQ, the EQ has been shown to reliably differentiate adults with ASD from typicals.

RITVO AUTISM AND ASPERGER'S DIAGNOSTIC SCALE

The Ritvo Autism and Asperger's Diagnostic Scale—Revised (RAAD-R; Ritvo et al., 2011) is an 80-item self-report questionnaire designed to assist clinicians in diagnosing adults who are suspected to have ASD and who have normal or above IQ. The questions assess ASD symptoms across the language, social relatedness, and sensory–motor domains and are rated using a Likert scale. It is meant to be filled out by the individual, but in the presence of the clinician (not to be a mail-in or online tool). It has been shown to be very accurate in discriminating among adults with ASD, those without ASD, and those with other DSM diagnoses. A shortened version containing 14 items, the RAADS–14 Screen, is much easier to administer and has shown promise as a screening tool (Eriksson, Anderson, & Bejerot, 2013) in adult outpatient settings.

SOCIAL RESPONSIVENESS SCALE

The Social Responsiveness Scale, Second Edition (SRS-2; Constantino & Gruber, 2012) has versions for all ages; the adult version has both a self-report 65-item question-naire and an other-report 65-item questionnaire. It measures the quality and severity of social functioning impairments and is compatible with DSM-5 criteria. As a stand-alone instrument, it may not discriminate between ASD-specific social impairments and the social communication deficits that can be found in other psychiatric disorders such as SAD (South, Carr, Stephenson, Maisel, & Cox, 2017) or psychotic disorders. To address these concerns, Sturm, Kuhfeld, Kasari, and MacCraken (2017) have developed a shorter version of the SRS that has 16 items and may be a more precise measure of ASD-specific social impairment—clinicians may want to keep track of further improve-ments in the development of that tool. In the meantime, the SRS-2 should be included as part of a comprehensive assessment including other assessment methods, as it can enrich the diagnostic by providing measures of the severity of impairment across sev-eral domains of social functioning.

Diagnosing Comorbid Mental Health Problems

While the therapist is assessing the patient for the symptoms of ASD, he or she must also attend to symptoms of other DSM-defined disorders. It is usually a mental health problem other than the ASD, per se, that brings a person into a psychotherapist's office. Often the individual reports some prior diagnosis(es) he or she has received. These should be considered and investigated. Sometimes these diagnoses are inappropriate for the current situation, especially if arrived at by a clinician in the distant past who was struggling to explain an odd clinical picture that did not fit neatly into any DSM category, given that the diagnosis of AS and recognition that ASD could occur with-out ID was not widespread until 1994. These diagnoses are either nonspecific, such as "atypical mood disorder," "atypical anxiety disorder," "psychotic disorder not other-wise specified (NOS)," or "autistic-like," or they are specific but do not fit the symptom picture as well as ASD; examples include schizoid personality disorder, schizotypal personality disorder, borderline personality disorder, undifferentiated schizophrenia, or schizoaffective disorder.

The following sections outline strategies for assessing the most common comorbid conditions observed in an outpatient clinical setting. It should be noted that these sec-tions are not meant to provide a comprehensive set of instructions on how to assess for each of the DSM-defined disorders in general. I assume that readers who are already practicing psychotherapy have developed their own strategies for exploring these issues with their patients. Other resources provide more details about each of these clinical problems, and the reader will be referred to some of them in the appropriate sections. The *principles* behind assessing these comorbid mental health disorders are the same for people with ASD as they are for any patient. Here I present the special considerations and modifications in technique that one should keep in mind for patients on the autism spectrum.

As you explore each of the areas below, remember the guidelines for interviewing patients with ASD that were presented earlier: pace yourself, learn to speak their language, and be respectful in the face of seemingly odd behavior.

Anxiety Disorders

Individuals with ASD are subject to chronic stress because they process information in unique ways and must, as some patients have described, "work harder" just to appear "normal." Often aware of their processing difficulties, they compensate with a hyper-vigilance directed toward the behavior of others and small changes in their environment. Due to problems with EF, they often must put extra energy into the simplest planning and organization tasks, which may lead to excessive worrying or obsessional thinking. A history of failure in the social and sexual domains may lead to avoidance behavior. It is easy to imagine how all of the above-listed experiences make people with ASD more likely to develop any of the anxiety disorders listed in DSM-5.

The possible presence of a comorbid anxiety disorder must be considered when planning treatment. Administering one or a combination of the Beck Anxiety Inventory (BAI; Beck, 1990; Beck, Epstein, Brown, & Steer, 1988), the State–Trait Anxiety Inventory (STAI; Spielberger, Gorsuch, Lushene, Vagg, & Jacobs, 1983), or the Multidimensional Anxiety Questionnaire (MAQ; Reynolds, 1999) early on can serve as preliminary screening instruments. Outlined below are the most commonly observed anxiety disorders, as defined by DSM-5, and guiding questions for exploring them with patients on the autism spectrum. Remember that these patients need very literal, specific questions about the factors surrounding their problems. Without that quality of questioning, they may underreport certain phenomena. The reader is referred to Barlow (2001) for a comprehensive description of anxiety disorders, theories explaining them, and current treatment approaches. (For more information about the overlap between anxiety disorders and ASD, see Bejerot et al., 2014; Maddox & White, 2015; Maisel et al., 2016; Swain et al., 2015; Tsai, 2006; White et al., 2012.)

SPECIFIC PHOBIA

Is the patient avoiding situations that are more specific than the areas discussed under agoraphobia? Is the avoidance not better accounted for by the sensory problems that can be part of ASD? For example, if a person is avoiding the dentist because of hypersensitivity to the noise of the equipment but is not afraid of the dentist or any other part of the procedure, then it is not a phobic response. Theoretically, this person would go to the dentist if the aversive noise could be contained. In another example, a man with ASD reported an intense fear of flying, which did meet criteria for a specific phobia because it was not related to sensory issues, was recognized as unreasonable by him, and was infringing on his leisure time and social opportunities.

SOCIAL ANXIETY DISORDER (SOCIAL PHOBIA)

If the patient is avoiding social situations because of a belief that scrutiny or negative evaluation by others will be likely, and that fear or avoidance is interfering with the attainment of a goal or is causing distress, these symptoms should be assessed further for possible SAD diagnosis. As mentioned in Chapter 1, disentangling the effects of core ASD symptoms from the development of a comorbid SAD is particularly difficult. Especially when one considers the DSM-5 criterion that says, "the fear or anxiety is out of proportion to the actual threat posed by the social situation" (American Psychiatric Association, 2013, p. 203)—for these patients the possibility that others really will evaluate them negatively, reject them, or say things to embarrass them is more likely than for a typical, socially competent person. So, the fear and avoidance is not based on an irrational belief in these cases. In fact, we now know that a large portion of people with ASD do have high social motivation and a wish to connect with others, and that subset of the ASD population is more likely to experience high levels of social anxiety and avoidance. For these individuals, a comorbid diagnosis is often warranted. For example, if a person begins to develop social communication skills through intervention and becomes more competent in being able to demonstrate interaction skills, yet their avoidance persists because of overwhelming anxiety, that patient needs intervention for SAD as any non-ASD person would receive.

PANIC DISORDER

Does the patient report intense episodes of anxiety? Does the patient or family report frequent *meltdowns*? This is a term used in the autism spectrum community to refer to episodes of sudden decompensation marked by the onset of high arousal, behavioral detachment, and/or physically aggressive behavior. These episodes are usually preceded by a situation that is experienced as extremely stressful and can have a number of causes and courses, but some are true panic attacks as defined by DSM-5. Patients may report classic panic symptoms if asked about them, even if they use idiosyncratic words to describe their feelings. For example, one young man reported that during such an attack, he felt nauseated, had a pain in his chest, believed he was going crazy, and had "mushy legs."

AGORAPHOBIA

Is the patient avoiding important activities or responsibilities outside of the home? Do the people around the patient complain about noncompliance with certain expected activities, such as medical appointments, grocery shopping, class attendance, or using particular modes of transportation? Does the patient refrain from going places alone or seem overly reliant on a family member to accompany him or her on outings? Does this problem go beyond the avoidance that might be expected because of ASD (e.g., avoidance of social situations) or a comorbid depressive disorder (e.g., loss of motivation)? I was working with one patient, a 20-year-old college student with ASD, for a whole year before realizing agoraphobia, as part of a panic disorder, was present. Her repeated "skipping" of classes had appeared to be related to the major depression she was experiencing at one point during the year, but when her depression remitted and she continued to miss classes, a reassessment yielded more information supporting the new diagnosis. Apparently, she had experienced several panic attacks in the past and was afraid it would happen again. I (to my own embarrassment) had never inquired about it, and the patient did not see the relevance to her problem and so never thought to report the experiences to anyone.

GENERALIZED ANXIETY DISORDER

Does the patient suffer from persistent worry? The patient may directly report chronic worrying as a problem, or the therapist may infer it from the patient's behavior. For example, does the patient perseverate about a problem, bringing it up repeatedly even after it appears to have been solved? Again, the arousal symptoms are difficult to assess in these patients who are so prone to regulation problems. Nevertheless, does the patient's persistent worries seem to be linked to restlessness, fatigue, difficulty concentrating, irritability, muscle tension, or sleep problems?

Obsessive–Compulsive and Related Disorders

As mentioned in Chapter 1, the repetitive and stereotyped patterns of behavior that are part of ASD can easily be confused with OCD and related disorders (hoarding disorder, trichotillomania, and excoriation disorder) in adults seeking treatment. Nevertheless, there are cases where one or more of these disorders are present as comorbid diagnoses. See Anholt and colleagues (2010) and Kaur and colleagues (2016) for more information about how the symptoms of ASD and OCD can overlap, yet be distinguishable as two comorbid conditions in some individuals. Below are guidelines for assessing for the presence of OCD, hoarding disorder, trichotillomania, and excoriation disorder in adult patients.

OBSESSIVE–COMPULSIVE DISORDER

Does the person have obsessions, which are thoughts, images, or urges/impulses that are unwanted? Does the person have compulsions that are repetitive behaviors or mental acts that he or she feels driven to carry out? Do these behaviors or mental acts have the intent to reduce or prevent harm or neutralize a threat? Are these obsessions or compulsions not explained by the individual's ASD? For example, does the preoccupation with a particular topic seem to be unwanted by the person? If the individual is enjoying the excessive time spent on the topic and is making no attempt to suppress the thoughts, then he or she does not meet criteria for OCD. However, if the person is experiencing the thoughts as intrusive and feels the related behaviors (compulsions) are driven or distressing, then OCD could be considered. I have observed that when OCD is present as a comorbid condition, it is common for the compulsions to have a social component and involve other people. These include the need to tell, ask, request, or demand information or reassurance from others. Observations from a caregiver may be necessary if the individual does not report a concern about this problem but is showing signs of distress while performing rituals (i.e., OCD with the *poor insight* specifier defined in DSM-5).

HOARDING DISORDER

Though considered a distinctive phenomenon in DSM-5, hoarding disorder was historically categorized as a manifestation of OCD. While some features of ASD could have the consequence of a person collecting and amassing large quantities of objects related to a special interest, the massive amounts of items needed to significantly impede access to living areas is usually seen more in hoarding disorder. A person with ASD may have a huge collection of baseball cards or unique cartoon-art pieces, for example, but the collecting is focused only on objects related to the interest and the items are not clogging access to every room in the residence or making every piece of furniture unusable, as would be observed in hoarding disorder. A person with ASD could also end up with a lot of clutter in his or her residence if EF problems are severe enough to make housekeeping tasks too challenging. If that is the reason for the accumulation, there would be very little distress if someone came in and cleaned up, unlike hoarding disorder, which would be marked by extreme distress when objects are discarded. Nevertheless, a comorbid diagnosis of hoarding disorder can be considered if a person with ASD has demonstrated all of the criteria of hoarding disorder, which represents behaviors more excessive than what would be explained by ASD alone.

TRICHOTILLOMANIA AND EXCORIATION DISORDER

Both of these body-focused disorders were newly added to the OCD-related category in DSM-5. Trichotillomania (hair pulling) was previously considered an impulse-control disorder and excoriation (skin picking) did not appear in any previous DSM. Discussed together here as potential comorbid diagnoses in ASD, both involve body-focused repetitive behavior that is distinguishable from the repetitive motor symptoms of ASD and can also appear as part of a separate but comorbid condition. Does the patient have visible signs of hair loss or skin lesions? If so, how does he or she respond to inquiries about these visible signs? Does he or she acknowledge hair pulling/skin picking, and if so, does he or she report having attempted to stop it? To distinguish these behaviors from the stereotyped motor movements of ASD, the distress caused by the behavior and desire to stop doing it is more often connected to trichotillomania and excoriation disorder, but not as often with ASD stereotypies. Also, age of onset is usually during or soon after puberty for trichotillomania and excoriation disorder, whereas ASD stereotypies are present since early childhood. So, if a person who meets criteria for ASD reports that hair-pulling or skin-picking behaviors developed during adolescence or later, and he or she finds these behaviors distressing and undesirable, then an additional diagnosis of one of these body-focused OCD-related disorders should be considered.

Trauma- and Stressor-Related Disorders

Traumatic verbal assaults, threats, and physical assaults are not uncommon in the backgrounds of adults with ASD. Sadly, their unusual behaviors draw unwanted attention from predatory people in schools or communities. A lack of education about sexuality increases the risk of many types of aversive sexual experiences, ranging from embarrassment during a desired encounter all the way to the trauma of an unwanted encounter, such as a rape. These types of major stressors make people with ASD vulnerable to trauma-related disorders, especially posttraumatic stress disorder (PTSD).

POSTTRAUMATIC STRESS DISORDER

Has the person experienced a traumatic event in his or her history? Begin by asking about the types of situations any patient could have experienced, such as an accident, physical assault, or sexual assault. If the individual denies all of these experiences, consider the likelihood that the patient has suffered repeated mistreatment by others at a far greater frequency than typical people. The school histories of many adults with ASD include daily episodes of verbal teasing, taunting, and threatening and/or physical assaults by peers. DSM-5 defines a traumatic event as exposure to "actual or threatened death, serious injury, or sexual violence" (American Psychiatric Association, 2013, p. 271). For many people with ASD, the repeated episodes of mistreatment that is so often part of their histories involve all those types of threats. Their difficulty understanding social norms and expectations affects their knowledge about sexuality, and many have histories of traumatic sexual experiences. Is the person bothered by intrusive memories or images of such events? Is the person avoiding reminders of these events? Although difficult to differentiate from the ER problems observed in ASD (King, 2010), the clinician should still investigate whether the person is experiencing problems with overarousal in relation to the other symptoms listed above.

Mood Disorders

As described in the earlier chapters, adults with ASD are predisposed to mood disorders from genetic, neurobiological, and psychosocial perspectives. Once the diagnosis of ASD has been established, the therapist should assume high risk for mood symptoms and should include questions in the assessment aimed at eliciting them in case they are present but not being reported clearly by the patient. Special considerations for assessing mood disorders in people with ASD are described below. DSM-5 has divided bipolar disorders and depressive disorders into two different sections, which represents a change from the historical umbrella category of "mood disorders" capturing both phenomena, so the two subsections to follow represent the disorders covered by two separate chapters in DSM-5. More comprehensive overviews of the theories and treatment of mood disorders can be found in Beck, Rush, Shaw, and Emery (1979); Frank (2005); Gotlib and Hammen (2014); Ingram, Miranda, and Segal (1999); and Persons and colleagues (2000). (For more detailed information on the overlap between mood disorders and ASD, see Buck et al., 2014; Matson & Williams, 2014; Matsuo et al., 2015; Skokauskas & Frodl, 2015.)

DEPRESSIVE DISORDERS

A major depressive episode is often the event that motivates a person with ASD to seek treatment. The chronic stress described above can "wear down" people to the point where they believe they are helpless. At that point they lose hope that they will achieve one or more of their life goals, and the classic symptoms of depression can set in. At intake, they may state that they are experiencing sadness, hopelessness, loneliness, feelings of worthlessness, problems concentrating, fatigue, insomnia, or suicidal ideation. For others, the report is made by family members who have observed withdrawal from activities, irritable mood, sleep difficulties, loss of previously attained skills (e.g., self-care), and suicide threats. Again, keep in mind the unique communication style of the patient and remember that he or she may need to be asked specific and literal questions in order to elicit these types of experiences. Also consider that some of the problems inherent in an ASD can mimic depressive symptoms, such as appearing socially aloof/withdrawn, difficulty regulating affect, and disordered sleep. If the problems have been present and stable since childhood and are not accompanied by an equally stable sad mood, then they are more likely to be part of the core disorder of ASD. However, if the problems have a recent or marked onset and represent a change in the person's usual way of functioning, then major depression should be pursued further. The Beck Depression Inventory—Second Edition (BDI-II; Beck, 1996) can be a useful screening instrument as well as a tool to measure progress, should depression become a target in the treatment plan. If you are convinced that depressive symptoms are currently or historically at play, the final diagnosis will depend on the severity of the symptoms and the history of other mood episodes in order to arrive at *major depressive disorder* (with modifiers about severity, chronicity, features, and state of remission) or *persistent depressive disorder* (dysthymia). If the patient is currently experiencing a depressive episode but has a history of manic or hypomanic symptoms, further exploration of a possible bipolar disorder should be conducted, as described in the next section.

BIPOLAR AND RELATED DISORDERS

As mentioned, some features of ASD can mimic mania or hypomania. These features include ER problems, disordered sleep, and intense goal-directed activity related to a special interest. As specified in DSM-5, manic or hypomanic symptoms must represent an *abnormal* display of behavior that is not characteristic of *that person's* usual way of functioning. Those criteria help the clinician rule out mania or hypomania as an explanation for stable patterns of behavior that have been present across the lifespan as part of the ASD symptom picture. It is rare for a patient to come to my outpatient psychotherapy office in a florid manic state. However, a portion of people with ASDs have relatives with bipolar disorders, and there is some preliminary evidence that people on the autism spectrum may be genetically predisposed to bipolar disorder (DeLong & Nohria, 1994; Joshi et al., 2013). A history of these symptoms must be explored, even if they are not being displayed at the time of intake. Some patients may come in for treatment after their manic symptoms have been stabilized pharmacologically, in which case the treating psychiatrist will become an important part of the treatment planning process. Only after looking at the severity and course of symptoms with the history of depressive episodes can a final diagnosis of *bipolar I, bipolar II,* or *cyclothymic disorder* be made.

Personality Disorders

Assessing for the presence of a personality disorder (PD) is complicated when a patient already has a well-established ASD. DSM-5 considers the presence of an ASD as a rule-out for only two of the 12 PD listed in that volume: schizoid and schizotypal personality disorders. This leaves the possibility open for diagnosing any of the other 10 PDs as comorbid conditions for adult patients with ASD. Why would it be necessary to add another diagnosis to explain problems related to dysfunctional interpersonal behaviors if we already have an explanation in ASD? I am prone to argue that it is not. In fact, some patients who have been previously diagnosed with PD demonstrate an "enduring pattern of inner experience and behavior that deviates markedly from the expectations of the individual's culture" (DSM-5 criterion for PD; American Psychiatric Association, 2013, p. 646), which can be explained better by ASD, and the PD can be ruled out.

My reluctance to add a PD diagnosis comes from my strengths-based approach with patients, which is part of a tendency not to want to "overpathologize" the personalities of people with ASD. Despite this bias, I occasionally find it necessary to include a PD when describing a patient with ASD. I add this diagnosis when the impairment in the interpersonal functioning of the individual seems out of proportion to the level of social-cognitive impairment (the core deficit in ASD) and is interfering with the person's ability to engage in the learning process of therapy. For example, a person with ASD alone may make offensive comments because he or she is simply lacking social information. Once that person receives the correct information about social norms and how to read nonverbal cues, he or she will be motivated to stop the behavior because he or she never wanted to offend. On the other hand, a person with ASD who receives the proper information, understands it thoroughly, and continues to choose the offensive behavior, with the intention to offend, is exhibiting interpersonal problems that cannot be explained totally by the ASD diagnosis.

The decision to give a PD diagnosis is subjective because it is impossible to know with certainty all the etiological pathways leading up to the dysfunctional interpersonal relationships observed in a patient. It is easy to hypothesize that an individual with ASD is vulnerable to the very factors thought to be instrumental in the development of PD in the *typical* population: neurodevelopmental deficits, negative social–emotional experiences, and a failure to learn coping skills. Special considerations for assessing PD in people with ASD are given below. In the interest of space, I present each disorder as part of the cluster to which it belongs. For a more thorough overview of PD, see Young (1999) or Beck, Freeman, Davis, and Associates (2004). (For more detailed information on the overlap between ASD and PD, see Duijkers, Vissers, Verbeeck, Arntz, & Egger, 2014; Lugnegård et al., 2011.)

CLUSTER A PERSONALITY DISORDERS

Individuals with Cluster A personality disorders—paranoid personality disorder, schizoid personality disorder, and schizotypal personality disorder—appear *odd* or *eccentric*. Paranoid personality disorder is the only one that can be considered in this cluster for a patient meeting criteria for ASD because DSM-5 gives ASD diagnostic precedence over the other two. Adults with ASD very often have histories of being mistreated by peers and members of their communities. They may appear paranoid because they have developed a *reasonable* mistrust of others. A diagnosis of paranoid personality disorder would be appropriate only if the suspicion and mistrust were out of proportion to the actual negative experiences the person has had with others.

CLUSTER B PERSONALITY DISORDERS

Individuals with Cluster B personality disorders—antisocial personality disorder, borderline personality disorder, histrionic personality disorder, and narcissistic personality disorder—appear *dramatic, emotional,* or *erratic*. The ER and social cognition problems that are part of ASD can mimic these disorders. A Cluster B disorder should be considered only if, according to the clinical judgment of the therapist, the symptoms go above and beyond what would be expected for ASD. One rough way to make this differentiation is by assessing skills *and* intent. People with ASD may have a pattern of doing things that are unkind, uncaring, offensive, or even harmful to other people. However, if these are mistakes made by people who are unable to extract the information they need from their environment in order to act in more considerate ways toward their fellow humans, and are doing these things *without the intent* to harm, then this behavior can be explained solely by considering the core deficits of ASD. However, if a person with ASD continually chooses to hurt or offend others even after he or she understands the consequences of his or her actions and has *demonstrated the skills* necessary to handle things in alternative ways, then a Cluster B personality disorder can be considered.

CLUSTER C PERSONALITY DISORDERS

Individuals with Cluster C personality disorders—avoidant personality disorder, dependent personality disorder, and obsessive–compulsive personality disorder— appear *anxious* or *fearful*. All of the Cluster C disorders represent personality *styles* that are commonly observed in people with ASD. These patterns of relating seem to be learned coping strategies that these individuals acquire to manage their ASD symptoms. Once again, these diagnoses should be considered only if they are so pervasive and extreme that they interfere with the individual's capacity to learn new information or alternative coping strategies in his or her current life. I have observed the presence of comorbid avoidant and dependent PD in individuals with ASD more often than any other PD. The tendencies to avoid interpersonal involvement or to avoid making life decisions are to be expected, to some extent, in individuals with ASD because of their core problems and learning histories. However, there are times when those patterns are out of proportion to the patient's skill deficits and persistent in the face of new learning opportunities.

Sexual Problems

As mentioned earlier, adults with ASD are prone to a variety of problems or reported distress around sexual functioning. When these issues are present, they are often interwoven with the core deficits and other mental health problems discussed in this chapter. The sexuality education and support needs of adolescents with all types of developmental disabilities, including ASD, have traditionally been neglected (Attwood, 2007; Hénault, 2005; Koller, 2000; Matich-Maroney, Boyle, & Crocker, 2005; Murphy & Elias, 2006; Nichols & Blakely-Smith, 2010), so individuals enter adulthood ill prepared to negotiate this complex domain of life. In order to effectively intervene when an adult is struggling with some aspect of sexual functioning, we must first understand what factors contribute to *sexual well-being* in the lives of people on the spectrum (Byers & Nichols, 2014; Byers, Nichols, & Voyer, 2013; Byers, Nichols, Voyer, & Reilly, 2013). Fortunately, some researchers have begun to focus more on these factors, and the initial findings are that many adults with ASD living in the community report positive sexual experiences and are able to be in satisfying sexual relationships (Byers, Nichols, & Voyer, 2013; Byers, Nichols, Voyer, & Reilly, 2013). Because adults on the spectrum can and do enjoy this important part of a quality life, when they are struggling with some aspect of it, therapists need to pay attention to the problem as they would any other mental health issue.

Before deciding whether a DSM-defined sexual disorder is present, it is helpful to view the sexual problems of adults with ASD along a continuum, as illustrated in the model described by Matich-Maroney and colleagues (2005). These authors discuss developmental disabilities more generically, but their approach to conceptualizing sexual problems is applicable to adults with ASD. They define clinical issues and commensurate intervention needs across four levels of complexity, beginning with the most basic and ending with the most complicated. These are *lack of sexual knowledge, impaired interpersonal skills, sexual disorders,* and *sexually offensive (illegal) behaviors.* Using this framework, therapists would first consider whether the presenting sexual problem is simply a *lack of sexual knowledge,* as some adults with ASD may be lacking factual information about anatomy/physiology, sexually transmitted diseases, abuse prevention, gender expression, and societal norms about social–sexual conduct. The next question would be if the presenting sexual problem is a manifestation of impaired *interpersonal skills.* Adults with ASD, because of social-cognitive deficits, may lack skills necessary to date, initiate an intimate relationship, or manage the demands of a committed relationship. This would obviously lead to dissatisfaction and frustration in the sexual domain of functioning, but does not warrant a comorbid diagnosis of a *sexual disorder.* However, if the problems are not fully accounted for by a lack of knowledge or skills, then the DSM-5 sexual disorders may be considered, as outlined below. In a smaller number of cases, *sexually offensive behaviors* may be involved.

I don't appreciate that most sexual issues seem to be connected to lack of information and poor social skills. It's bypassing sensory issues, and implies that NT teenagers grow with healthy sex views which is not true for females

SEXUAL DISORDERS

Adults with ASD may experience any of the DSM-5-defined *sexual dysfunctions* (disorders of ejaculation, erection, orgasm, arousal, interest, desire, or sexual pain), *gender dysphoria,* or *paraphilias* (voyeuristic, exhibitionistic, frotteuristic, sexual masochism, sexual sadism, pedophilic, fetishistic, or transvestic disorders). When assessing a possible paraphilia in an adult with ASD, it is important to consider that the behavior displayed may be *counterfeit deviance.* This term was used first by Hingsburger, Griffiths, and Quinsey (1991) to describe behavior that is topographically similar to a paraphilia but is actually a manifestation of deficient education or experience during sexual development, as mentioned above. These factors include lack of information about sexual expression, poor social skills, and limited opportunities to interact in typical ways with same-age peers. Depending on the experience of the individual therapist, the patient may be referred to an expert for further assessment and/or treatment.

SEXUALLY OFFENSIVE BEHAVIORS

Whether an adult is engaging in illegal sexual behavior because of a lack of information or skills or, in rarer cases, because of a comorbid paraphelia, the risk of arrest and incarceration is significant (see Attwood et al., 2014; Lerner et al., 2012). Unfortunately for the former group, the criminal justice system is universally intolerant of sexually offensive behavior, whether it is counterfeit or bonafide deviance. Increasing numbers of adults with ASD are at risk for arrest as the Internet has become accessible to so many people (Attwood et al., 2014). It has developed into a primary source of pornographic material, dating services, and opportunities to interact with potential sexual partners. This medium can be appealing to someone who might be shy or intimidated in face-to-face social situations, but it is also more dangerous because it is much easier to unknow-ingly make an illegal mistake, leading to very severe counsequences (e.g., downloading pornographic material that contains content that is illegal to possess or share; setting up a date to meet a potential sexual partner with someone who, unbeknownst to the adult with ASD, is underage). If a therapist is assessing a patient with ASD, when taking a sexual history it is critical to inquire about Internet use and the types of materials or encounters being sought there. An adult patient with ASD who has never been arrested can be educated about the risks and a legal crisis can be averted.

If a treatment-seeking adult with ASD already has been arrested, the assessment and treatment planning is best carried out by an expert in sexuality and forensic issues, ideally someone who is also familiar with ASD. Unless the therapist has that back-ground and experience, a referral to a qualified clinician is warranted.

Sleep–Wake Disorders

Sleep problems are commonly reported by adults on the spectrum and their families, though it is not listed as a symptom or associated feature of ASD in DSM-5. While we still do not know whether sleep disturbance is a consequence of core ASD impairments, there is some evidence suggesting that people with ASD may have atypical or disturbed sleep patterns, even when they are not experiencing noticeable sleep problems (Baker & Rich-dale, 2017; Limoges, Bolduc, Berthiaume, Mottron, & Godbout, 2013; Limoges et al., 2005). The field of sleep disorders in general is in flux, which is reflected in the many changes between DSM-IV (American Psychiatric Association, 1994) and DSM-5 (American Psy-chiatric Association, 2013) in terms of how the problems are classified and labeled. For the present purposes, any of the disorders listed in DSM-5 can be diagnosed as a comorbid disorder if all of the criteria are met, as ASD is not a rule-out for any of the 10 sleep–wake disorders listed. While there is no research on behavioral sleep interventions designed exclusively for adults with ASD suffering from sleep disorders, the sleep interventions that have been shown to work for typical adults can be offered to adults with ASD, as long as the symptoms are not better accounted for by a comorbid anxiety or mood disorder.

Substance Use Disorders

Adults on the spectrum who are seeking treatment for mental health problems should be screened for substance use disorders (SUD) at intake, something that has tradition-ally been overlooked in this population (Butwicka et al., 2017; Clarke, Tickle, & Gillott, 2016), despite evidence that ASD is represented in treatment-seeking samples with SUD at a higher rate than in the general population (Butwicka et al., 2017; van Wijngaarden-Cremers, 2016). While the use of alcohol or cannabis is appealing as a stress manage-ment strategy or social facilitator for a person facing the daily difficulties of living with ASD, the impairments associated with ASD are worse during the course of substance use (Sizoo et al., 2009). For this reason, the treatment plan will need to include inter-ventions to address this issue if it is present, as efforts to treat the other problems for which the patient is seeking treatment will be compromised by the effects of an active SUD. Therapists trained in substance use treatment may provide the intervention, or the patient may be referred elsewhere for concurrent or primary treatment before other mental health and ASD-related problems can be treated.

Suicidality

Suicidality may not present the same way in people with ASD as in the typical population, and does not only occur during a course of depression (Segers & Rawana, 2014). Therefore, screening strategies should be present for all intakes in this population, as a universal precaution, and should be periodically repeated throughout the course of treatment because it may be more difficult to detect in patients with autism. An additional challenge for the therapist is that some adults with ASD will experience what Attwood (2007, 2015) calls a *suicide attack*. Attwood (2015) describes this as " . . . the sudden onset of intense negative emotion paired with a spur-of-the-moment decision to make a dramatic end to life" (p. 154). These attacks are unanticipated by the individuals, and if the attempts are thwarted and they survive, they very quickly return to a state that involves little to no suicidal thoughts or plans. This is very disturbing to the individuals, their loved ones, and their therapists, as they imagine how a fleeting emotional state can quickly lead to death. Interestingly, the research field on suicidality in the general population has begun to examine related phenomena, as the *fluid vulnerability theory* (Rudd, 2006) suggests that the manner in which people make transitions from suicide thought to suicide action is nonlinear and dynamic, requiring mental health practitioners to rethink traditional approaches for understanding and assessing suicidality in their patients (see Bryan & Rudd, 2016).

Assessment of Strengths and Resiliency Factors

Adult patients with ASD who have chosen to enter psychotherapy are survivors. The older they are, the longer they have lived with myriad problems in an overwhelming world and without any good explanation as to why the simplest things in life are such a struggle for them. When I hear their stories, I am often surprised by the persistence of some to keep trying to improve their lives, despite an immeasurable amount of pain. When I first started working with these patients, I often felt the urge to ask, "How the hell did you manage to come this far?"—but I did not necessarily say that out loud. Over the years, however, I have learned that questions like that are crucial parts of the intake interview; the information yielded from this line of inquiry is invaluable in the treatment planning process. These questions serve as an intervention for some patients because while answering them, they view themselves from new perspectives.

My interest in the resiliency of my patients has led me to the field of positive psychology, which includes the scientific study of positive subjective experience and positive individual traits (Seligman & Csikszentmihalyi, 2000). As a refreshing shift away from studying pathological conditions, positive psychology researchers seek to understand human strengths and resiliency factors, which are strikingly relevant to the incredible lives of courage and perseverance I have seen in my patients. Even when people are struggling and seeking help from a therapist, positive psychology can be practiced—Seligman and Peterson (2003) suggest therapy should be about embracing "both healing what is weak and nurturing what is strong" (p. 313).

What Strategies Has the Patient Learned to Compensate for Deficits?

Most patients have made adaptations in their lives to minimize the impact of particular deficits, even if they are not able to articulate them easily. For example, one man had learned that the social demands of his job depleted his energy so much that he could not socialize successfully on Friday nights. For years, he had gone out on Friday nights but was withdrawn and tense. However, if he went out on Saturday nights, he was more relaxed and able to focus on the people with whom he was socializing. He had therefore made the wise adaptation to schedule social events on Saturday nights and to keep Friday nights free for a solitary relaxing activity.

To What Extent Does the Patient Use Natural Self-Observation to Learn?

Some patients are quite good at telling the therapist what they have noticed about themselves and how they have tried to make changes based on their observations. In the example above, it was the man's self-observation that had allowed him to realize he was sullen on Friday nights and more socially engaging on Saturday nights. I have noticed that the cliché about wisdom coming with age holds true for adults with ASD. The older they are, the more they have managed to learn and change on their own. Some of the most innovative ideas have come from patients who were well into their 40s or 50s when they were first diagnosed with ASD. These individuals had to live a long time without any intervention for their problems and were left to figure out a lot on their own. The therapist can elicit these adaptations and use them as building blocks for the treatment plan.

In What Healthy Lifestyle Practices Does the Patient Engage?

Is the person attentive to healthy eating? Does the person exercise regularly? Does the person use meditative, spiritual, or religious practices to relax? Any aspects of the person's lifestyle that are health promoting (but not obsessive, which must be assessed) should be highlighted and reinforced.

In What Adaptive Ways Does the Patient Cope with Stress?

How does the person recognize stress? What does he or she do to reduce tension? Some people use their special interest (e.g., aviation, model railroading, astronomy) as a means of reducing stress and increasing relaxation. Although family members are sometimes concerned about the immersion in a subject as being obsessive, and rightly so, care should be taken to preserve the activity, even if the amount of time spent on it is reduced in order to make room for other necessary tasks of daily living.

In What Ways Has the Patient Been Successful in Relationships?

Many adult patients have made one or two friends, if not more, by the time they enter treatment. These patients should be asked to reflect on aspects of those friendships in order to understand what they are doing right. One 19-year-old man told me about two friends he has had since grade school. As a college student, he and these friends continued to get together every week. When asked what these friends liked about him, he said, "I haven't the slightest idea." A full session of exploration led him to finally realize that they liked the same activities he did (the latest video games). He also reported that they appeared to laugh a lot when he made jokes—an observation that had not meant anything to him until I focused on it, leading to the conclusion they must like his sense of humor.

What Are the Patient's Talents, Interests, and Hobbies?

Individuals with ASD often have very focused interests in one or more topics or activities. In its most extreme form, this phenomenon is considered a "symptom" (e.g., in DSM-5, "fixated interests that are abnormal in intensity or focus"; American Psychiatric Association, 2013, p. 50). But if expressed in moderation (meaning the person is able to make room for practicing necessary tasks of daily living), the person's interest can provide him or her with a powerful link to self-sufficiency and life satisfaction. Imagine a successful person whom you really admire. Do you think that person could have achieved what he or she did without intense interest and focus in the area of success? Helping patients with ASD preserve the pursuit of their interests and talent is a crucial part in any treatment plan, so the therapist must devote some part of the assessment to learning about that aspect of each patient's life.

How Does the Patient Use Humor?

For reasons already reviewed, many patients report some difficulty understanding other people's jokes or knowing when someone is joking versus not joking. However, they can be quite adept at making jokes, and their unconventional view of the world contributes to a "quirky" sense of humor that many typical people will enjoy. Once a therapist and patient have achieved a certain level of familiarity with each other, humor can be used during therapy sessions to reinforce the learning process. Any patient who has a natural, preexisting enjoyment of humor brings an important strength to social situations as he or she gets better at reading other people and practicing the right timing of jokes.

What Are the Likable Features of the Patient's Personality?

Therapists should remain objective with all patients, of course. However, with patients who have social skill difficulties, the therapist can use his or her own personal reactions to the patient as a gauge for how others are probably reacting to him or her in the real world. The style of interacting in the therapist's office is a behavioral sample of what might be going on when the individual interacts with peers. Do you like this person? If so, what is it about his or her personality that you find appealing? Where is the patient on the dimensions of extroversion–introversion, optimism–pessimism, humorous–humorless? Whether or not one person likes another is a rather subjective decision. Nevertheless, whatever characteristics you like about the patient, there is a good chance that at least some other people would like those features, too. Therefore, those characteristics should be highlighted. Also, the factors that may be blocking others from seeing these characteristics should be explored so that their reduction can be incorporated into the goals of the treatment plan.

What Is the Quality of the Patient's Social Support?

People with ASD tend to have less social support than typical people. Nevertheless, there is great variability within the ASD population in terms of the quality and quantity of their relationships. Keep in mind that quantity does not guarantee quality; any relationship can be helpful and/or a source of stress for the person. Questions about this area should include:

- Is there a spouse or significant other? Does the patient perceive that person as supportive?
- Does the patient see friends regularly? Does the patient perceive these friends to be supportive?
- Are there parents involved? Does the patient perceive them to be supportive?
- Are there siblings involved? Does the patient perceive them to be supportive?
- Does the patient belong to any community-based groups, such as clubs, sports leagues/teams, religious groups, support groups? How does the patient perceive the relationships with the people in these groups?
- Does the patient have any social service staff involved in his or her life, such as case managers or supportive living staff? Are they viewed as helpful, unhelpful, or intrusive?

Creating the Problem List and Setting Preliminary Goals

The goal-oriented approach of CBT is explained to the patient from the very beginning of the intake process. By the end of the assessment phase, the therapist and patient should be able to identify the key areas of the person's life that are most problematic and therefore most in need of change. The patient is asked to generate goals by describing what he or she hopes to change. Some patients with ASD are subject to stating expectations that are too concrete or extreme. A tendency toward all-or-nothing thinking and problems with EF (e.g., planning) means that the therapist has to be active in helping to phrase the patient's objectives in attainable terms. Here is an example of a discussion that came from the intake of a man in his mid-30s who was diagnosed with ASD only a few months before coming in for treatment. These types of discussions usually happen at the end of the first or second intake session.

THERAPIST: Just to summarize, now, you have come here to address problems with anger and getting disappointed with other people. You also want to learn more about your recent diagnosis of ASD. What would you like to see change? In other words, how would life be different for you in, let's say, 6 months, if you could change something?

PATIENT: I want to stop people from ruining my day and making me feel like a loser. I also want to stop being hard on myself.

THERAPIST: OK, so you want to see if there is a way for you to be less upset by the interactions you have with other people and also to feel more confident in yourself around other people?

PATIENT: Absolutely.

THERAPIST: Notice I changed the wording a little bit. You said you wanted to stop people from ruining your day and making you feel like a loser. Because those people will not be here with us during our sessions, we won't have much control over them. But we will have access to your perception of them and your reactions to them, so that is why I suggested that we look for a way for you to manage that differently so that you will not be so upset by them.

PATIENT: Yeah. I don't want to feel like a loser. If you could help me control that feeling, I would not get so upset, I think.

THERAPIST: We can definitely work on that. You can learn strategies to challenge that "loser" idea about yourself. Do you think that would also help you to be less hard on yourself, which is the other goal you mentioned?

PATIENT: Yes. Yeah, I am extra hard on myself because I am trying not to be a loser. So, yeah. It's all connected . . . definitely all connected.

Note that the therapist gave an explanation when she changed the wording of the patient's objective. This is an important way to maintain respect for the patient while building trust.

Once the therapist and patient agree about the most pertinent problems on which to work, they can begin to form hypotheses about the factors contributing to those problems, and those hypotheses will ultimately provide a rationale for the interventions chosen. Gardner and Sovner's (1994) biopsychosocial case formulation model provides a multifactorial way of thinking about patients' problems. Designed to assess severe, aberrant behavior in individuals with ID, their approach was meant for a population quite different from adults with ASD. However, I have found their grid format useful and have adapted it as a worksheet for conceptualizing therapy cases (Figure 3.1). The vulnerability model for mental health problems in ASD, which was introduced in Chapter 2 (Figure 2.4), serves as the outline for hypothesis generation. By the end of the initial assessment, the therapist should be able to list the problems on this sheet and then apply the vulnerability model to explain the unique way in which factors are interacting to produce the problems for this patient.

Chapter Summary and Conclusions

This chapter covered the key strategies for conducting an intake with an adult patient and gathering the necessary information to make a diagnosis and define the target problems for treatment. A thorough assessment lays the foundation for the case conceptualization that will lead to the individualized treatment plan. Chapter 4 outlines this process, illustrating the utility of a case formulation worksheet.

| Name: | Gender: | Age: | Marital Status: | Religion/Ethnicity: | Occupation: |

Living Situation: _____

Reason for Referral: _____

Referral Source: _____

Psychotropic Medications: _____

Prescribing Physician: _____

Problem List:	Diagnosis:	Goals:
1.	1.	1.
2.	2.	2.
3.	3.	3.
4.	4.	4.
5.	5.	5.

Causal or Maintenance Factors	Hypothesis	Hypothesis-Based Interventions	Outcomes
Medical			
Core Problems of ASD Social Cognition Emotion Regulation Sensory–Motor Regulation Executive Function			

(continued)

FIGURE 3.1. Case formulation worksheet.

Schemas			
Self			
Others			
World			
Future			
Origins			
Activating Event			
Behavior			
Antecedents (A)			
Consequences (C)			
Strengths and Resiliency Factors			

Potential Obstacles to Treatment:

1.

2.

3.

Prevention Strategies for Obstacles:

1.

2.

3.

FIGURE 3.1. (continued)

CHAPTER 4

Individualized Case Formulation and Treatment Plan

The purpose of this chapter is to present a case formulation worksheet to help the therapist form hypotheses about presenting problems and choose evidence-based interventions that are driven by the formulation. Hypothesis generation is the most crucial step in the treatment of any problem, and the more complex the problem presentation is, the more important it is to put great effort into this stage. Because ASD in adulthood is a complex problem, the formulation process is illustrated in detail in this chapter. If the therapist can make educated guesses about what is causing or maintaining the patient's problems, then the decisions about which interventions to try first can be made more easily. Persons and colleagues (2000) discuss the importance of combining nomothetic and idiographic bases when formulating cases. They describe how to generate hypotheses based on empirically supported theories about the presenting problem (nomothetic) and to individualize them according to the unique set of factors that is influencing the patient in his or her life (idiographic). This method allows the therapist to avoid "shot in the dark" approaches that patients with complex problems have often, unfortunately, experienced in their previous treatments. Weston and colleagues (2016) recommend taking a formulation-driven, individualized approach when using CBT with ASD, given the heterogeneity of the symptom pictures presented. This chapter demonstrates how the therapist can create an individualized (idiographic) model to explain the problems of the adult patient with ASD, and then use that model to choose treatment approaches.

Case Formulation

Case Formulation Worksheet

The case formulation worksheet introduced at the end of Chapter 3 (Figure 3.1) serves several purposes. It is more than just a form that needs to be filled out; it is a framework for *thinking* about the case. It can be viewed as a tool to cue the therapist to ask a wide variety of questions and to consider multiple causes for the presenting problems. The model worksheet was designed to be comprehensive, so it includes many questions about causal factors. Some clinicians may find it complicated or "user-unfriendly" for that reason. While some readers who use it as a training or practice model may use it exactly as it is presented here, others may streamline it or design their own. Some may keep the form in front of them from the beginning of the intake session on, whereas others may be able to adopt a mental representation of the model. Regardless of therapist style, a multitude of internal and external factors must be considered to explain the problems of adults with ASD before a comprehensive treatment plan can be designed.

The worksheet is used throughout the chapters ahead to repeatedly illustrate the multifactorial approach that is encouraged when treating adults with ASD. Figure 4.1 presents the worksheet again with added instructions for each section. The general (nomothetic) model of vulnerability to mental health problems in ASD was presented in Chapter 2 and is not reiterated here. However, the "Causal or Maintenance Factors" listed on the left-hand side of the worksheet serve as a "cheat sheet" for remembering the major components of that model. Before this sheet can be filled in, a thorough assessment must be completed. As described in Chapter 3, the therapist will use several assessment approaches across multiple sessions before this phase can be completed.

Using the Worksheet to Formulate Bob's Case

The case of Bob, introduced in Chapter 1, is used to illustrate this tool, and his case formulation is shown in Figure 4.2. He was chosen because of the multiple comorbid conditions he had along with his ASD, which is typical when treating this population. The intervention, outcome, and goal sections are deliberately left blank to emphasize the need to have a comprehensive set of hypotheses *before* deciding on interventions.

Basic Background Information

The top section of the worksheet should be filled in with relevant demographic information, as the example shows for Bob. Psychotropic medications and the physician prescribing them are included as a reminder to consider them while generating hypotheses.

Problem List

Underneath the demographic information, the problem list and diagnosis should be written out before hypotheses are generated. Logically, it is important for the therapist and patient to be clear on what the problems are before they can be explained by hypotheses. The problems should also be listed in order of priority, with the first one being the most acutely disruptive to the patient's life.

To briefly review, Bob came into therapy because of what his family reported as an extreme reaction to the World Trade Center disaster. He lived on the outskirts of New York City and watched TV coverage of the events all day on September 11; he did not suffer tangible loss from the attacks, nor did anyone he knew. Nevertheless, he began to

(*Text resumes on page 123.*)

Name: _____ Gender: _____ Age: _____ Marital Status: _____ Religion/Ethnicity: _____ Occupation: _____
Living Situation: _____
Reason for Referral: _____ Referral Source: _____
Psychotropic Medications: _____ Prescribing Physician: _____

Problem List:
1.
2.
3.
4.
5.

Diagnosis:
1.
2.
3.
4.
5.

Goals:
1.
2.
3.
4.
5.

Causal or Maintenance Factors *Consider all of the following when generating hypotheses.*	Hypothesis *What factors may be causing or maintaining the problems listed above? Explain how they contribute to the presenting problems.*	Hypothesis-Based Interventions *What intervention should be built into the plan to minimize each factor?*	Outcomes *What is the expected outcome? Describe how it will contribute to the attainment of a goal (indicate which goal by writing the number).*
Medical	*How might medical or psychopharmacological issues be causing/maintaining problem(s)?*	*Which cognitive–behavioral interventions will help coping or compliance with medical issues?* *Which referrals to medical professionals are needed?*	*How will the medically related interventions help attain the global therapy goals?*
Core Problems of ASD Social Cognition Emotion Regulation Sensory–Motor Regulation	*How might core/associated ASD impairments be causing/ maintaining problem(s)?* *How might social–cognitive deficits be causing/maintaining problem(s)?* *How might ER issues be causing/maintaining problem(s)?* *How might sensory–motor regulation issues be causing/ maintaining problem(s)?*	*Which skill-building or coping strategies will compensate for core deficits?* *What referrals to adjunctive therapies (speech, occupational therapy) might be needed?*	*How will the skill-building, coping, or adjunctive interventions help attain the global therapy goals?*

(continued)

FIGURE 4.1. Guidelines for generating hypotheses and planning treatment.

Executive Function	How might EF deficits be causing/maintaining problem(s)?		
Schemas			
Self	How does schema about self cause/maintain problem(s)?	What strategies will modify maladaptive schemas?	How will the schema-changing interventions help attain the global therapy goals?
Others	How does schema about others cause/maintain problem(s)?		
World	How does schema about the world cause/maintain problem(s)?		
Future	How does schema about the future cause/maintain problem(s)?		
Origins	What are the historical origins of schemata?		
Activating Event	What large- or small-scale events activate distorted thinking?		
Behavior	How are the patient's overt behaviors causing/maintaining problem(s)?	What strategies will modify antecedents and consequences of maladaptive behavior in order to bring about behavioral change?	How will the behavioral interventions help attain the global therapy goals?
Antecedents (A)	What are the antecedents for these behaviors?		
Consequences (C)	How are consequences causing/maintaining behavior?		
Strengths and Resiliency Factors	What strengths and coping strategies of the patient have served as protective or resiliency factors?	How can the patient's strengths and talents be optimized and used as tools for the intervention plan?	How will the utilization of the patient's strengths and talents help attain the global therapy goals?

Potential Obstacles to Treatment:

1.

2.

3.

Prevention Strategies for Obstacles:

1.

2.

3.

FIGURE 4.1. (continued)

Name: _Bob_   Gender: _M_   Age: _29_   Marital Status: _S_   Religion/Ethnicity: _Jewish_   Occupation: _Unemployed_

Living Situation: _House w/parents_   Referral Source: _Evaluating psychologist_

Reason for Referral: _To address severe symptoms of anxiety and depression trigged by World Trade Center disaster_

Psychotropic Medications: _Prozac, Effexor, and Geodon_   Prescribing Physician: _Dr. Jones (psychiatrist)_

Problem List:	Diagnosis:	Goals:
1. Obsessions—intrusive thoughts about terrorist attacks, worrying about impending acts of terrorism 2. Compulsive behavior—perseverative questioning of family members about terrorism 3. Depressed mood (BDI = 51)—extreme irritability, hopelessness, poor self-worth, recurrent thoughts of death 4. Avoidance of self-care—negligence of diabetes regimen, dependence on parents in all activities of independent living 5. Social isolation—premorbid social skill deficits	1. Obsessive–compulsive disorder w/fair insight 2. Major depressive disorder; recurrent severe 3. Autism spectrum disorder, Level 1 severity w/o intellectual or language impairment (Asperger's disorder) 4. R/O–dependent personality disorder 5.	1. 2. 3. 4. 5.

Causal or Maintenance Factors	Hypothesis	Hypothesis-Based Interventions	Outcomes
Medical	Unstable blood sugar levels could contribute to mood instability. The rigors of caring for diabetes are chronic stressors. Original diagnosis with the disease at age 21 was traumatic.		
Core Problems of ASD Social Cognition	Difficulty attending to nonverbal communication of other people, difficulty with perspective taking, flat affect, and poor expression of own mental states and needs. All deficits contribute to misattributions that result in social anxiety and anger and reinforce negative schema about others.		

(continued)

FIGURE 4.2. Generating hypotheses for Bob.

Emotion Regulation	Negative thoughts and distressing emotions are unacceptable and are suppressed; uncertainty is intolerable.
Sensory–Motor Regulation	Mild tactile sensitivity may affect self-care.
Executive Function	Planning and organization deficits make basic independent living tasks overwhelming and reinforce negative schema about self. Cognitive rigidity makes adaptation to change very difficult.
Schemas Self	"I am helpless and powerless." "I cannot take care of myself." "I am defective." "I should not have negative thoughts or feelings."
Others	"Others must take care of me." "Others must protect me from harm." "People are usually out for themselves." "People are not trustworthy."
World	"The world is an unsafe place." "The world gives people what they deserve."
Future	"The future is full of danger that is unpredictable." "I will never be normal."
Origins	Bob was aware that he did not function the same way as other students in elementary school (due to a learning disability). A sense of not fitting in made him feel vulnerable. Peers were unkind to him due to his behavioral differences. He relied on his parents to advocate for him, but in adolescence began resenting them for not protecting him from stressors. The trauma of the diabetes diagnosis strengthened his belief that his parents were failing him, because they could not protect him from the disease.

FIGURE 4.2. (*continued*)

(continued)

Activating Event	Small scale—any situation that Bob perceives to include pressure to take care of self, pressure to achieve social success, reminders that parents may not be able to take care of him. Large-scale precipitants—9/11, which reactivated the traumatic aspects of his diabetes diagnosis 8 years before, triggering beliefs that others should be able to protect him from all bad things and that they have failed him.
Behavior Antecedents (A) Consequences (C)	1. Repetitive questioning of family members; seeking reassurance about terrorism. 　A—Intermittent exposure to TV or Internet reports about 9/11 and increased anxiety. 　C—Reassuring statements by family members, which result in temporary reduction in anxiety. 2. Social withdrawal/passivity 　A—Social situations where Bob is uncertain about the other people and/or how he should behave; lack of conversation skills. 　C—Anxiety reduction results from withdrawal; passivity relieves pressure. 3. Verbally aggressive behavior (sudden outbursts of anger toward others) 　A—Social situations where Bob attributes negative intent to another person's behavior and escape is not possible; lack of assertiveness skills. 　C—Other people act hostile toward Bob and reject him, reinforcing negative schema about others.

FIGURE 4.2. *(continued)*

121

Strengths and Resiliency Factors	Bob is bright, articulate, has enjoyed writing and believes he expresses himself best that way, can use humor as a coping strategy, and has formed positive connections with some people. He was also active in a bowling league and frequently played tennis prior to 9/11.	
Potential Obstacles to Treatment: 1. 2. 3.	Prevention Strategies for Obstacles: 1. 2. 3.	

FIGURE 4.2. *(continued)*

experience extreme anxiety within the first several days following the attacks. He questioned his family members repeatedly about the event, how it could have happened, and whether it would happen again. These episodes of grilling questioning occurred between 10 and 20 times each day and were accompanied by insomnia, frequent angry outbursts, a loss of motivation to take care of personal hygiene and grooming, neglect of diabetes regimen (diet, exercise, daily blood sugar readings, insulin shots), and a sense of hopelessness about the future. He had a history of previous depressive episodes as well as problems with interpersonal relationships and social skills. The referring psychologist had mentioned the possibility that Bob's developmental history was indicative of an ASD. Although all of the problems were seen as equally important, on the worksheet they were broken down into five categories, prioritized from most acute to the more chronic. The problem list for Bob was:

1. *Obsessions*—intrusive thoughts about terrorist attacks, worrying about impending acts of terrorism
2. *Compulsions*—perseverative questioning of family members about terrorism
3. *Depressed mood* (BDI = 51)—extreme irritability, hopelessness, poor self-worth, recurrent thoughts of death
4. *Avoidance of self-care*—negligence of diabetes regimen, dependence on parents in all activities of daily living
5. *Social isolation*—premorbid social skills deficits

Diagnosis

Here the therapist provides the diagnosis of the presenting problems in DSM-5 terms (American Psychiatric Association, 2013). Though the original case formulation was done at a time when DSM-IV-TR (American Psychiatric Association, 2000) was in use, the DSM-5 is used here to make the illustration more current. The diagnoses are listed in an order that places the disorder with the most acutely disruptive problem first and more chronic, long-standing problems after.

Bob's symptom presentation initially suggested PTSD because he indeed experienced the events of 9/11 as traumatic and showed some of the symptoms of PTSD (diminished interest in activities, estrangement from others, sense of foreshortened future, sleep difficulties, irritability, hypervigilance). However, PTSD was ruled out because his intrusive thoughts did not involve a reexperiencing of the events of that day; he was not having intrusive memories or images of the things he saw or heard on 9/11. Rather, he was preoccupied with the possibility that the country was going to be attacked again, and that his personal safety might be threatened. These thoughts about harm coming to himself and his family met criteria for obsessions in that they were recurrent, intrusive, and recognized by Bob as irrational on some level; he described his awareness that everyone around him was frightened by the events of 9/11 and that it was realistic to have some concern, but he noticed that other people were able to function despite their worries. He believed that his fears were excessive because they were interfering with his ability to function, and he wished he could make the thoughts stop. He did not show signs of magical thinking. He attempted to neutralize them by engaging in a questioning ritual with his family members in which he was demanding reassurance from them. His distress would increase if his family members were unavailable or refused to answer his questions, leading to anger outbursts involving yelling and cursing. The questioning behavior met criteria for a compulsion under *obsessive–compulsive disorder*. The specifier "with fair insight" was also applied. His depressed mood qualified as a major depressive episode, accompanied by diminished interest in activities, insomnia, psychomotor retardation, loss of energy, and feelings of worthlessness. He also had recurring thoughts of death, but they were related to the impending terrorist attacks. The current severity (BDI = 51) and his history of at least two previous episodes (at ages 21 and 26) led to the diagnosis of *major depressive disorder* with recurrent and severe specifiers. The third diagnosis, *ASD, requiring support for deficits with social communication (Level 1), requiring support for restricted, repetitive behaviors (Level 1), without accompanying intellectual or language impairment*, came from a review of his developmental and social history and administration of assessment tools that were available at that time (e.g., Australian Scale for Asperger's Syndrome; Attwood, 1998). From at least preschool age, his parents recalled problems Bob had in social interaction, such as poor eye contact, lack of social reciprocity, odd facial grimaces, and problems making friends. He also adhered rigidly to routines and would become highly distressed whenever there were changes in the schedule. He had some associated features, such as motor clumsiness, excessive memory for details, tactile sensitivity (would not wear certain clothes), and high pain tolerance. Although these symptoms changed in form through the years, they carried over into his adulthood.

Bob was extremely dependent on his parents in every area of functioning and, at the time of the intake, was not responsible for any aspect of managing himself. This situation could be expected, given the severity of his other symptoms. However, there were indications that he had been overly reliant on his parents' help even before the current episode of anxiety and depression. The therapist had questions about a possible *dependent personality disorder* but could not make the diagnosis with confidence because it was difficult to differentiate acute from chronic symptoms, given the complexity of the presenting clinical picture. The decision was made to assess PD at a later date if improvement could be achieved for the acute anxiety and depression. This diagnosis was therefore preceded with a "rule-out" indicator.

As mentioned, the diagnoses are listed in an order that places the most acutely disruptive problems first, but not necessarily in order of importance or the chronological order of onset. The diagnosis of ASD, for example, would appear first if I made the list in order of occurrence across Bob's lifespan.

Hypothesis about Causal and Maintenance Factors

All the major categories of factors that could be maintaining mental health problems in adults with ASD are listed on the left side of the form: *medical, core problems of ASD, schemas,* and *behavior.*

MEDICAL

Medical factors are mentioned first because of the importance of ruling out physical causes of emotional and behavioral problems for any new psychotherapy patient. All medical issues should be considered in terms of the role they may be playing in the current presenting problems. Of course, nonmedical psychotherapists will not intervene directly on medical issues, but it is still important to think about the powerful impact these issues can have in terms of perpetuating and maintaining the problems that will be addressed in therapy.

The section devoted to hypotheses about medical factors maintaining Bob's presenting problems begins with consideration of the role of diabetes in his state of being. At the physical level, mood instability could be exacerbated by blood sugar fluctuations. Psychologically, the daily tasks that must be devoted to caring for the disease were overwhelming to Bob. These included following a diet, exercising, taking blood sugar levels twice a day, and injecting insulin. From a historical perspective, receiving the initial diagnosis of diabetes 8 years before had been traumatic to him, and he had not ever successfully adjusted to it.

CORE PROBLEMS OF ASD

Bob has difficulty attending to, and making use of, the nonverbal communication of other people—that is, a problem with social cognition. He often misses important information that others convey nonverbally, and therefore he misattributes their behavior. These misattributions feed his perspective-taking problem, in that he has difficulty imagining what another person may be thinking or feeling. For example, if his mother is in a hurry in the morning because she is running late for her job, Bob interprets her spending less time than usual on his breakfast as a rejection of him. He misses the cues she gives about her own lateness, such as watching the clock, walking quickly through the house, and frantically searching for her keys, and assumes that she is slighting him for some other reason. This problem impedes his ability to form satisfying relationships because other people assume he is selfish, and he assumes he is being rejected, even when he is not. There are obvious implications for his depression, as well, which is discussed further in the section on schemas. ER factors include nonacceptance of emotion and intolerance of uncertainty. While these cognitive issues fit into the schema factors to be mentioned shortly, his ASD-specific cognitive rigidity plays a central role. His parents expressed concerns that, even before 9/11, Bob dressed in a sloppy way and never liked to wear neat clothing. However, tactile sensitivities that were evident since early childhood (seemingly odd clothes preferences) suggested that he only feels comfortable in well-worn cotton garments. Finally, EF deficits, seen in poor planning and organizational ability, cause daily living tasks to be overwhelming for him, especially the diabetes regimen. Cognitive rigidity is central here again, as his difficulty changing mind-sets impede his ability to adjust to changes in his routine or environment.

SCHEMAS

Bob's presenting problems were being maintained by a number of maladaptive schemas that he had developed throughout his life and that were influencing his mood, thoughts, and behavior. They are outlined here:

- *Self*: "I am helpless and powerless"; "I cannot take care of myself"; "I am defective"; "I should not have negative thoughts or feelings."
- *Others*: "Others must take care of me"; "Others must protect me from harm";

"Others must prevent me from having distressing thoughts or feelings"; "People are usually out for themselves"; "People are not trustworthy."

* *World*: "The world is an unsafe place"; "The world gives people what they deserve."
* *Future*: "The future is full of danger that is unpredictable"; "I will never be normal."

Origins. As a child with learning and developmental problems, Bob knew he was different from his siblings and peers from an early age. As a special education teacher herself, his mother was his advocate with the school system. Bob saw her efforts as "pushy," and he often felt that she pressured him to be "normal." His father went through bouts of depressed mood and made negative and pessimistic comments about many different things, including Bob's academic and social progress. Bob came to resent the mixed messages he got from both parents. His odd mannerisms and lack of social skills led to victimization and bullying from peers throughout his school years. The diagnosis of diabetes reinforced his belief that his parents have failed him because they are supposed to protect him from all negative things. The responsibility that it placed in his hands (the rigors of the self-care for diabetes) overwhelmed and angered him, and he blamed his parents for the situation. He avoided adult responsibilities and risks because he was not confident that he could succeed at an independent life, but also because he was afraid that if he did succeed, his parents would be "too happy" and expect too much. In addition, he believed that he could protect himself from any further mistreatment, such as the type he had suffered in school, by acting belligerently toward people who tried to interact with him.

Schema-Activating Events (Stressors). Exposure to the news media was the most immediate schema-activating event, and it triggered thoughts about danger, helplessness, and a need to be taken care of. Bob did not seek out media coverage, but would encounter it inadvertently if he overheard it when others in his family were watching or listening to news. Small-scale activating events that existed before and after 9/11 included any situation that involved pressure to take care of himself or to achieve social success; these would activate his maladaptive schemas that all fit a theme of helplessness, dependence on others, and a simultaneous mistrust of others. The large-scale precipitant for the current anxiety and mood episode was the World Trade Center disaster, which reactivated the traumatic aspects of an earlier major event—his diabetes diagnosis. Both events activated a schema that others must protect him from harm, accompanied by his belief that others are not trustworthy, as evidenced by his parents' failure to protect him from diabetes and "the government's" failure to protect him from terrorist attacks.

BEHAVIOR

Bob's immediate behavioral problem—compulsive questioning of family members about terrorism—was being reinforced in a classic cycle of OCD. The antecedent was exposure to news media. His passive approach to consuming news information led to his stumbling on information without having planned it. Bob was only catching "snippets" of information on TV and the Internet, but these were enough to activate the cycle as follows: He would receive a small amount of information from the news media → have repetitive intrusive thoughts about impending terrorist attacks → experience an increase in anxiety → seek out parents for information and reassurance by asking them repeatedly about the likelihood of future attacks → receive various reassuring statements (consequence) from them → experience temporary relief from anxiety (a consequence that negatively reinforced the questioning behavior) → experience a recurrence of intrusive thoughts → experience an increase in anxiety → seek out parents . . . and the cycle would repeat again. His angry outbursts also fit into the cycle; he would scream and curse at his parents if they did not provide the types of reassuring statements he was seeking.

Strengths and Resiliency Factors

Bob is bright, articulate, and has enjoyed writing in the past. He even thought of becoming a journalist at one point while he was in college. Bob can use humor as a coping strategy and can form positive connections with some people, as evidenced by the enjoyment he anticipates when he knows he will be visiting his two young nieces. He also has some friends. Before 9/11, he participated on a bowling league and played tennis on a regular basis.

Summary of Bob's Formulation

After completing the list of hypotheses, it is always helpful to pause and summarize the conceptualization in a concise statement that represents a more cohesive way of thinking about the case: Bob's obsessions about impending acts of terrorism are being triggered by his unplanned, intermittent exposure to news media. His passive approach to consuming news information contributes to his sense of helplessness; instead of seeking out reliable sources of information, the way most adults do, he waits until he overhears or stumbles on bits of information. His belief that his parents should protect him from all bad things leads him to turn to them in order to gain reassurance, which he does through a compulsive questioning ritual. When they answer his questions, his anxiety is temporarily alleviated and the questioning compulsion reinforced. When his parents attempt to refrain from answering, he uses angry outbursts and threats to get them to comply—and this compliance reinforces his aggressive approach. His depression is maintained by a sense of helplessness that he feels, not only in the wake of 9/11 but also about having diabetes, being unemployed, and having a long history of social failures.

Bob has had ASD-related learning deficits since early childhood, including problems with (1) reading and interpreting the behavior of others, (2) expressive communication, and (3) planning and organizing tasks. These problems have contributed to his struggle to get along with people and make friends and have also made it harder for him to learn to take care of himself as he reached the age at which most people seek independent living. His diabetes diagnosis at age 21 exacerbated these issues because he viewed himself as incapable of handling it; he could not manage the responsibilities of self-care, nor could he accept that his parents could not protect him from the disease. These factors have contributed to his view of himself as defective and incapable, and his view of others as untrustworthy and "out for themselves." ER is difficult for him because he believes that negative thoughts and distressing emotions are unacceptable and need to be extinguished, and that uncertainty is intolerable. His belief that people get what they deserve in this world contributes to his blaming himself for being defective, but also blaming his parents for having "produced defective offspring" and then failing to protect their child. In that sense, he believes they deserve to be "saddled" with him and to continue attending to his every need. Bob's passive approach to life ultimately reinforces his belief that he is helpless and perpetuates his frustration about his life not moving forward. His cognitive rigidity makes it more difficult for him than typical people to modify his maladaptive schemas so that he can adapt to change.

Treatment Plan

After hypotheses are generated for the possible contributing factors, interventions can be specified. The more care and thought that is put into the formulation, the easier it should be to choose therapeutic strategies designed to directly target the hypothesized causal factors. The goals should be set at the same time and represent the measurable ways in which the presenting problems are expected to change. The outcomes represent the specific changes that each intervention elicits toward the more global goal attainment.

A Philosophical Word about Change and ASD: "Don't Throw the Baby Out with the Bathwater"

Before continuing to discuss the use of the treatment formulation worksheet, it is worth spending some time considering the philosophy of change that one may carry through the treatment planning process. It is important for therapists to think about the vision they share with the patient for the quality-of-life improvements that are expected, as well as ideas about what parts of the patient's lifestyle are worth preserving. Therapy goals address both of these, but they must be consistent with a more global view of the patient's life. Before the goals can be made realistic, the therapist and patient must together consider the following broad questions: What *can* be changed? Are those things that *should* be changed? Which things *should not* be changed? Which things are *not possible* to change? How can those things be coped with and accepted?

I have developed a general philosophy about change for adults with ASD that is based on a need to decrease distress while preserving and building strengths. Recalling the quote from the mission statement of the Global and Regional Asperger Syndrome Partnership (GRASP) that was offered in the Introduction to this book, adults with ASD are expressing their desire to "maximize the talents . . . harness the unique capabilities and celebrate the accomplishments . . . minimize the damage . . . [and] reduce the harm caused when our behavior diverges from non-autistic norms" (2003, p. 3). At the beginning of treatment for any adult with ASD, I hope that the symptoms that are causing distress can be reduced, that relationships can become more satisfying, and that any obstacles to the patient's achievement of personal life goals can be reduced. In order to create a treatment vision, I consider how the person is functioning along three crude dimensions. This is a value-driven idea that is based on my personal experience with these patients.

Satisfied	↔	Dissatisfied
Likable	↔	Unlikable
"Normal looking"	↔	"Weird looking"

The first dimension, *satisfaction,* refers to the subjective sense of well-being a patient feels about major areas of life functioning, including relationships, occupation, and self-sufficiency. Most patients who come into therapy wish for more satisfaction in at least one of these areas.

The second dimension, which refers to *likability,* is not always a problem for patients with ASD, but most are looking to improve in this area because they have experienced alienation in their pasts. Likability refers to the possession of characteristics that typical people in the patient's own culture/society would find appealing (this an obvious oversimplification of a complex issue). Examples of appealing characteristics include showing interest in others, attempting to share experiences with others, exhibiting talent or intelligence, expressing and responding to humor, and respecting other people's rights. Conversely, *unlikable* characteristics that others typically find unappealing include ignoring others, saying hurtful or offensive things to others, expressing self-pity, appearing humorless, practicing poor hygiene, or doing anything that infringes on another person's rights.

The third dimension is deliberately defined in lay terms because it is an estimate of how much typical people would judge the person to be *"normal looking"* or *"weird looking."* This dimension refers to the extent to which a person would blend into a crowd as opposed to exhibiting characteristics that would make him or her stand out. Examples include idiosyncratic habits, mannerisms, unusual voice quality, unusual phrasing, unique wardrobe choices, and uncommon favorite topics or hobbies. Although such behaviors may draw attention, they do not directly affect others in a destructive way. In other words, even at their weirdest, these "quirks" are basically harmless to others. Patients with ASD vary quite a bit from one another in terms of where they fall on this dimension (i.e., how obvious their idiosyncrasies are).

When patients come into therapy, they are usually looking to move themselves closer to the left side of all three dimensions: toward *satisfaction, likability,* and *"normalcy."* However, as mentioned previously, they are not all impaired to the same degree. The worst-case scenario would be seen in a person who is dissatisfied with most domains of life, unlikable to most people, and weird looking. Despite the variability among individuals with ASD on these dimensions, many people, including patients, assume that the second and third dimensions are the same thing—that being weird means being unlikable, or that being unlikable means being weird. It is important to discuss this issue during the goal-setting stage of therapy because patients who have self-awareness about their peculiarities may say, "If I am weird, then no one will ever like me." However, I believe that this is an erroneous assumption and have observed that these dimensions work fairly independently. It is true that the behaviors that make someone unlikable may sometimes overlap with the things that make them appear weird, but if a person is likable, his or her weird quirks will be tolerated more easily by others. In fact, the more likable a person is, the more his or her quirks will be seen as charming or endearing. Likewise, if a person is relatively normal looking but not very likable, he or she is less likely to find satisfaction in his or her life.

For these reasons my vision for a patient is usually focused more on the first two dimensions. The quality of life can be improved for a person if he or she can find satisfaction in the interpersonal and work domains of life, and if he or she can change behavior enough to be more likable. I am much less concerned about weirdness if the first two objectives can be achieved. A person who is normal looking and has few quirks but is also nasty, self-absorbed, withdrawn, pessimistic, and humorless is not going to do as well as a person who is very weird looking, eccentric, and quirky but has an interest in other people, shares their talents and intelligence, seeks to share experiences, has an optimistic attitude, and enjoys humor. I rarely focus on changing eccentricities as long as they do not interfere with life satisfaction and the connections the individual desires to make with others.

I usually share this three-dimensional philosophy with patients who are concerned about their ASD diagnosis and what it means for prognosis. In fact, when patients express concern that their weirdness is going to get in their way, I usually say, "We are shooting for life satisfaction and to be likable–weird. If you can learn how to be more comfortable with people and to help them be comfortable with you, then you can afford to be quite weird. Likable–weird is better than unlikable–normal."

One example is the case of Andrew, a 32-year-old man who has a degree in culinary arts and works as a manager in a gourmet food shop. He came to therapy looking for help with his lack of social relationships and depressive symptoms. In the treatment planning stages, he raised a concern about one of his hobbies, which was model railroad building. He was a passionate and talented model railroad builder and was active in several related clubs and organizations, but he was ashamed of this hobby and would not share this information with anyone he met socially. He believed it was weird and that it would be the basis of rejection if he was with new acquaintances or on a date, and he wondered whether therapy should focus on helping him find more "normal" hobbies. He had a long history of being rejected by others and was afraid to have these experiences repeated. I did not agree with Andrew's goal because he appeared to be making the wrong attribution for his social failures. I had observed, over several meetings with him, that he almost always had a scowl on his face, never smiled, and made repeated negative remarks that would be perceived as self-pitying by most people (he was ultimately diagnosed with persistent depressive disorder [dysthymia]). Although he was correct in his assessment of model railroad building as an unusual hobby, it was probably not the reason he had been rejected in the past; the rejection he experienced was probably because others perceived him to be negative and self-absorbed.

I shared the three-dimensional model with Andrew to prioritize the therapy objectives. I emphasized that, in addition to decreasing depressive symptoms (to become more *satisfied*), he would also need to learn self-awareness about the impact of his verbal and nonverbal behavior on others (to become more *likable*), which was more important than the type of hobby he had (*weird*). It was explained that people are not likely to reject him for being a model railroad hobbyist if he projects a pleasant disposition and shows genuine interest in others; people would rather spend time with a pleasant but eccentric model railroad builder than a sour, negative person with a conventional hobby. If anything, his model railroad activity needed to be preserved and encouraged because it had the potential to serve as an important bridge to more social success for two reasons: The first was that his talent was very impressive (he showed me pictures of his work) and would likely bring admiration from others, and the second is that his involvement was a great source of enjoyment for him and provided natural mood enhancement—and a better mood would make it easier for him to practice the new social skills he would be learning in therapy.

In sum, intervention planning and goal setting should be preceded by some thought about the global philosophy the therapist and patient share about change. Because ASD is interwoven with the individual's personality and brings with it unique qualities and talents, the therapist must be careful not to try to inadvertently eliminate aspects of the person's lifestyle that are positive and adaptive. This section began with the idiom "Don't throw the baby out with the bathwater," and ends with one as a final word of guidance: "If it ain't broke, don't fix it."

Using the Worksheet to Choose Interventions and Set Goals

While keeping in mind the global vision that the therapist and patient share, the next step is to fill in the "Hypothesis-Based Interventions," which brings attention back to the case formulation worksheet. Each idea the therapist has about what factors might be contributing to the presenting problems and the mechanism by which those factors are occurring leads to an idea about how to intervene. The "Goals" section should be filled in with the list of overall, quality-of-life improvements that are hoped for by the end of treatment. These are more global statements about change. The "Outcomes" represent the *mechanisms* by which interventions will lead to the attainment of goals. This in-between step must be specified because each intervention may not be the *only* one necessary to achieve a goal. Because each problem is often driven by *multiple factors*, there may be more than one intervention specified in the treatment plan toward one goal. For example, the goal of decreasing depressive symptoms may require activity scheduling for one reason, social skill improvement for another reason, and cognitive restructuring for yet another reason, depending on the individual needs of the patient. Each intervention will work toward the goal through a different mechanism, *each* of which needs to be monitored.

Bob's completed treatment plan is shown in Figure 4.3. Again, his case is used to provide instructions on how to use the worksheet. Considering the hypotheses outlined for Bob's problems, I formed a cohesive conceptualization of his problems, which allowed me to build a global vision for change. This vision influenced the goals, intervention design, and expected outcomes. This process is outlined in the following section.

Goals

The goals should be listed in priority order in terms of the immediacy of the need for change. Mirroring the problem list, the issues that are most disruptive or pose the greatest threat to health or safety should drive the choice for the highest-priority goals.

In Bob's case, *reducing the obsessions and compulsions* were the highest priority. *Decreasing depressive symptoms* was a close second. Not only were they the most disruptive at the time of intake but the OCD symptoms were "obscuring the view" for me; I could not get a clear sense of the severity of the other problems (dependency and

(Text resumes on page 136.)

Name: Bob	Gender: M	Age: 29	Marital Status: S	Religion/Ethnicity: Jewish	Occupation: Unemployed

Living Situation: House w/parents

Reason for Referral: To address severe symptoms of anxiety and depression triged by World Trade Center disaster

Referral Source: Evaluating psychologist

Psychotropic Medications: Prozac, Effexor, and Geodon   Prescribing Physician: Dr. Jones (psychiatrist)

Problem List:	Diagnosis:	Goals:
1. Obsessions—intrusive thoughts about terrorist attacks, worrying about impending acts of terrorism 2. Compulsive behavior—perseverative questioning of family members about terrorism 3. Depressed mood (BDI = 51)—extreme irritability, hopelessness, poor self-worth, recurrent thoughts of death 4. Avoidance of self-care—negligence of diabetes regimen, dependence on parents in all activities of independent living 5. Social isolation—premorbid social skill deficits	1. Obsessive–compulsive disorder w/fair insight 2. Major depressive disorder; recurrent severe 3. Autism spectrum disorder, Level 1 severity w/o intellectual or language impairment (Asperger's disorder) 4. R/O–dependent personality disorder 5.	1. Reduce frequency of obsessions and compulsions 2. Decrease depressive symptoms 3. Increase self-reliance and independence 4. Increase quality and quantity of relationships 5.

Causal or Maintenance Factors	Hypothesis	Hypothesis-Based Interventions	Outcomes
Medical	Unstable blood sugar levels could contribute to mood instability. The rigors of caring for diabetes are chronic stressors. Original diagnosis with the disease at age 21 was traumatic.	Teach self-monitoring strategies for compliance with regimen and taking more active role in endocrinology appointments.	Increased sense of independence and control over diabetes, decreased stress (2, 3)
Core Problems of ASD Social Cognition	Difficulty attending to nonverbal communication of other people, difficulty with perspective taking, flat affect, and poor expression of own mental states and needs. All deficits contribute to misattributions that result in social anxiety and anger and reinforce negative schema about others.	Teach perspective-taking skills/reading nonverbal cues of others. Teach assertive communication.	Increased competence and confidence in social situations, less anger (4)

(continued)

FIGURE 4.3. Choosing interventions and setting goals for Bob.

Emotion Regulation	Negative thoughts and distressing emotions are unacceptable and are suppressed; uncertainty is intolerable.	Emotion education, using tools to teach the purpose of emotions and how to identify and label them.	Acceptance of Bob's own emotions (1, 2, 3, 4)
Sensory–Motor Regulation	Mild tactile sensitivity may affect self-care.	Reassess if self-care problems persist after depressive symptoms improve.	Increased number of tasks completed without help, decreased stress (3)
Executive Function	Planning and organization deficits make basic independent living tasks overwhelming and reinforce negative schema about self. Cognitive rigidity makes adaptation to change very difficult.	Design task management systems that are suited to Bob's learning style.	
Schemas Self	"I am helpless and powerless." "I cannot take care of myself." "I am defective." "I should not have negative thoughts or feelings."	Schema–Changing Techniques: Teach cognitive restructuring to modify maladaptive schemas.	Increased ability to challenge maladaptive automatic thoughts (2, 3, 4)
Others	"Others must take care of me." "Others must protect me from harm." "People are usually out for themselves." "People are not trustworthy."		
World	"The world is an unsafe place." "The world gives people what they deserve."	Use successes in other areas of treatment plan (e.g., successful completion of daily living tasks without help) as evidence that is counter to negative views.	Expression of new beliefs about self—"I am capable and competent"; and about others—"Others do not have to take care of me." (2, 3, 4)
Future	"The future is full of danger that is unpredictable." "I will never be normal."		
Origins	Bob was aware that he did not function the same way as other students in elementary school (due to a learning disability). A sense of not fitting in made him feel vulnerable. Peers were unkind to him due to his behavioral differences. He relied on his parents to advocate for him, but in adolescence began resenting	Teach cognitive restructuring to reappraise stressful situations.	Decreased perception of pressure, decreased stress (1, 3)

(continued)

FIGURE 4.3. (continued)

133

Activating Event	them for not protecting him from stressors. The trauma of the diabetes diagnosis strengthened his belief that his parents were failing him, because they could not protect him from the disease. Small scale—any situation that Bob perceives to include pressure to take care of self, pressure to achieve social success, reminders that parents may not be able to take care of him. Large-scale precipitants—9/11, which reactivated the traumatic aspects of his diabetes diagnosis 8 years before, triggering beliefs that others should be able to protect him from all bad things and that they have failed him.		Large-scale precipitants will no longer be viewed as having catastrophic impact on daily life (1, 3)
Behavior Antecedents (A) Consequences (C)	1. Repetitive questioning of family members; seeking reassurance about terrorism. A—Intermittent exposure to TV or Internet reports about 9/11 and increased anxiety. C—Reassuring statements by family members, which result in temporary reduction in anxiety. 2. Social withdrawal/passivity A—Social situations where Bob is uncertain about the other people and/or how he should behave; lack of conversation skills. C—Anxiety reduction results from withdrawal; passivity relieves pressure. 3. Verbally aggressive behavior (sudden outbursts of anger toward others) A—Social situations where Bob attributes negative intent to another person's behavior and escape is not possible; lack of assertiveness skills. C—Other people act hostile toward Bob and reject him, reinforcing negative schema about others.	1. Exposure + response prevention: • Assign Bob task of exposing self to news media in a scheduled, structured, and systematic way. • Have Bob monitor SUDs. • Instruct family to implement response prevention; provide them with a script for Bob's questions. 2. and 3. Teach perspective-taking skills/reading nonverbal cues of others and assertive communication (as mentioned above).	Bob will become desensitized to the news. Taking active versus passive role over consumption of current events information will increase sense of control and decrease need for parent involvement. (1, 3) Increased initiation of social engagement (2, 4) Decreased frequency of angry outbursts (2, 4)

FIGURE 4.3. (continued)

(continued)

Strengths and Resiliency Factors		Activity scheduling	Increased expression of talent and frequency of enjoyable activities (2, 3, 4)
Bob is bright, articulate, has enjoyed writing and believes he expresses himself best that way, can use humor as a coping strategy, and has formed positive connections with some people. He was also active in a bowling league and frequently played tennis prior to 9/11.			

Potential Obstacles to Treatment:

1. Bob's belief that others are untrustworthy and his reliance on hostile behavior to protect himself may interfere with building a working relationship with the therapist. It may be worsened by his tendency to misinterpret what others are doing and saying to him.

2. Bob's planning and organization deficits may interfere with managing the tasks of therapy.

3. Bob's belief that he is helpless and incapable may interfere with his taking an active role in the therapy process; he may remain passive and avoid doing exercises and homework.

Prevention Strategies for Obstacles:

1. Assume a slow pace; use a lot of reflection and validation in the early sessions.

2. Break down tasks into small subtasks; accompany verbal instruction with visual aids.

3. By assigning tasks that are small and manageable (described above), the probability of Bob's willingness to try may be increased.

FIGURE 4.3. (continued)

135

social difficulties). I was eager to get the OCD symptoms "out of the way" so that a clearer picture of premorbid functioning could come into view. It was assumed that the chronic problems he had prior to 9/11 had set the stage for the acute and severe OCD and depressive episodes. The third and fourth goals, to *increase self-reliance/independence* and to *increase quality and quantity of relationships,* were more important ones to work on in the long run. These would improve overall quality of life for Bob and minimize his risk for future acute episodes of anxiety and depression.

Hypothesis-Based Interventions and Outcomes

The hypotheses about the factors causing or maintaining problems should drive the choices for interventions. Whenever possible, the literature for evidence-based thera-pies should serve as a resource for the therapist. By breaking down the problems into causal components, the therapist is led to more options about how to help. In Bob's case, like all of the cases discussed in this book, labeling him as "an adult with ASD" is not that helpful for treatment planning. However, based on the multiple causal factors that are thought to be contributing to his dysfunction, one can find evidence-based strate-gies in the literature to use for people who are suffering from OCD, have maladaptive schemas maintaining depressive symptoms, or have social skill deficits that contribute to social anxiety.

The process of choosing interventions and specifying expected outcomes is described using Bob's worksheet, starting at the top of the last two columns and work-ing down.

MEDICAL

Bob's diabetes played a major role in his functioning. Because he was already being treated by an endocrinologist with whom he and his family were satisfied, no referrals were necessary. He did need to take more responsibility over the care of his disease, however. Teaching self-monitoring skills as well as encouraging a more active role in scheduling and participating in his quarterly endocrinology visits would be part of the psychotherapy plan. The outcome was hoped to be an increased sense of control over the disease that he continued to feel so helpless about, even 8 years after being diagnosed. This intervention would be one of several treatment components that would contribute to decreasing depressive symptoms (Goal 2) and increasing independence (Goal 3).

CORE PROBLEMS OF ASD

Bob's problems with nonverbal communication, which had been evident since child-hood and were symptomatic of ASD, would be addressed by using published curricu-lum materials designed to teach perspective taking and nonverbal cue reading (e.g., Winner, 2000, 2002). He would also be taught how to express his feelings and needs to others through assertiveness training. It was hoped that these social skill improvements would increase his competence and confidence in social situations. However, this was thought to be a long-term objective and would be included in session agendas only after more acute symptoms of depression and anxiety began to improve. At that point, these strategies were intended to increase the quality and quantity of his relationships (Goal 4).

ER problems would be addressed by offering emotion education, using tools to teach the purpose of emotions and how to identify and label them. This would provide Bob with the prerequisite skills for later efforts toward acceptance of his own emotions, which would enhance his ability to participate in the other treatment strategies geared toward Goals 1–4.

It was unclear how much of a role Bob's historical tactile sensitivity was playing in his current self-care problems, especially given that his severe depression could have been causing some of the neglect. It was therefore decided to reassess that issue only if self-care continued to be a problem after other parts of the intervention plan proved to be successful.

Bob also needed help in the areas of planning and organization and therefore would be given task management systems that were more suited to his learning style. He had shown more responsiveness to visual, pictorial representations of ideas in sessions, so creating tools for self-direction based on his visual preference became an intervention target. The outcome was hoped to be an increase in the number of tasks of daily living completed without help from others. This outcome would increase his self-reliance and independence (Goal 3).

SCHEMAS

Schema-changing techniques would begin with cognitive restructuring through use of the thought record. It would be important to implement schema-related strategies simultaneous with other parts of the treatment plan because success in those other areas would provide evidence to Bob that would counter some of his maladaptive schemas. For example, if he began to show some success in taking care of his diabetes regimen, it would provide evidence against the schema about self that said, "I am helpless and powerless" and "I cannot take care of myself." These changes would also help him reappraise situations that he had previously found stressful. The outcome would be increased ability to challenge maladaptive automatic thoughts and increased expression of new beliefs about himself and others, such as "I am capable and competent" and "Others do not have to take care of me." These changes in his basic belief system would contribute to all of the therapy goals, especially decreasing his depressive symptoms (Goal 2), increasing his self-reliance and independence (Goal 3), and increasing the quality of his relationships (Goal 4).

BEHAVIOR

The first task of therapy would be to implement an exposure plus response prevention approach for treating OCD. The conceptualization of Bob's OCD in terms of a vicious cycle would be explained to him. He would be taught to use a 10-point subjective units of distress (SUDs) and told to watch a news program once each day, preferably the same show at the same time each day. He would thereby be exposed to somewhat unpredictable and anxiety-producing news stories, but he would be consuming a more systematic and balanced view of current events. This strategy would also give him more control over how he received such information. He would be asked to rate his SUDs before and after each program and to bring his tally sheets to therapy. He would also be keeping thought records, as mentioned in the section on schema-changing techniques. His family members would be invited to a session for instructions on how to refrain from answering Bob's questions; they would receive a script dictating how to respond to him if he began his obsessive questioning. Finally, Bob would be instructed to self-monitor the frequency of his questioning of others. As an outcome of exposure plus response prevention, it was expected that he would become desensitized to the news (or at least less distressed by it) and would take a more active role in consuming current events, thereby needing his parents less in this domain. All of these tactics would help decrease his obsessions and compulsions (Goal 1) as well as increase his self-reliance (Goal 3).

The social skills that were mentioned previously, which would be taught to help Bob compensate for core deficits in social cognition, will also help ameliorate his tendency to withdraw and engage in angry outbursts. If Bob can more easily read others and has a wider repertoire of verbal responses from which to choose, he will feel more competent and confident in initiating social engagement and will be less likely to use hostility and anger as a self-protective strategy. These skills will help decrease depressive symptoms (Goal 2) and improve his relationships (Goal 4).

STRENGTHS AND RESILIENCY FACTORS

As part of the task management approaches that would be taught to Bob to help him plan and organize better (mentioned previously), he will be taught how to use activity scheduling to bring pleasant events back into his life. This is a well-established strategy for decreasing depressive symptoms (Goal 2), but it will also increase his expression of talent, thereby increasing self-sufficiency (Goal 3) and opportunities to practice new social skills toward improving relationships (Goal 4).

Potential Obstacles to Treatment and Prevention Strategies for Obstacles

The final step in treatment planning is to project pitfalls and to make provisions for them. Every therapist knows that treatment always involves unexpected twists and "curveballs" that are thrown by patients or the people in their lives; unfortunately, these cannot be avoided. Nevertheless, the more the therapist can predict, based on known risk factors, the better prepared both therapist and patient can be to cope with obstacles.

In Bob's case, several factors could work against the therapy process. The first was his difficulty forming relationships with people, which originated with his belief that others are untrustworthy. He would obviously make that assumption about me. His use of hostile and belligerent behavior as self-protection would make it difficult for me to express empathy and validation, the building blocks of trust. Also, his problems in reading nonverbal cues and tendency to misinterpret what is said by others may trigger more angry responses. All of these problems would be addressed by proceeding at a slow pace and using a lot of reflective statements at the beginning. By reflecting and asking for clarification, I would be less likely to misinterpret what Bob was saying, and I would also be learning his style of communication. It was hoped that Bob would feel validated and begin to trust me.

A second problematic area was Bob's planning and organization deficits. I was concerned that the task-oriented nature of CBT would overwhelm Bob, in the same way that his diabetes treatment and other self-care responsibilities did. Again, a slow pace would minimize the likelihood of this undesirable outcome. Extra time would be needed to break down tasks into manageable pieces and to provide ample in-session instruction and practice for the use of homework tools.

Finally, Bob's schemas about himself as helpless and incapable, paired with his idea that others should take care of him, had the potential to interfere with his willingness to take an active role in therapy. If he were to carry these assumptions into sessions, he may view me as yet another person who should do things for him. He may also avoid doing exercises and homework for the same reason. It was hoped that the slow pace and effort put into making tasks manageable would prevent this problem.

Chapter Summary and Conclusions

This chapter described a framework for conceptualizing cases and planning treatment. A worksheet was presented as a suggested tool for going through this process with adult patients who have ASD. The case of Bob is used to illustrate how to design a treatment plan for patients with multiple comorbid conditions: how to generate hypotheses based on empirically supported theories about the presenting problem (nomothetic bases) and to individualize them according to the unique set of factors that is influencing the patient in his or her life (idiographic bases). A philosophy of change was presented for adults with ASD that allows sources of distress to be minimized and unique characteristics, talents, and sources of enjoyment to be preserved and encouraged. The next chapter presents more details on how to provide psychoeducation and orient the patient to the treatment process.

CHAPTER 5

Psychoeducation and Orientation to Treatment

The process of orienting a patient to treatment begins with the initial phone contact and continues through the intake, assessment, and treatment planning sessions. The previous two chapters addressed some of the issues encountered when establishing rapport and creating a collaborative partnership with the adult patient who has ASD. As mentioned, many of the guidelines presented were not original and are likely to be standard practice for most experienced clinicians working with any adult population, whereas others were specific to adults on the autistic spectrum. This chapter presents additional orientation guidelines that are unique to working with patients who have ASD. Two areas are covered: One section focuses on how to provide psychoeducation to patients regarding the ASD diagnosis itself, and the second section presents ways to inform patients about what to expect from the therapist and the cognitive-behavioral approach.

Psychoeducation

Explaining ASD

Most patients with ASD have questions about the syndrome, whether they were diagnosed recently or not. Many patients who meet criteria for ASD without ID would have previously been diagnosed with *Asperger syndrome,* and a subset of them have heard the latter term and wonder how that fits into their current situation. Some who were diagnosed prior to 2013 will identify their diagnosis as Asperger syndrome, and may express confusion or even anger about the change in terminology represented by the publication of DSM-5 (American Psychiatric Association, 2013). It is important to spend time at the beginning of therapy helping the patient understand the autistic spectrum, in general, and then figuring out the specific ways in which it is affecting him or her in life. Many patients have had experiences with professionals who misdiagnosed them and therefore may have feelings of resentment or mistrust. Extra time can be spent with those individuals discussing the purpose as well as the limitations of diagnostic labels.

140

The factual information about ASD should be presented to the patient in a modality that matches his or her preferred learning style. The therapist should keep a library of materials in the office to aid in the process. The following list includes the different approaches and tools therapists can use:

- Present DSM-5 criteria and discuss what each symptom means.
- Review the term *Asperger's disorder* or *Asperger syndrome,* explaining how different classification systems use different terms to describe similar issues (e.g., ICD-10 [World Health Organization, 1992], older versions of DSM).
- Review the evidence provided in Chapter 1 that the change in DSM terminology may have very few negative consequences in day-to-day life for most adults.
- For those who enjoy reading scientific or technical textbooks, assign one of the overview books listed in the Appendix for professionals.
- For those who prefer books for laypeople, assign one of the books in the Appendix that provides a comprehensive overview with less technical jargon.
- Assign a book that contains an autobiographical account of autism or ASD. The Appendix provides a list of books whose authors are on the autism spectrum.

It is noteworthy that people with ASD usually respond positively to this process. As mentioned, one of the only domains in which many of them have been successful is academic, so they are often enthusiastic about learning. Many are bright people who enjoy acquiring new facts. Those who have that attitude will quickly read and understand material the therapist recommends and will come to session with many questions about it. Others will conduct extensive library or Internet research and read beyond the therapy assignments. Those who have EF problems that interfere with follow-through between sessions may still actively participate in discussions about psychoeducational material within sessions.

Positive Reactions to the Diagnosis

At times, involved family members may discourage discussions about ASD for fear of adding to the patient's negative view of him- or herself. However, I have observed that most adults who are receiving the diagnosis and psychoeducation for the first time report a sense of relief. For example, one 46-year-old man said, "I always knew something was wrong and that I did not fit in with other people. I felt like an alien—a freak. Now I understand what the problem is and it all makes sense to me now." Another man in his mid-50s said, "I have been living my life with an invisible ball and chain attached to my ankle. Now that I can see it, I think I have done pretty damn well, despite it!" Most of these patients have known something "wasn't right" throughout their lives, and many of them made attributions for their struggles that were much worse than the explanation that comes from an ASD diagnosis.

Negative Reactions to the Diagnosis

Even though the initial reaction to the ASD diagnosis for most patients involves relief, a subgroup absorbs and assimilates the information over time in an unfavorable way. Contrary to the family fears mentioned above, the diagnosis does not make them feel any *worse* about themselves than they ever did. However, they may use it to support a preexisting negative self-schema. Those who had schemas about self that involved themes of inferiority and defectiveness, for instance, may distort the facts about ASD in order to make it fit with their belief system. Or they may selectively attend to pieces of information that focus on the deficits involved in ASD and ignore facts about strengths, potential benefits, or factors contributing to a good prognosis.

One strategy that therapists can use to minimize this phenomenon is to ensure that the patient understands what ASD is from the beginning of the psychoeducation stage. This can be done by checking in frequently with the patient as he or she consumes the educational material. If a reading assignment is given, then part of the next session should be spent having the patient describe what he or she understood about what was read and also to *interpret* what it means to him or her. This strategy gives the therapist the opportunity to clarify any material that was misunderstood and to dispel any myths to which the patient may be subscribing.

Some patients demonstrate that they understand the material during the psychoeducational phase of therapy, but later on in treatment, they show signs of having "drifted" away from the facts and begin to distort what they learned. This shift can be handled in the same way that any cognitive distortion would be handled in CBT. Having the patient generate a list of beliefs about ASD and the evidence that either supports or refutes each belief is one example (these strategies are covered in more detail in Chapter 7).

Connecting the Patient with Resources

Benefits of Network Involvement

In addition to assigning books as educational material, the therapist can also refer the patient to a wide variety of organizations and associations that are devoted to autism spectrum issues and that offer some combination of annual conferences, regional support meetings, and newsletters. In addition, numerous online news groups, blogs, and support networks have become more prevalent in recent years. A large community of adults with ASD keep in touch with one another, mostly through electronic communication, and engage in ongoing and lively dialogues about the latest research and news about ASD. Some have developed a strong sense of belongingness through this process, which has had a beneficial effect on their self-image and social support quality. This community has been described by some as a subculture, and they refer to themselves affectionately as "Aspies" or "Spectrumites" and to people not on the spectrum as "neurotypicals" or "NTs," and promote mutual understanding and acceptance in the spirit of "neurodiversity."

The Appendix includes a list of organizations and groups that should be considered. Of course, a therapist is wise to investigate any resource before recommending it to a patient, remembering that different patients will respond to material in different ways at different times. No matter which organization(s) the patient accesses, it is important for the therapist to check in with the patient from time to time to monitor the ways the involvement is helping and also to watch for warning signs that it is causing distress. I have found that involvement in a group that is well suited to the patient's style is usually beneficial, but there are some caveats of which therapists should be aware so that they can be minimized. These are discussed below.

Caveats of Network Involvement

The first potential problem involves an issue mentioned in the previous section on negative reactions to diagnosis. Some individuals who have negative self-schemas involving themes of defectiveness and inferiority may be prone to misunderstand or distort information they receive from organizations and use it as evidence to support their preexisting belief. It is important for the therapist to elicit discussions about the information the patient is accessing. The patient should not be discouraged from utilizing these resources—rather, the therapy should be geared toward helping him or her reconceptualize the information and to make more adaptive use out of it.

The second problem that can arise out of a patient's involvement with networks and groups comes from the fact that interpersonal interaction is inherent in the process. Because ASD, by definition, includes problems with social interaction, some of the patients have interpersonal difficulties that are bound to play out there (i.e., online, on the telephone, in person), the same way they would in any setting. For instance, if a patient has a history of overattributing negative intent to others, he or she will eventually have that problem with a peer in an ASD resource network. If a patient has a history of cursing loudly in the face of disagreement, that person is likely to do that to someone in an ASD support group. As these issues arise, it is again important for the therapist not to discourage involvement in the various associations and support networks. Rather, it is more important to use these real-life examples to build the patient's interpersonal skills.

Disclosure

During the psychoeducational process, it is common for patients to ask whether they should tell others about their diagnosis. Disclosure is a highly sensitive issue and has many implications that are individual to each patient. Some patients may benefit from reading the book *Ask and Tell: Self-Advocacy and Disclosure for People on the Autism Spectrum* (Shore, 2004). The editor, Stephen Shore, and all chapter authors are people on the autism spectrum who address this issue from a number of perspectives and offer many practical suggestions.

I am reluctant to give patients direct advice about disclosing their diagnosis. However, I do provide a general list of questions with a patient who is struggling with dilemmas about whether to tell friends, relatives, employers, coworkers, or dating partners. These questions are outlined below. Figure 5.1 presents the questions on a worksheet for use by a patient.

1. *"Why do you want this particular person to know about your diagnosis?"* If the patient does not have any answer for this question, it should be explored in session so that he or she can formulate a clear idea about it. Sometimes there may be problems in the relationship that the patient thinks would improve if the information were shared. Other times the patient believes that sharing this information with someone very close to him or her, just as they would any type of personal information, will add to the intimacy of the relationship.

2. *"How do you think it will improve your interactions with this person if he or she knows about your ASD?"* Again, the patient should be able to answer this question before proceeding further. Without a clear idea, the patient is not as likely to achieve the desired effect by disclosing.

Name of the person to whom you may disclose your diagnosis: _____

Please answer each of the questions below.

1. Why do you want this particular person to know about your diagnosis?
2. How do you think it will improve your interactions with this person if he or she knows about your ASD?
3. Are you prepared to ask this person to support you in a different way because of this new information? ____ Yes ____ No If yes, list below the things he or she can do to be more helpful to you.
4. What are the risks of telling this person?
5. If the person is someone with whom you are not very close (e.g., a coworker), are there other ways you could ask for specific types of help and support without telling him or her about your ASD?

FIGURE 5.1. Disclosure worksheet.

3. *"Are you prepared to ask this person to support you in a different way because of this new information? If so, can you be <u>specific</u> with this person about how he or she can be more helpful to you?"* When a patient is hoping that an interpersonal problem will improve with the disclosure, it is important for him or her to be able to explain *how* he or she expects things to change with the recipient of the disclosure. This approach requires an ability to be assertive in asking the other person for specific actions or accommodations. Otherwise, the recipient of the information may not know how he or she should use the information. Assertiveness is often a weak ability in these patients, so practice may be necessary in session.

4. *"What are the risks of telling this person?"* The better the patient knows the person he or she is going to tell, the easier it is to answer this question. However, when the recipient of the disclosure is not someone who is known well (e.g., an employer or coworker), it is harder to predict the reaction. It is therefore important to help the patient anticipate negative reactions so that specific plans can be made (sometimes including behavioral rehearsal) for how to handle them.

5. *"If the person is someone with whom you are not very close (e.g., a coworker), are there other ways you could ask for specific types of help and support without telling him or her about your ASD?"* If the patient believes it would be too uncomfortable or risky telling a boss or a coworker, for example, an alternative plan can be made. It is sometimes possible to ask for accommodations or supports without disclosing the diagnosis. One man with ASD who was stressed by various work issues figured out that he would be less stressed if he had a different break schedule. Instead of taking the conventional 1-hour lunch break with two 15-minute breaks, he preferred to take six 15-minute breaks throughout the day. He needed frequent but short trips outside for fresh air in order to maintain good concentration. He decided to ask his boss for this modification without mentioning his ASD, deciding to disclose his diagnosis only if his boss did not grant his initial request. Ultimately, he was allowed to take the breaks the way he preferred. When presented with the request, the boss only showed momentary mild interest in *why* it was being made. The patient simply said, "Oh, it just helps my concentration." The boss said, "It makes no difference to me, as long as your work gets done." This patient was surprised that he could simply ask for a change and relieved that he did not have to share his personal information with his boss at that time. Granted, things do not always work out so nicely, but it is always worth a try before revealing personal information that some patients find embarrassing.

Orientation to Treatment

Once the individual begins to see that there is an explanation for many of the struggles he or she has encountered, the motivation to find out how therapy is going to help usually increases. The orientation to treatment serves to answer that question by educating the patient about the reasonable expectations he or she can have for the therapist and the therapy as well as the responsibilities the patient is expected to hold. In addition, the rationale for CBT and the cognitive model are explained as a foundation for the individualized treatment plan, which has been collaboratively designed by the therapist and patient. Chapter 4 described how the therapist and patient work together to formulate goals; that phase is also part of the orientation process. This section provides additional guidelines for establishing a relationship and explaining the rationale for treatment.

Establishing and Maintaining a Working Relationship

It goes without saying that a good working relationship is crucial for any course of psychotherapy to be effective, regardless of the therapist's orientation or the nature of the patient's presenting problem. However, because ASD involves difficulty with interpersonal interaction, there are some unique factors that therapists working with this population must take into consideration. Many of the social-cognitive deficits and behavioral differences that have negatively impacted these patients' relationships with other people will present themselves in therapy. However, by following the guidelines presented in this section, therapists can minimize the interference of these factors with relationship development. Some of the suggestions made in Chapter 3 regarding the initial interview are presented again here, among strategies to be practiced throughout the life of the relationship. Guidelines are provided on how to set clear expectations, set a realistic pace, use language effectively, validate the patient's experiences, and provide constructive feedback. Keep in mind that these approaches work most of the time for most patients. However, Chapter 10, which discusses obstacles to treatment, covers more details about what to do when these strategies do not work.

Setting Clear Expectations

One of the difficulties people with ASD report is that they often do not know what to expect from others, and/or they do not know what others expect from them. Their uncertainty and confusion about this aspect of social situations contributes to their anxiety. It is therefore important for the therapist to pay special attention to how roles are explained at the onset of treatment.

Most therapists in general practice give patients some type of consent document to sign at the beginning of treatment, which may be called a "therapist–patient agreement," a "contract," or a "consent to treatment" form. No matter which format the therapist uses, it applies to all patients, regardless of population, and contains information about roles and expectations. For patients with ASD, a discussion about the document after they have read it can serve a role clarification function.

The therapist can start by reviewing the basic information that already appears in the formal intake and consent documents. The therapist should mention each point and ask the patient to summarize what he or she understood about it and whether he or she has any questions. These issues would include:

- Confidentiality and its limits
- Cancellation and fee policies
- Therapist accessibility in between sessions/emergency contact information
- Therapist policies and limits regarding telehealth modalities (use of telephone or videoconference tools for sessions)
- Record-keeping practices

Again, reviewing these issues with new patients is good standard practice for any therapist. However, extra time should be spent ensuring that the adult patient with ASD understands it accurately. The literal mindedness of some can lead to misinterpretation of certain policies, for example. For others, a lack of assertiveness or social language problems may preclude them from initiating questions about areas of the document they do not understand. People with this problem, however, usually ask questions if the therapist directly elicits them during a point-by-point review of the document.

Once the patient understands the procedural consent-to-treatment issues described above, the therapist can present expectations that are based on his or her own style and philosophy of therapy. Of course, these expectations will be individual to each therapist, but the presentation should be based on a general assumption that people with ASD process information in unique ways. The objective is to be as clear and explicit as possible, remembering that patients with ASD may not infer some points that other adult patients would readily assume. The formula presented below offers a conceptual framework for setting expectations.

I [therapist] am going to behave in this way and do these things _____

during sessions for these reasons: _____. I *will not* do

these things _____ for these reasons: _____.

I will also expect you [patient] to do these things _____

during/between sessions _____ for these reasons: _____.

Finally, I will expect that you *will not* do these things _____

for these reasons: _____.

This is not meant to be a script but rather a tool for ensuring that the therapist remembers to cover each and every point. The therapist should never assume that the patient will infer or generalize any one piece of information from another, no matter how articulate or intelligent he or she may be.

I offer the following role definitions to my patients—that is, these are the phrases that I use to "fill in the blanks" in the formula presented above. Remember that these are just examples coming from one therapist, and that each therapist will have different points to make, depending on his or her style and philosophy. The principle that *should not vary* from therapist to therapist, however, is that points should be made as *explicit* as possible to the patient.

THE ROLE OF THE THERAPIST

- "I will be a *facilitator* in our sessions. This means that I will ask you a lot of questions that require you to think about a lot of different things. I will also ask you to try new things, but they will always be based on ideas that come from you, and I will always give you a rationale. I *will not be an authority figure*. This means I will not give you orders, commands, or advice that you do not ask for (unless I believe you are at risk to harm yourself or someone else). I am your *partner* in trying to improve the things you want help with, but I am not your *boss* who is here to tell you what to do.

- "It is my responsibility to *provide information and resources* to you. I will share facts about your problems and treatment options that are based on research. I will refer you to the sources of that material. I will be honest with you when I do not know the answer to one of your questions, and will do my best to either find the answer for you or point you in the direction of finding it yourself. I *will not* make decisions for you. I can help you evaluate information you receive or options you are considering, but will not try to tell you what to think or do. If I share my personal opinion about some information we are discussing, I will clearly identify it as such, by saying, 'This is my personal view on this issue,' or 'This is my bias—other professionals may disagree with me about this.'

- "I will *provide you with direct feedback* about the impact your actions or words have on me. I assume that the way you relate to me bears some resemblance to how you are relating to others in your life. Because you are coming here to improve your interpersonal skills, it will be important for us to use our relationship as a means of practicing new skills you may work on. People in the natural environment generally do not give direct feedback in social situations, even if they are forming a negative impression. It may seem unnatural to you, and it may make you feel uncomfortable, but I will sometimes interrupt our conversation to share an observation with you—sort of like a 'freeze-frame' of a film or video. I will either tell you that something you did had a positive impact or that something you did had a negative impact. *I will not judge or criticize you.* My purpose is to provide information, which you may not get from people in your day-to-day life, about the impression you are making."

THE ROLE OF THE PATIENT

- "I expect you to be as *honest and open* as you can be about your thoughts, feelings, and experiences as they relate to our goals, including your impressions about me and the way the therapy is going. I hope you will *question* things that do not make sense to you or with which you do not agree. I hope that you *will not* keep ideas or feelings to yourself that relate to our work. Sometimes patients withhold their thoughts or feelings because they do not think it is their place to question things, or they think they should accept unconditionally the things that the therapist says. As I mentioned earlier, we are partners in trying to solve your problems, which means I cannot do a good job without your input and opinions.

- "I expect that you will play an *active role* in your therapy. This means you will attend regularly scheduled sessions and adhere to the frequency of meetings that we agree to, as per your treatment plan. It also means you will engage in exercises in session with me and complete homework in between sessions. As mentioned before, I will not assign you anything that does not make sense to you, so again, you will need to tell me the truth if you do not understand something. I hope you *will not be passive* in therapy—that is, I hope you *will not sit back* and wait for the therapist to "fix" the problems you have. The progress you make will depend on the energy you put into this process. If at any point, I think I am working harder than you, I am going to tell you that so we can revisit our goals and expectations.

- "I expect you to become an *observer of yourself.* This means that you are willing to pay attention to your actions, thoughts, and feelings as if you were an objective bystander and to report your observations to me. This may sound odd to you now, or you may have learned to do this already throughout your life. If you do not know how to do this yet, I will teach you as we go along. If you do know how to do it, I will rely heavily on your skill in this area in order to help you. What goes along with this is a willingness to *critique* yourself. This means that you are willing to think about things from a new perspective, to explore alternative ways of handling things that are different from how you have handled them in the past, and to accept feedback from others. This *does not* mean that you are *judging* yourself or *criticizing* yourself in a nonproductive way. Productive critiquing leads to positive change, whereas nonproductive criticizing leads to shame and avoidance."

The role expectations outlined may be presented all at once or shared bit by bit across several sessions. They should also be repeatedly reinforced throughout the course of treatment. Helping the patient to *take control* of important aspects of the therapy is crucial. Many patients with ASD do not believe that they have power over many parts of their lives, or they do not have the confidence to initiate more control or decision making. It is hoped that the *active role* they take in the therapy process will serve as practice for real-life situations. However, if that expectation is not explicitly stated for them at the beginning of treatment, they may be confused or annoyed by the therapist's attempts to activate them.

Setting a Realistic Pace

CBT has the potential to offer typical people with anxiety and mood disorders a short-term treatment option. However, therapists who have years of experience practicing CBT (but not necessarily with ASD) have learned that change takes place more slowly when patients have complex problems and multiple comorbid conditions. This assumption can be made when offering CBT to patients with ASD; the treatment is still time limited, but not necessarily as short term as it would be with typical adults. As this book has emphasized throughout, the problems associated with ASD are determined by multiple factors that have long histories. The patient must learn skills that represent brand new ways of thinking and behaving, and old maladaptive behaviors are extinguished only when the new skills can replace them. EF problems and cognitive rigidity may limit how much can be accomplished within a session. Change is a very slow process that requires repeated practice and reinforcement. Therapists who are accustomed to working with complex problems will have no trouble making this adjustment. However, novice therapists or those who have treated more "neat and clean" cases of anxiety or depression may need to pay special attention to setting realistic time frames for goal attainment when working with patients with ASD. There is no formula for determining how long treatment of a patient with ASD will take. It depends on the severity of comorbid psychopathology, the patient's resiliency factors, and the number of changes the patient is hoping to make by the end of treatment. Discounting cases where treatment ended before goals were attained, my shortest-term ASD case was 1 year. The longest-term case has been ongoing for 23 years at the time of this writing.

Using Language Effectively

All of the points made here were already mentioned in Chapter 3 in the section about intake interviewing. However, it is worth repeating them because the ongoing working relationship is dependent on the verbal communication between the therapist and the patient. Because of the unique ways in which some people with ASD use language, the therapist needs to take extra steps to ensure that he or she understands what the patient means to say. The therapist should make ample use of reflective statements and paraphrasing to check with the patient about his or her intended message. The therapist must be constantly aware that the patient may take words and phrases very literally, so the therapist should also prompt the patient to paraphrase what the therapist said in order to confirm that the intended information has been conveyed. When appropriate, the therapist may adopt some of the patient's words and phrases for concepts discussed in session in an effort to develop a shared language. This effort conveys the therapist's willingness to accept the patient's uniqueness and a desire to understand how he or she sees the world.

Validating the Patient's Experience

Validation strategies are, to some extent, practiced by any effective therapist, regardless of orientation. Therapists who practice CBT strike a balance between providing structure and offering a "listening ear" with validation. The therapist may need to spend more time providing validation to a patient with ASD than he or she would other adult patients, however, for two reasons. One is because of some of the language issues presented above. It may take longer for the therapist to figure out why a patient is in distress, for example, if the patient cannot use expressive language to effectively convey a problem. It is not uncommon to observe a patient coming into session in an agitated state, struggling to find the words to describe why he or she is upset. It might take me the entire session to find out what had triggered the emotional arousal—and only then can I provide the validation that is so crucial. The other reason extra time and attention must be paid to validation is because the patient often has a poor social support network. The long history of struggles and traumatic experiences that is so common to these patients is exacerbated by the fact that they have rarely had anyone to talk to about it. The validation that people typically get from natural supports such as friends and family is not as available to many patients with ASD. The therapist cannot replace those supports, and it is hoped that the patient will be able to build a better social network as functioning improves. However, in the meantime, the patient will be more receptive to the structured components of CBT if he or she is also supported by a validating atmosphere in sessions. This need for validation requires that the therapist remain somewhat flexible because sometimes a preplanned agenda has to be put aside if the patient has had a particularly upsetting experience before the session.

Providing Constructive Feedback

Therapists working with adults who have ASD must be willing to give them direct and immediate feedback about their behavior at the appropriate time. This guideline may seem to contradict what was just said about validation, as some therapists may perceive this practice as being critical of the patient. However, if the therapist is conveying validation to the patient during times of distress, then the patient is more likely to trust the therapist and to be more open to the direct feedback at other times. Also, it was mentioned in Chapter 3 that the therapist should not confront patients on their socially inappropriate behaviors during the intake. However, once the treatment plan is under way and some degree of rapport has been built, the therapist can use the relationship as a "practice field." If any of the treatment goals involve improving interpersonal or social skills, then those skills can be taught using the ongoing interaction between the therapist and the patient.

For example, some people with ASD have a problem with excessive talking. They may repeat the same point four or five times, even after their communication partner has given nonverbal cues that he or she has heard them. If that behavior turns out to be one of the targets for social skill improvement, then the therapist is obligated to inform the patient when he or she displays that problem in session. People in the natural environment are not as likely to give direct feedback but *are* likely to convey annoyance or disapproval indirectly, and ultimately to avoid and reject the patient. Here is one way the therapist could phrase feedback about this topic:

> (*interrupting the patient*) "I am sorry, but I am going to interrupt you for a minute. You were beginning to make a point that you just made very clearly, and you did say it twice. Did you notice that you were beginning to say it for a third time?"

The patient may answer this question in a number of different ways, depending on his or her particular problem. Not only does this intervention provide in vivo feedback that would not commonly be found in the patient's natural environment, but it opens up a dialogue that helps both patient and therapist understand better what is maintaining this behavior. Here is another way the therapist could facilitate this process:

> "Did you notice that when you were presenting your point the first two times, that I was nodding my head up and down and saying, 'umm hmm'? What do you think I was trying to tell you by doing that?"

Because the therapist must go against his or her own societal norms of courtesy, it may feel like he or she is being "rude" to the patient when this intervention is practiced. However, using a nonjudgmental tone in conjunction with a previously established trusting relationship with the patient will minimize the discomfort the patient may feel. In fact, some patients have expressed gratitude for this feedback because, though they have had an awareness that they were "missing something," no one ever told them what it was. One patient said, "When I am around a group of people, I always feel like I have come into a room where everyone is playing a game that they already know, but I don't. I want to enter the game, but nobody will stop and tell me what the rules are." Through most of their lives, in an ironic twist of conventional courtesy, they have been rejected without being given any clues about why. It is therefore an important part of the therapist's job to step out of the role of being "polite" in order to give the patient the feedback that is so crucial to learning and changing.

Providing a Rationale for Treatment

The treatment plan provides the rationale for each proposed intervention because the hypotheses about problem behaviors have led the therapist to choose the strategies. As mentioned several times before, this plan should be designed with the help of the patient, and the information on the case formulation worksheet should be familiar to the patient by the time treatment is under way. During the psychoeducational phase described earlier in this chapter, the patient receives information about the core deficits of ASD, how they are affecting him or her, and what interventions will help improve those problems. However, additional time is usually warranted to help the patient understand the rationale behind CBT, in general, and the way in which the traditional cognitive model applies to his or her specific case.

Describing CBT

The therapist should briefly explain what CBT is, starting with an overview of its history and assumptions. I use a large dry-wipe board or easel pad when presenting this information to patients because a combination of verbal descriptions with pictures can ensure understanding. Borrowing some concepts from Dobson and Dozois (2010), I usually explain the model this way:

> "CBT refers to a collection of therapeutic techniques that have been developed by mental health professionals over the past 50 years to help people with depression, anxiety, and stress, but *not* specifically for ASD. The assumptions behind CBT are:
>
> 1. Cognitive activity (thoughts, images, and perceptions) affects mood and behavior.
> 2. Cognitive activity can be dysfunctional at times. Sometimes people make errors in their thinking or distort their perceptions of things. *All people* do this *sometimes* for different reasons. Some people do it a lot, which can lead to ongoing problems with mood and behavior.
> 3. Cognitive activity can be monitored and altered.
> 4. Desired behavior change can be brought about through cognitive change.
> 5. People are active learners, not just passive recipients of environmental events; they create their own learning environment.
> 6. CBT treatment goals center on creating new adaptive learning opportunities to overcome cognitive dysfunction."

For therapists who include mindfulness-based strategies in their CBT approach, a general overview of mindfulness and acceptance concepts may be introduced at this point, as well. Chapter 8 details how strategies found in acceptance and commitment therapy (ACT), dialectical behavior therapy (DBT), and mindfulness-based stress reduction (MBSR) can be applied in a CBT treatment plan for adults with ASD. Because all include mindfulness and acceptance as core components, at the orientation phase these concepts can be introduced as follows, which are borrowed from Hayes and Smith (2005) and Harris (2008):

Over the past 20 years, CBT has evolved to include some additional assumptions about the things that cause suffering in human beings and contribute to anxiety and depression. Some of these concepts are counterintuitive, or seem to be against conventional wisdom on how to solve problems and feel better. Keep that in mind as you hear more about these ideas that inform some of the strategies we may be including in your treatment plan:

1. Pain is by nature unpleasant, yet it is inevitable across the course of a lifetime. Attempts to get rid of pain or avoid it may amplify it and cause even more pain, transforming it into suffering.

2. Acceptance involves learning to resist the urge to escape pain when it arises. It *does not* mean people should embrace and celebrate unpleasant events, negative thoughts, or painful emotions but rather to learn to continue to be active in meaningful ways *even when* a painful experience is present.

3. Mindfulness is a way of paying attention to experiences that may be different from what people are accustomed to. Mindfulness practices are rooted in the teachings of Eastern religions and have existed for thousands of years, but applied in secular ways in modern mental health practice. People can learn to become more aware of how they direct their attention and to become more observant of things that are happening right now, in the immediate present, including environmental and internal (thoughts and feelings) events.

The therapist should ask the patient to explain what he or she understood each point to mean before moving on. Using pictures and diagrams can help illustrate points with which the patient seems to be struggling. For example, using the approach suggested by Carol Gray (1994), I draw a cartoon "thought bubble" above a stick figure to illustrate cognitive activity and a cartoon speech bubble right next to it, while saying, "In here are all of the thoughts, images, or perceptions that we have inside our heads, which may not be the same as the things we say out loud" (see Chapter 7, Figure 7.4).

Explaining the Cognitive Model

By continuing to use drawings and pictorial representations of the ideas being presented, the therapist can introduce Beck's (1976) cognitive model of mental health problems. I usually draw the diagram that is presented in Chapter 2, Figure 2.3, in order to introduce the concept of how schemas (core beliefs) influence mood, thoughts, and behaviors. I then fill in the diagram with specific information about the patient, to help illustrate how the cognitive model explains some of his or her problems. Chapter 7 provides a case example of this process. I have observed that patients with ASD seem to grasp the cognitive model quickly, once it is presented in a modality that suits their learning style (e.g., pictures for a visual learner). Its logical, cause-and-effect quality seems to appeal to the need, experienced by so many of these patients, to understand and follow rules. In this sense, patients with ASD are ideal candidates for CBT.

Chapter Summary and Conclusions

This chapter began with guidelines for helping patients understand their ASD diagnosis, with precautionary suggestions for preventing dysfunctional use of the information. Strategies for orienting the patient to treatment came next. The unique issues faced by therapists while they build a working relationship with patients who have interpersonal difficulties were addressed. Finally, an approach for introducing the rationale for CBT and helping the patient begin conceptualizing his or her problems using the cognitive model was described. The next chapter discusses the actual implementation of CBT with patients who have ASD.

CHAPTER 6

Intervention

Increasing Skills to Address the Core Problems of Autism Spectrum Disorder

This chapter presents options for interventions that can be offered to adult patients with ASD. Chapter 2 introduced a general framework, or nomothetic formulation, for understanding the way ASD affects adults and the factors that can lead to mental health problems (illustrated in Figure 2.4). Chapter 4 described a case formulation approach that allows a therapist to apply the nomothetic formulation to conceptualizing an individual adult patient, thereby producing an idiographic hypothesis-based treatment plan. The interventions that are chosen by the therapist should be based on both the nomothetic and idiographic formulations explaining the patient's presenting problems. The three chapters ahead are meant to provide ideas and resources to therapists in order to ease this decision-making process and guidance on how to carry out the techniques through the use of case examples. This chapter focuses on strategies for teaching *social* and *coping* skills that address the core problems of ASD, Chapter 7 explores the use of a traditional cognitive therapy approach to treat comorbid mental health problems, and Chapter 8 offers methods to improve ER ability for help with core ASD issues and comorbid conditions.

Review of Nomothetic Formulation

A brief review of Figure 2.4, the nomothetic formulation of mental health problems in ASD, serves as an introduction to the interventions that are discussed ahead. Each set of factors in this model represents a possible point of intervention for a therapist. It is assumed that when a person with ASD presents with anxiety or depression, it is an outcome of many variables that have interacted with one another throughout his or her history up to the point of intake. The idea that the mental health problem has resulted from this process is illustrated by placing *anxiety* and *depression* at the bottom, or end, of the diagram. Through the assessment and case formulation process, however, the therapist must "look back" in the patient's life in order to conceptualize the developmental processes that led up to the current issues. This diagram "tells the story" by mapping out this course.

The core problems of ASD, grouped as problems with processing *information about others, information about self,* and *nonsocial information,* appear at the top or beginning of the diagram, suggesting that they have been present since early life and have affected the way the individual has learned, behaved, and interpreted his or her world. This process is represented in the middle of the diagram, where *behavioral differences* and associated *social consequences,* as well as *self-management* difficulties and associated *daily living consequences,* have led the person to experience *poor social support* and *chronic stress.* Beck's (1976) theory regarding the role of schemas in the development and maintenance of mental health problems in the general population can be used to describe the mechanism by which the problems inherent in ASD could lead to anxiety and depressive disorders. The diamond shapes in Figure 2.4, representing schemas about self, others, world, and future, are placed at the points in this developmental process where the individual may have acquired maladaptive beliefs.

When a therapist is designing a plan for an adult with ASD, considering the nomothetic model, there are generally two types of objectives that lead to two categories of interventions. There are those that aim to increase competencies and skills in order to improve relationship and occupational functioning, which have been impaired by the symptoms of ASD. These are the issues listed in the top-to-middle region of Figure 2.4. Then there are those that aim to decrease symptoms of other comorbid mental health problems, such as anxiety and depressive disorders, the issues listed in the middle-to-bottom region of the diagram. This chapter presents the former, and Chapter 7, the latter. Chapter 8, which covers mindfulness-based CBT approaches, describes interventions that may have utility in targeting both by addressing ER problems. This division is made for the sake of conceptual clarity. However, in real practice, an individualized treatment plan that is formulated in the way described in Chapter 4 will almost always have strategies for both skill building and symptom reduction, and the therapist will likely deliver these interventions in coordination with each other. Maddox and colleagues (2016) and White and colleagues (2013) have shown, for example, that treating both ASD social impairments simultaneous to treating comorbid anxiety helps adolescents with ASD make improvements in both domains of functioning. The individualized treatment plan helps the therapist prioritize and integrate these goals within each session.

"Habilitation" for Core Problems

Chapter 2 outlined the core deficits that have been shown to be present in people with ASD. The case formulation worksheet described in Chapter 4 should help the therapist generate hypotheses about how these deficits might be contributing to the presenting problems at the point of intake. It is my assumption that these core deficits, for practical purposes, can be viewed as *skill deficits.* ASD is, after all, a *developmental disability.* By definition, this means that adults with the syndrome have failed to acquire certain skills that others their age have been able to learn by a given point in life. Logically, if someone is missing a skill, that person needs to be taught either that skill or a compensatory strategy.

The idea of building skills that were *never learned* is often referred to as *habilitation* in the field of adult developmental disabilities—that is, within the network of professionals who provide services to adults with intellectual disability, autism, and cerebral palsy. This model assumes that people with disabilities can learn new skills throughout the lifespan. The objective is to ensure that these individuals become as self-sustaining as possible by giving them a multitude of learning opportunities. This philosophy is similar to the rehabilitation approach that may be found among professionals who treat traumatic brain injury or stroke victims, with the only difference being that in rehabilitation, a patient is trying to *regain lost skills* that he or she previously possessed. In habilitation, on the other hand, a patient is trying to *learn brand-new skills* that he or she never before possessed.

I emphasize this point here because any therapist who is working with adults with ASD should not assume that a skill not yet learned *cannot* be learned. It is better to start off assuming that a patient's missing skill was not acquired because the individual could not learn it in a *typical* way, but that he or she may be able to learn it in an *atypical* way. The opportunities that were not provided by the natural environment can be provided in the psychotherapy setting. Sadly, several patients have reported being told either directly or indirectly by professionals that it is too late in life for them to do anything about their ASD and that early intervention (i.e., aggressively teaching skills to children between infancy and the preschool years) is the only way to change the course of the syndrome. There is no question that early intervention has the greatest impact on a person and will do so in the shortest amount of time. However, I have a lifespan developmental perspective on ASD: even one new skill acquired at one point in an adult life can improve the way that a person experiences his or her world. In that sense, the intervention affects the course of development from that point on, no matter how old the person might be.

This chapter presents intervention choices for addressing the skill-building needs of adults with ASD. These skill-related needs are divided into two broad categories that encompass the most common needs seen in this population: *social skills* and *coping skills*. Referring back to Figure 2.4, these intervention categories are meant to address the problems listed in the middle boxes. Teaching social skills addresses the *behavioral differences* with their *social consequences*. Likewise, teaching coping skills addresses the *self-management* difficulties with their *daily living consequences*. Because these issues are considered to be part of the pathway to the development of mental health problems, building skills in these areas serves as a prevention strategy. These skills would help any person with ASD, even if there were no comorbid mental health problems present. Including these skills in the treatment plan of a person who does have comorbid anxiety or depression can be considered part of a relapse prevention approach. In fact, many of the strategies described in this chapter will likely be recognized by readers as behavioral components of traditional CBT.

There is one important consideration to keep in mind as the following skill-building strategies are described. Many of these techniques were not designed for the psychotherapy setting, but were developed by professionals from other disciplines for use by rehabilitation specialists (speech therapists, occupational therapists) or special education teachers. Nevertheless, they lend themselves well to CBT because teaching is a crucial role for a therapist practicing with a traditional cognitive-behavioral orientation. This is not to say that a psychotherapist can be a substitute for the other disciplines mentioned, however. If a patient is in need of a comprehensive social language interven-tion plan or sensory–motor skill plan, a referral to a qualified speech or occupational therapist is necessary for a more specialized approach to these issues.

Increasing Social Skills

Of course, all patients with ASD have some difficulty with social interaction, as it is a crucial component of the diagnostic criteria. In most psychotherapy cases, all involved parties (patient, supporters, referral sources) will agree that the individual is in need of "social skills training." However, the interventions that are warranted for a particular patient may not be clear—the term *social skills* can mean many different things to differ-ent people and vary by stage of development. Adaptive expressions of sexuality and the development of healthy intimate relationships are key facets of social skill development in adults that may not be named by a referral source, for instance. Adults with ASD vary greatly among one another in terms of the severity and quality of the interaction problems they have. Some may make gross errors with the most basic rules of courtesy (e.g., speaking too loudly in a restaurant, cutting to the front of a ticket line, repeat-edly interrupting a conversation partner), whereas others have mastered simple eti-quette but may struggle with subtler social rules (e.g., how to initiate a friendship with a coworker, how to respond to the criticism of a college professor, or how to maintain a healthy sexual relationship).

Gutstein and Sheely (2002) offer a useful way of defining the social difficulties seen in ASD. They divide social skills into two categories. *Instrumental skills* are a set of spe-cific behaviors, such as making eye contact, greeting with a handshake, smiling, turn taking, or starting a conversation—what laypeople would call "being polite." These behaviors are considered instrumental because they are used by one person to get another person to provide something; one is using another person as an instrument for getting a need met or as a means to a specific end. *Relationship skills,* on the other hand, are those that involve observing the social environment, rapidly processing emotional information, and then using it as a reference point for determining actions, all toward nurturing an ongoing relationship with another. These processes were described in Chapter 2 under *social cognition.* Gutstein and Sheely emphasize that instrumental skills are necessary but not sufficient for making and maintaining friendships. Only through the more dynamic relationship skills can a person learn to share genuine joy, collabo-rate to solve novel problems, cooperate in a joint creative effort, or reach shared goals with another. Although instrumental skills can be taught, rehearsed, and memorized as discrete behaviors, relationship skills can be achieved only by learning to *process social information* in a flexible and dynamic way. For adults, these skills are not only important in pursuing friendships but also for the development of healthy sexual relationships.

When setting goals for psychotherapy, I find it useful to conceptualize instrumen-tal and relationship skills separately. However, I break them down further into *four* categories of skills that can be specifically targeted in therapy with adults, and each level represents an accumulation of previous levels of skill. Listed in order of most basic to most complex, they are (1) increasing instrumental skills; (2) increasing the fund of knowledge about social norms; (3) increasing dynamic "people-reading" skills, or improving social cognition; and (4) increasing assertive communication skills.

Increasing Instrumental Skills

Surprisingly, many adult patients with ASD demonstrate a repertoire of socially *appropriate* behaviors that are evident upon first meeting them. However, some may need to spend time building a larger base of these while learning more complex interaction skills, such as the ones required in a romantic or sexual relationship, for instance. The types of skills that fall into the instrumental category are discrete behaviors that can be scripted, rehearsed, and memorized. They include smiling, eye contact, polite phrases (including "please" and "thank you"), greetings, conversation starters, and telephone skills. Also included might be "scripts" for how to complete a transaction with a bank teller, postal worker, store clerk, doctor's office staff, or service/repair professional (e.g., plumber, electrician). They allow the person to get things accomplished that involve other people (as long as nothing unexpected occurs). These skills make the individual generally likable to people when dealing with them on a superficial level.

I have observed a trend in my caseload regarding instrumental skills. Roughly speaking, it seems that the older a patient is, the more likely it is that he or she has learned many instrumental behaviors and can recognize the right time and place to use them. Some have actually reported that they have used their logic or memorization to gradually build a large collection of polite things to say and do. For example, one woman in her mid-50s told me that, some time in her 30s, she had noticed that her coworkers tended to smile and talk a lot when making reference to their own children. This observation led her to conclude that asking people about their children was something that made them willing to talk. Because she wanted to converse with people at lunchtime, she added questions about children to her repertoire of conversation starters.

I rarely teach these skills in isolation but do so within the context of teaching social norms or social inference, issues covered in the next two sections. Nevertheless, an example is provided below to illustrate how an instrumental skill can be targeted as the therapist is giving a patient a strategy for using eye contact in a more adaptive way. Notice that the rationale for building the skill is presented first, and then the strategy is provided.

Bob's comprehensive treatment plan was presented in Chapter 4 and appears in Figure 4.3. He had multiple presenting problems, only one of which involved social skills (Problem 5). His plan involved many interventions; his acute anxiety and depression were addressed in his earlier sessions, leaving social skills as a lower priority. The following discussion took place in a session where social skills were just beginning to be addressed, after his acute anxiety and depression symptoms had improved.

First the rationale was explored.

PATIENT: People tell me I have poor eye contact. My parents are always telling me that people will like me if I make better eye contact. It's gotten to the point that it's all I can think about when I meet someone new. I become obsessed with the fact that I am not making eye contact.

THERAPIST: Why do you think that it is important?

PATIENT: I guess people think you are weird if you don't make eye contact. That's what my parents keep telling me.

THERAPIST: I noticed that you do make some eye contact with me. Is it something that you do sometimes but not others?

PATIENT: Yeah. It just feels strange to me. When I look at someone in the eye, it feels too intense. It almost hurts if I look too long. Like looking into the sun. I have to look away.

THERAPIST: Is it harder to do when you first meet someone?

PATIENT: Oh, definitely. It's much worse. I guess because I am nervous. If I am not nervous, I can do it a little bit. But still not for long.

THERAPIST: Yeah. I noticed that when you look at me, it is only for brief moments. I think you have good timing, though, and I think we might be able to build on that. I will explain that more in a minute. But first, let's try to figure out why people think eye contact is so important.

PATIENT: I have no clue. I just know it counts as a point against you if you don't do it right.

THERAPIST: What if I gave you a hint and told you that it is a tool for communication? You were a communication major in college, so how could you apply your knowledge to this problem?

PATIENT: I do not get that. Are people sending secret messages to each other with their eyes? That is bizarre.

THERAPIST: Well, sort of. When I look at you while you are talking, what am I telling you, even though I am not talking at that moment?

PATIENT: Oh. That you're listening to me.

THERAPIST: With my eyes? How?

PATIENT: I don't know. All I know is that I would not think you were listening if you did not look at me. If you looked out the window or something. Then I would be afraid you were not listening.

THERAPIST: Do you think that is important?

PATIENT: Well, yeah.

THERAPIST: Why?

PATIENT: If you did not listen to me, I would think you don't give a crap about me.

THERAPIST: OK, then. You answered a big part of the question. To use what you just said, people look at each other to signal that they are listening, which also conveys the message "I do give a crap about you."

PATIENT: OK. So, if I don't look at a new person I meet, that person thinks that I don't give a crap about them?

THERAPIST: Bingo.

PATIENT: Hmm. I thought it just made me look weird. But you're saying that I am sending people the wrong message.

THERAPIST: Right. Now I am going to ask you another question. How do you know that I am looking at you? You just said that you know I look at you while you are talking. But how did you find that out about me?

PATIENT: Because I look at you sometimes. I can see it. Even out of the corner of my eye I can see that you are looking at me.

THERAPIST: OK. So, we already talked about the importance of my looking at you to convey a message to you. Now we are talking about you looking at me in order to pick up that message. What would happen if you did not look at me at all during our sessions? Would you even know where I was looking? How would you know that I wasn't staring out the window?

PATIENT: Well, I wouldn't know.

THERAPIST: So, then you look at me to gain information.

PATIENT: I never really thought about that. I don't do that on purpose, but I see what you are saying.

THERAPIST: What is the point? In other words, what is another reason people look at each other and make eye contact, if the first reason is to *convey* a message?

PATIENT: I guess it is to *receive* a message.

THERAPIST: Right. Can you summarize by listing the two biggest reasons a person will look at another person's face, or make eye contact, while conversing?

PATIENT: One is to send the message that you are listening, and one is to see if the other person is sending a message—to receive the message.

THERAPIST: Exactly.

PATIENT: But what do I do about my problem that I feel like it is too intense? I told you that when I do look, the eye contact is so intense and I have to look away. How am I going to get over that?

Here the strategy is introduced.

THERAPIST: Think about the two reasons you just gave me for making eye contact. Do you have to stare continuously into someone's eyes in order to accomplish those two things?

PATIENT: No. I guess not. But what should I do?

THERAPIST: Other patients have told me that they have the same problem as you. It puts them on "sensory overload" to look directly into other people's eyes. So, I can share with you some of the strategies that they have learned that have helped them to feel more comfortable with this aspect of communication.

PATIENT: What, force myself to stare until I get used to it?

THERAPIST: No. I don't even think that would work—I actually think *that* would make you look weird!

PATIENT: Well, then what?

THERAPIST: I mentioned to you a few minutes ago that you are using some eye contact with me, and I said that "your timing is good." You are already practicing a skill that we can build on. I noticed that you use a lot of glances and make momentary eye contact. You often do this to punctuate certain things you are saying while you are talking. You also tend to look at me whenever I accentuate a point or pause between sentences while I am talking.

PATIENT: OK. I guess I do.

THERAPIST: I remember that you said you have enjoyed writing, right?

PATIENT: Yeah. I haven't done it lately. But I do like it.

THERAPIST: Think about how you use punctuation when you write. Pay special attention to commas and periods. What are they for?

PATIENT: They mark pauses or endings.

THERAPIST: OK. I want you to close your eyes and listen to me say something. Imagine the words being typed on a page and picture in your mind where you would put a comma or a period. (*Reads a brief paragraph from a book.*) Did you get an image of it?

PATIENT: Yeah, I think so.

THERAPIST: OK. Now, open your eyes and listen to me read it again. This time, I want you to give me a brief glance of eye contact at each point where there is a comma or period.

PATIENT: This is so odd. But OK.

THERAPIST: (*Reads the passage again while keeping the patient in the line of sight.*) That was great. You did it perfectly. How did it feel?

PATIENT: Very awkward.

THERAPIST: That's because it is awkward. I'm asking you to do something brand-new that will not feel natural at first. But with repeated practice, like anything new that you learn, it will get easier. Now let's do the same thing again, only I want you to say something to me. First close your eyes and say something while imagining the commas and periods. Then open your eyes and say it again, giving me momentary glances at those points.

This exercise was repeated several times across several sessions until the patient reported that he was using it in social situations. This strategy serves to teach the patient an isolated instrumental skill that was not acquired early in life the way it would be for a typical person. This is not a substitute for what early intervention provides to a young child on the autism spectrum because what an adult learns is likely to be qualitatively different from what a toddler learns through skill training. Bob is not likely to ever sustain long continuous eye contact with other people. However, he does not need to, especially because he finds it aversive, in order to succeed in exchanging important messages with other people through the strategy presented here.

Increasing the Fund of Social Knowledge

Increasing the patient's fund of social knowledge involves giving him or her information about social norms and codes of conduct that tend to be "unwritten"—that is, are not generally taught through explicit means. Typical people acquire this knowledge through inference as they grow and develop. These inferences are based on observation of other people and the accurate perception of nonverbal feedback that is given when a norm is violated; formal instruction is not usually needed. For example, typical people "just know" how far away to stand from someone while talking in the hallway at work or at a cocktail party, without ever having been given explicit, formal instructions on what the norm is (approximately 18 inches or arm's length), or "can just sense" when somebody is flirting with them and "just know" how to reciprocate. People with ASD, on the other hand, need more explicit instruction on such norms in order to learn them.

Although these skills do overlap with the instrumental skills mentioned earlier, building this fund of knowledge requires more abstract thinking ability. It is through discussion of social norms that the thoughts, beliefs, and expectations *of others* begin to be explored with the patient. Instrumental skills, as mentioned, can be memorized and performed successfully without any knowledge of what the other people in the environment are thinking. For example, patients can learn to smile and say, "Nice to meet you" when introduced to new people and can repeat the performance flawlessly every time, without having any idea why they are doing it. In order for the skill to be acquired, it is not necessary to know, for example, that people practice this behavior to make each other feel comfortable or to make a positive impression on each other.

Learning about social norms and rules, however, though requiring instrumental skills as a prerequisite, also requires an ability to imagine the expectations of others, which is the beginning of the social inference process. After all, many social rules exist only in the minds of the people in one's culture and society, as most are not written down anywhere. Of course, there are some written rules within one's society, including laws, religious rules, or secular codes of conduct that can be found in etiquette books. Beyond that there remain hundreds, maybe thousands, of rules that govern peoples' behavior that are not explicitly stated by any particular source.

Several commercially available tools for teaching these rules to adults with ASD are listed in the Appendix. One is a book called *The Hidden Curriculum: Practical Solutions for Understanding Unstated Rules in Social Situations* (Myles, Trautman, & Schelvan, 2004), which is described below.

The Hidden Curriculum

The Hidden Curriculum (Myles et al., 2004) includes a list of more than 400 statements about the social norms and expectations of people in a multitude of social settings. Some are very elementary instrumental skills that might be found in traditional etiquette books, such as this example:

"Always chew your food with your mouth closed."

However, many are more obscure norms that typical people know but are less likely to state explicitly. People with ASD often miss many pieces of this type of information, even those with high IQs. It may be surprising to the reader to learn that a bright, articulate person would need to be told the following:

"If you are around people who are not invited to a party you are going to attend, do not discuss the plans in front of them."
"When other seats are available in a movie theater, leave a space between yourself and a stranger."

I continue to be dismayed by the paucity of social information some of these patients possess relative to their intellectual functioning level. Family members and other supporters express frustration over this deficit and often make comments such as "Come on. How could he *not* know that by now?" I have come to adopt a motto regarding the knowledge of social norms in patients with ASD, which I occasionally have to remind myself about as well as members of the patient's support system. The saying is "Assume nothing; explain everything."

An example of one way the *Hidden Curriculum* (Myles et al., 2004) can be used is illustrated by the case of Rose, the 37-year-old woman with ASD who lived in a group home, introduced in Chapter 1. As a brief review, her social behavior was particularly immature, given her age and IQ. This immaturity had caused her to be fired from two different jobs that would have otherwise been quite manageable for her. As part of her treatment plan, the therapist had identified "increase understanding of social norms" as one goal. The *Hidden Curriculum* was introduced to her in one session, which caused her to protest. She glanced at the book and said, "This is for babies. I don't need this." The therapist knew that Rose did enjoy making jokes, using humor, and playing games, however. She tried to appeal to those qualities by approaching her again with the book, with the idea that it could be looked at "just for fun." This is how the discussion went:

THERAPIST: How about if we just read a couple of these each week, and you can tell me if each one makes sense or not; if you agree with the rule or not.

PATIENT: Don't I have to agree with all of them?

THERAPIST: No. Some of them may seem silly to you. Some of them are too easy and some of them are strange. Some of them will make us laugh. You can tell me which ones seem ridiculous to you, and we can discuss them.

PATIENT: OK. Can you read one to me now?

THERAPIST: OK, how about this one? (*Deliberately picks one that will appeal to Rose's sense of humor.*) "Pajamas should not be worn outdoors."

PATIENT: (*laughing*) That is ridiculous! Everyone knows that.

THERAPIST: Well, *someone* didn't know it, or else it would not be in this book.

PATIENT: Really? Well *I* know that! Read another one, please. This is funny.

This activity continued in the weekly sessions. Although other therapy goals were also being worked on, about 10 minutes of each session were spent reading these social rules. Eventually, Rose did not understand some of the rules, and she was willing to engage in a dialogue with the therapist about the rationale behind them. Here is a discussion that took place several weeks after the first one, while reading rules from the book again. Notice that the therapist uses Socratic questioning to get the patient to come up with the rationale behind the rule.

THERAPIST: Here is another one: "If you are eating at a friend's house and you don't like what is being served, say, 'Just a little bit please; I'm not very hungry' instead of 'I don't want anything—I don't like that.'"

PATIENT: I'm not eating what I don't like! No way!

THERAPIST: You don't have to eat it. But don't tell them you don't like it.

PATIENT: Why not? I think I should ask them to get me something I like.

THERAPIST: Has your mother ever had people over for dinner while you were there?

PATIENT: Yeah. All the time. She cooks a lot.

THERAPIST: Have you ever heard a guest tell her they did not like the food?

PATIENT: No.

THERAPIST: No? Why do you think that is?

PATIENT: Because she cooks good food. And she would get pissed if someone said that!

THERAPIST: Why? Let's go back to what you said you would do if you did not like the food at someone's house. Don't you think a guest has the right to ask your mom to give them something they like?

PATIENT: It takes my mother all day to make the food. They should eat it.

THERAPIST: But if someone doesn't like it . . .

PATIENT: I told you. My mom would get *pissed* if someone told her that.

THERAPIST: Because it took her all day to make it?

PATIENT: Yeah.

THERAPIST: Do you think it's possible that whenever *anyone* has people over to eat, that they have to put some work into preparing the food?

PATIENT: I guess so.

THERAPIST: Do you think anyone who has put work into preparing food would get pissed if the guests rejected it?

PATIENT: I guess so.

THERAPIST: Could that be the reason this rule is in this book?

PATIENT: Yeah, but I still think people should serve me what I like.

THERAPIST: Of course, we all prefer to eat what we like. When we go to restaurants we get to pick what we like because we are *paying* for it. But when you are at someone's house, they are giving you the food for free. That means you don't get to pick.

PATIENT: Hmm. Well, don't you think a good friend makes sure they have everything you like in their house already?

THERAPIST: You tell me. When was the last time your mother had people over?

PATIENT: Saturday.

THERAPIST: How many people were there?

PATIENT: I don't know. About 10.

THERAPIST: What did she make?

PATIENT: Lasagna. It was really good. Ummmmmm.

THERAPIST: Do you think she called up each one of them beforehand and asked them for a list of the things they like and things they don't like? Ten people? Ten lists?

PATIENT: No. That's ridiculous. She doesn't have time for that.

THERAPIST: OK. You just said that good friends make sure they have all of your preferred foods on hand. Does that mean your mother does not have time to be a good friend? She does not have time to find that out about each of her friend's food preferences?

PATIENT: She *is* a good friend because she is cooking all day to give them good food!

THERAPIST: But we're back to the same question again. What if one person out of the 10 who came over Saturday night happens to dislike lasagna?

PATIENT: They should shut up and eat it!

THERAPIST: Isn't that what this rule is saying we should all do?

PATIENT: OK, OK. I get the point. I guess I forgot that other people work hard at preparing food before I come over. I never thought about it because I didn't see them do it. But I guess they do it before I come over. OK. OK. I get it.

Rose demonstrated a problem that many people with ASD have, which is generalizing information. Typical people understand this rule because they can naturally generalize an experience they have had personally (e.g., watching Mom work hard on meal preparation) and assume that others must go through the same thing when preparing meals for guests even though it is not directly observed. Rose had never made that connection, however, until she received explicit guidance through that logic process. It would be easy for people to label Rose as selfish and uncaring about others. However, once she made the connection between her mother's hard work and the work of others, she accepted the rule.

The Social Narrative

The social narrative provides a useful tool for moving away from hypothetical situations into using real-life scenarios that may be problematic for a patient. A story is cowritten by the therapist and the patient that integrates *new social information* with the *patient's current perspective* on the situation. A formula for designing such a narrative is found in the Myles and colleagues *Hidden Curriculum* (2004) book mentioned above. Instructions can also be found in the Social Stories™ approach offered by Gray (1995, 2015).

Although the stories vary greatly according to the age, functioning level, and learning style of the patient, all can be used to teach social norms that will be personally relevant to the patient. Most will include a description of the situation that is currently causing a problem, information about the patient's current subjective experience of the situation, information about how others feel and react, and what prompts the feelings and expectations of others in such situations. The expectations should be explained in a way that fits the information-processing style of the person and should include some direction for what the patient should *do* in such circumstances, based on the expectations of others. The therapist should avoid using language that is judgmental or critical about the patient's maladaptive behavior, however. In other words, the story should not be focused on telling the patient that his or her behavior has been wrong or inappropriate. Generally, the patient has already been told that numerous times, but has not been told why. The assumption behind this intervention is that the patient needs to be told *why* his or her strategy is not working or else behavior change will not occur.

This approach is hard to grasp without an example, so one is described here. Ted was a 19-year-old man who had been repeatedly asked to leave college classrooms and had been fired from several jobs because of his overtly intrusive behavior, which involved violating other people's "invisible boundaries." The most frequent complaint of others was that he would ask people he did not know very well whether they had any candy or gum to give him. He would persist with his question whenever someone denied having any to give. Although it was a relatively harmless behavior on one level, it annoyed people to the point of avoiding him or directly criticizing him in an unkind way. It also made him appear vulnerable in front of strangers, and I was concerned that he was risking exploitation by predatory members of the community. He had been told repeatedly by supporters (e.g., family members and teachers) that the behavior was inappropriate, but he did not seem affected by that feedback. I took advantage of an opportunity to write a social narrative with him when the location of sessions was to be incidentally changed from one location to another. The original location was a quiet, private, sole practitioner's office, but the new one was in a busy outpatient medical clinic. I was concerned that Ted would alienate everyone in the office on the first day there by asking other patients in the waiting room and office staff for gum or candy. Therefore, this scenario was chosen as the center of the story.

The following narrative was written in one session the week before the change in location was to occur. I sat next to the patient at a computer and alternated writing phrases. Whenever I used my words to describe the patient's thoughts or feelings, I used a hypothesis about what *might be* the patient's experience and checked it with him before settling on it. If I made a wrong assumption, the patient would let me know, and the wrong phrase would be erased. I was confident that the patient was able to discriminate between phrases that matched his experience, versus those that did not, as he appeared to put careful thought into each one before endorsing it or not. Whenever I wrote phrases that imparted social information to the patient, I would check to see whether he understood what was being said. If he did not understand or he disagreed with a norm, we would stop writing and discuss the rationale in more detail. With this process, the end product, presented below, included a relatively accurate assessment of the patient's perspective, which was integrated with new information about social norms and direction on what he should do in such situations.

> *I am going to see Dr. Gaus in a new place next week.*
> *I might get to the clinic early.*
> *I get nervous when I have to wait. I also get bored if I have to wait.*
> *I feel better if I eat a snack or candy.*
> *Sometimes there is candy in waiting rooms.*
> *Candy that is displayed in a dish on the coffee table or counter is for people to take. This is "public food."*
> *Candy that is not displayed publicly on the coffee table or counter is "private food."*
> *People keep "private food" in their drawers, cabinets, pockets, or purses.*
> *People feel offended when they are asked to give away their "private food."*
> *Sometimes when people feel offended, they hide those feelings.*
> *I will bring a book with me. If I have to wait, I can read my book.*
> *I will bring some Life Savers in my backpack. If I have to wait, I can eat some of my Life Savers.*

Interestingly, when I wrote the phrase "People feel offended when they are asked to give away their 'private food,'" the patient adamantly protested. I paused in the writing process and the following dialogue took place:

PATIENT: That is *not* true. You are wrong.

THERAPIST: What's wrong about it?

PATIENT: People don't feel offended. I have never seen that. You are wrong.

THERAPIST: How do you know they are not offended?

PATIENT: Because they always give me the gum or candy. I don't think they would give it to me if they were mad at me. Most people share their candy.

THERAPIST: Do you think that it is possible that people could give you the candy *even though* they are offended? Could people be offended but still give away their candy?

PATIENT: I can tell when people are mad. They usually curse at me or call me names. But those people don't give me their candy. They're mean, anyway. They probably have bad candy. (*Laughs.*)

THERAPIST: Do you think it is possible that there are types of annoyance that people are less dramatic about? I mean, are cursing and name-calling the only ways people show that they are offended?

PATIENT: I never noticed anything else. What do you mean?

THERAPIST: I mean that people sometimes feel annoyed inside but don't show it outside. In our society, it is usually considered rude to ask people to give away their private food. I know this is kind of confusing, but in our society, it is also considered polite to hide annoyed feelings from people whom you don't know very well. So, polite people will usually hide those feelings from you because they don't want to hurt your feelings. But they are still secretly annoyed as they give you the candy. It may lead some people to think you are rude or strange, but their politeness stops them from telling you that out loud. They will hand you their candy but will not want to be your friend and may even try to avoid you if they see you again on another day.

PATIENT: (*pause*) Hmm. I never really noticed that. People do avoid me sometimes, but I figure it's just because they are not nice.

THERAPIST: Well, we can certainly talk about that some more, maybe even in some other sessions. For now, though, would you be willing to consider that when people are offended, they sometimes hide those feelings?

PATIENT: Yeah, I guess so. I never thought about that before.

THERAPIST: OK. Then I will add a line to our story about that.

As you can see, this process serves not only as an intervention but also as an ongoing assessment. In this example, I gained more information about the way the patient perceived social situations that I may not have learned through other means.

On the day of the appointment, I called the patient at home and asked him to read this story out loud and to ask questions about any part that was still unclear. When he came to the appointment later that day, I was unable to observe him in the waiting room because I was in session. However, he was asked to evaluate his own performance when his session started, and he proudly reported success; he did not ask one person for gum or candy. His accomplishment was praised, and I was pleased at the effectiveness of the intervention. Nevertheless, after he left, I went around the office and queried staff about his conduct. They all corroborated his self-report. He had not asked anyone for gum or candy. However, he had asked them all for money, as he had spotted a vending machine in the building on the way in. On one hand this sounds like a humorous punch line to this case example. On the other hand, it serves as a powerful lesson about how literal minded these patients can be, and how skills taught in one context will not necessarily generalize to another. Needless to say, the next session was spent writing a social narrative about asking people for money!

Improving Social Cognition

Having good instrumental skills and a solid fund of social knowledge is, as previously noted, still not enough for social success. One must know *when to use* these skills; to be able to recognize which social encounters call for which instrumental behaviors and relate to *which social norms*. This type of knowledge is based on the ability to assess the social context of a situation, observe the verbal and nonverbal behavior of other people, infer their mental states, understand what is expected, and then carry it out. This is the most complex set of skills.

I often tell patients that I wish I could have ongoing video footage of all the social encounters they are having from day to day in the natural environment. This hypothetical footage could be used in session for discussions about the verbal and nonverbal communication between each patient and the people he or she encounters. Until I can figure out a way to make that happen, I must rely on other means of teaching patients how to "read" others and then use that information to come up with adaptive responses. For all patients, a combination of the following interventions is used to build these skills.

- Didactic presentation of commercially available materials.
- Retrospective discussions about encounters the patient reports having had between sessions.
- Behavioral rehearsal of planned encounters.
- Incidental feedback on the natural behavior displayed during interactions with the therapist.

No matter how basic or sophisticated the skills being taught are, multimodal teaching strategies will optimize learning. For example, if teaching a patient how to apply a new social norm that requires reading the nonverbal cues of others, using didactic presentation alone is not as likely to lead to behavior change if not combined with visual aids, rehearsal, and/or incidental feedback.

Several published teaching packages include useful tools for enhancing social cognition. They are listed and briefly described below. More detailed information about sources can be found in the Appendix.

- *Social Stories*™ (Gray, 1995, 2015). The author is an educator who developed this social narrative approach in educational settings for adolescents with ASD. It was already introduced in the previous section as a tool for teaching social norms. It is also used to enhance perspective-taking skills and to introduce the idea of inferring mental states of others.

- *Comic Strip Conversations* (Gray, 1994). This workbook comes from the same author who developed Social Stories, and it offers visual materials based on traditional comic symbols (e.g., bubbles above people's heads symbolizing thoughts), which can teach various social inference concepts to patients. This approach can be used for analyzing incidents that have already occurred or to prepare for and rehearse planned social encounters.

• *Mind Reading Software* (Cambridge University, 2004). This interactive software, created by a team headed by Simon Baron-Cohen, presents patients with a variety of real-life faces, gestures, body postures, and scenarios on the computer screen to teach them to infer mental states.

• *Social Literacy: A Social Skills Seminar for Young Adults with ASDs, NLDs, and Social Anxiety* (Cohen, 2011). This workbook and CD provides curriculum materials to teach a 12-week course to adults with social-cognition deficits how to become more skillful in managing the social demands of adult life.

• *Program for the Education and Enrichment of Relational Skills (PEERS®) for Young Adults: Social Skills Training for Adults with Autism Spectrum Disorder and Other Social Challenges* (Laugeson, 2017). This workbook provides the instructions to a therapist to deliver a 16-week intervention to adult patients and targets both social-behavioral and social-cognitive factors.

• *Inside Out: What Makes a Person with Social Cognitive Deficits Tick?* (Winner, 2000) and *Thinking about You Thinking about Me* (Winner, 2002). The author of both of these workbooks is a speech–language pathologist who has developed an excellent set of strategies that target the *cognitive dysfunction* believed to be responsible for the overt social behavior problems observed in people with ASD and related syndromes. She provides a multitude of worksheets and exercises that are well suited to teaching adults about social inference and perspective taking.

• *Asperger's Syndrome and Sexuality: From Adolescence through Adulthood* (Hénault, 2005). This book is a valuable resource for assessing social–sexual treatment needs and offers a set skill-building program aimed at increasing competency in the sexual domain of functioning.

The individualized treatment plan of a patient will direct which of these intervention strategies are chosen and how they are combined. As mentioned before, these abilities involve dynamic and flexible processes that cannot be taught as static, isolated behaviors. In that sense, the therapist should interweave these concepts into everything that is done in session, no matter what the topic of discussion might be, teaching patients through both direct and indirect means. Even if the therapist is talking to the patient about a financial problem, let's say, the impact that social-cognition issues may have had on the money problem can be in the back of the therapist's mind. Also, the way in which the therapist interacts with the patient during the money discussion can be guided by social behavior that the therapist is trying to model for the patient. The following description offers one example of how higher-level social-cognition skills can be taught directly.

Perspective-Taking Exercises

The case of Andrew was introduced in Chapter 4. To briefly review, he is a 32-year-old man who has a degree in culinary arts and works as a manager in a gourmet food shop. He came to therapy looking for help with his lack of social relationships and depressive symptoms. He has a passionate interest and talent in model railroad building, of which he is ashamed. I had determined that, among other issues, his extreme self-focus and sour-appearing expressions were probably contributing to his friendship and dating problems. Extremely poor perspective-taking skills were likely playing a role, as per the model put forth by Winner (2000, 2002). When I asked Andrew to describe several different scenarios in which he had been uncomfortable in social situations (e.g., at a bar with coworkers, "hanging out" with his brother's friends), I asked him to tell me a little bit about each person with whom he interacted. He knew almost nothing about any of them (e.g., their interests, family situations, personality traits). It appeared that he did not know how to focus on others and learn more about them, which is a basic skill necessary for relationship success. Granted, his depressive symptoms were also playing a role in this process, and that area was being addressed in the treatment plan through other means. To address the self-focus, I chose to use exercises in the *Thinking about You Thinking about Me* book (Winner, 2002). The following discussion shows how the idea was introduced to Andrew.

THERAPIST: Andrew, we have been talking quite a bit about how frustrated you are with your lack of social connections.

PATIENT: Yes. I am totally sick of it. I am sick and tired of being ignored.

THERAPIST: It sounds like you really have been ignored in a lot of the situations you told me about. It also sounds like you are quite nervous each time you are in a group of people.

PATIENT: I am. I just don't know what to do about it. How can I get people to notice me and see that I am a nice guy?

THERAPIST: Well, Andrew, I have to say that I found it interesting last week in our session that you were not able to tell me very much about your coworkers or your brother's friends. It seems as though in the time you have known them, you have not learned anything about them.

PATIENT: How can I? They have not given me the time of day!

THERAPIST: Have you given them the time of day?

PATIENT: What do you mean?

THERAPIST: It seems that they are ignoring you. But it also seems that you are ignoring them.

PATIENT: I don't understand.

THERAPIST: You want to become friendly with these people, but you have not done one of the things that people do when they want to get to know someone. They learn about them. How do you even know if you like them, or which ones you like, if you don't know anything about them?

PATIENT: I don't know.

THERAPIST: (*Remembers his culinary arts training.*) People are like food and wine. You have to figure out which kind you like. They are not all the same, and you won't like all of them.

PATIENT: Well, I don't think I can afford to be so picky.

THERAPIST: Well, maybe you won't be picky yet. But the process of *getting to know* someone is actually going to help you in more than one way. If you practice some strategies that I am going to suggest to you, there are two things that are going to change for you. One is that you will be so busy with the exercise I am going to give you that you will be less focused on yourself and therefore less nervous. The second is that you will actually appear more appealing to others because people enjoy the idea that someone else is interested in *them*. Let me show you a worksheet that will help with this. This is called the "Visual Web of What You Remember about Others." (*Shows the patient the worksheet from Winner, 2002, presented in Figure 6.1.*) This sheet gives you a framework for beginning to get to know someone. Think of one person in one of the groups you hang out with whom you would like to do this worksheet for this week.

PATIENT: How about Paul? I work with him every afternoon.

THERAPIST: OK. Write his name in the middle circle of this sheet. Then for homework, fill in the four boxes with the information requested.

PATIENT: Oh, I already know something for the types of food he likes. He loves Thai food.

THERAPIST: How did you know that?

PATIENT: I heard him tell a customer he was serving one time.

THERAPIST: Perfect. Write that down in the food box. Why do you think that just came to your mind now, and not last week when I was asking what you knew about these people?

PATIENT: I guess I'm in a different mind-set right now. I'm also less nervous. I can't think of things when I'm nervous.

THERAPIST: Well, that means you are using this sheet correctly already. It is supposed to simultaneously change your mind-set and reduce your anxiety. I think you are going to be good at this. OK, so this week you will finish this sheet. One thing to keep in mind is, do not approach Paul and "interview" him all at once. That may appear awkward. Rather, try to see how much you can learn just by continuing to listen to him talk to customers—for example, like the way you found out about his favorite food. Then occasionally ask him a question if you have free time with him.

PATIENT: So that's all I have to do this week?

THERAPIST: Yes. I will show you what we are going to do in the near future. (*Shows the patient the "Creating Files in Your Brain" worksheet from Winner, 2002, shown in Figure 6.2.*) This sheet shows you where we are headed. Each person in your social group will eventually be represented on this sheet—and hopefully in your memory because the goal is to create a "file" in your head on each person.

Andrew used these sheets for 6 weeks until he was more accepting of the idea that getting to know someone is a mutual process, in which each person is responsible for paying attention to each other.

In summary, this section presented strategies for social skill building in adults with ASD. Three levels of skill needs were described separately for the sake of conceptualization: *instrumental skills*, the *fund of social knowledge skills*, and *social cognition skills*. However, therapists generally teach all three types of skills in an integrated fashion, depending on the individualized case formulation for a given patient. Materials and

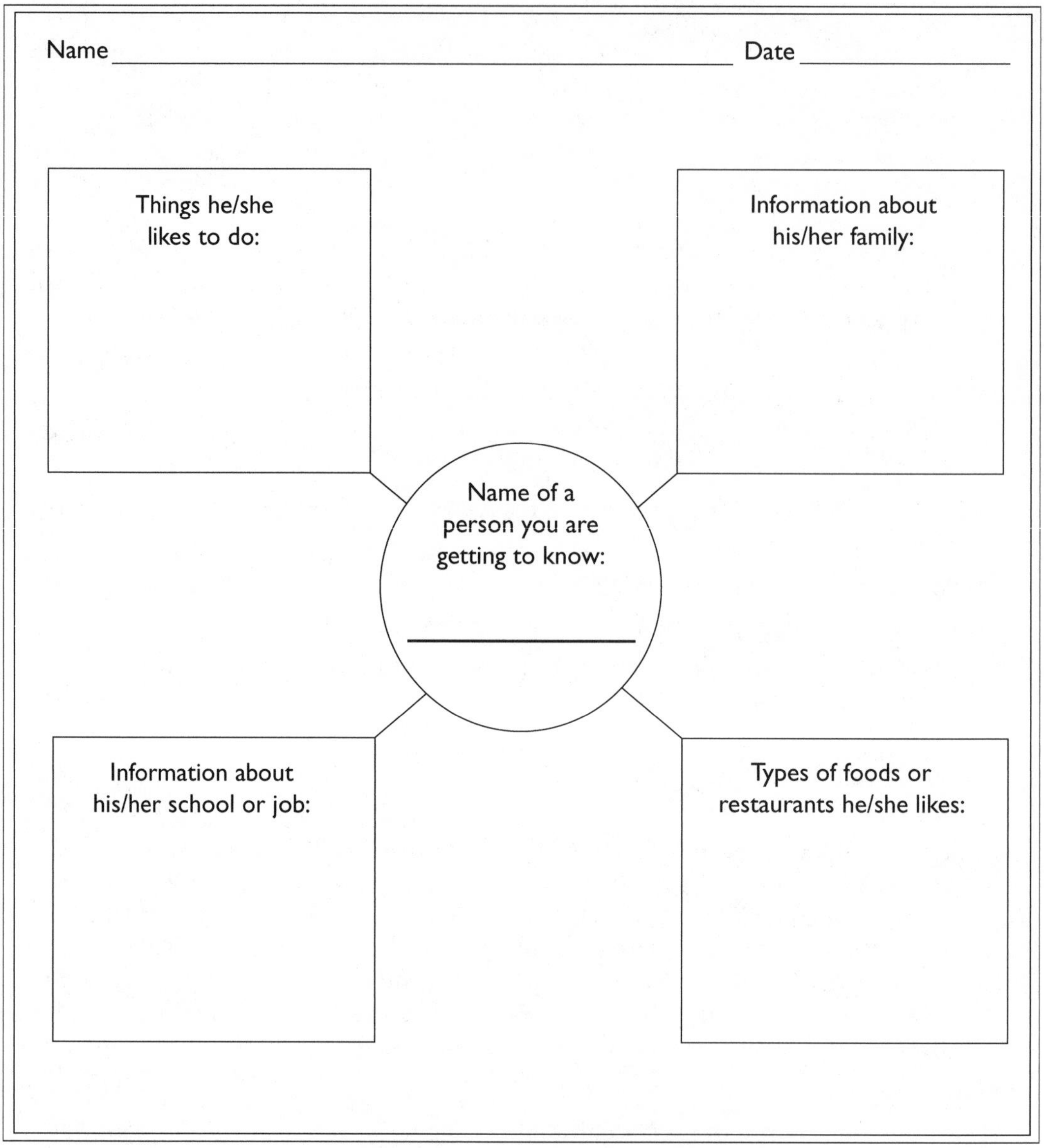

Name _____ Date _____

Things he/she
likes to do:

Information about
his/her family:

Name of a
person you are
getting to know:

_____

Information about
his/her school or job:

Types of foods or
restaurants he/she likes:

FIGURE 6.1. Worksheet: Visual web of what you remember about others. From Winner (2002). Copyright © 2002 Michelle Garcia Winner. Reprinted by permission.

Your brain holds all the information for what you think and know. Getting to know someone else means you have to store that information in a file in your brain. You have to work at remembering to put the information into your brain. Then the next time you see that person, you can brainstorm, which means when you think hard about that person, you will be able to open your file about them!

Below, brainstorm what you remember about the different people you have met in this group.

I remember 3 things about

_____

1. _____

2. _____

3. _____

I remember 3 things about

_____

1. _____

2. _____

3. _____

I remember 3 things about

_____

1. _____

2. _____

3. _____

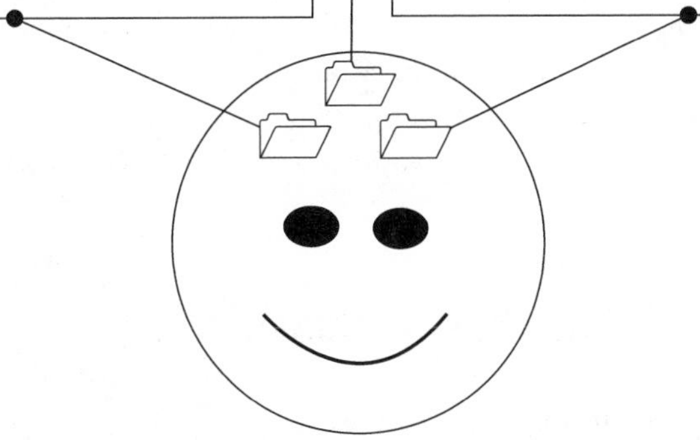

FIGURE 6.2. Worksheet: Creating files in your brain to remember about others. From Winner (2002). Copyright © 2002 Michelle Garcia Winner. Reprinted by permission.

resources that have been developed for this purpose were recommended. Although some of these published packages have been designed for different settings and age levels, case examples were used to illustrate how they could be applied in an adult psychotherapy context.

Improving Assertive Communication Skills

The last skill set addressed in this section is assertiveness, or the strategies people use to ask other people for things they need, and to say no or disagree with unwanted requests from others. For people with disabilities, the term *self-advocacy* is often used instead, and may be familiar to patients with ASD. When a person lacks these abilities, a sense of disempowerment and no control over one's life is a common experience. Improving these abilities allows for more opportunities to exercise choices and avoid exploitation by others. Assertive communication is a complex social skill and can be considered an important part of the social language and pragmatic skills that speech–language pathologists may work on with patients with ASD. Psychotherapists can also teach these skills through the wide variety of packages that have been published for typical adults. I find the approach offered by Linehan (2014) in the *interpersonal effectiveness* component of her *DBT Skills Training Manual* to be most useful. In line with Linehan's model, patients not only need to learn the skills but also gain an understanding of *why* they find it hard to be assertive. People with ASD may encounter obstacles that are different from other patients, but will still benefit from learning the strategies, once their unique barriers to practicing them are addressed.

As described in Chapter 2, adults with ASD have a higher rate of alexithymia (a deficit in the fund or accessibility of words to describe subjective mental states) than typical adults (Berthoz & Hill, 2005; Samson, Huber, & Gross, 2012). This could interfere with learning and practicing assertiveness communication because one must be able to first *recognize* an internal mental state, *acknowledge* that distress can be a signal for a need to initiate a change in the environment, and *differentiate* emotions from needs before *translating* the need into words as an assertive statement or request. Before embarking on such training, a therapist should assess for basic emotion identification ability and/or presence of alexithymia (e.g., using the TAS-20). If the patient is showing a deficit in this area, strategies to address those impairments can be implemented, as described in Chapter 8.

Increasing Coping Skills

In addition to the socialization problems discussed above, some symptoms of ASD create ongoing stress in an individual's life. Simple daily tasks and responsibilities are difficult to manage because of EF problems. Sensory input and emotional arousal are not easily modulated, making even the most mundane events overwhelming. Cognitive rigidity makes adaptation to change and unexpected events very challenging. For most patients with ASD, a portion of the treatment plan should be devoted to building coping skills so that stress can be managed more effectively (Gaus, 2011; Groden et al., 1994, 2006). The acquisition of coping skills enhances quality of life, supports the treatment of comorbid mental health problems, and prevents relapse of those comorbid conditions. In the spirit of Meichenbaum's (1985) stress inoculation model, different patients will need to learn different skills, depending on which factors are making them most vulnerable to stress, and the individualized case formulation will specify those factors for a given patient.

Rationale for Developing Compensatory Skills

Despite the fact that an ASD diagnosis in adulthood can bring some relief, it also brings many questions to mind about ability versus disability. During the psychoeducational process discussed in Chapter 5, patients often connect the symptoms with the nonsocial problems they have in carrying out the tasks of daily living and performing well at a job. They often ask, "How much of this problem can I change, and how much do I have to accept?" or "Which abilities can I learn, and which ones do I have to live without?"

The therapist does not have easy answers to these questions but can guide the patient through a self-assessment process, with the goal of gaining a better understanding of strengths and deficits. Although I support a strengths-based approach, I also value helping the patient come to a realistic understanding of his or her own limitations. The more clearly defined a deficit is, the easier it is for the patient to come up with a way to get around the inherent obstacles. This circumvention can be very difficult, however, because so many of the deficits are subtle in their presentation. Receptive language processing problems, EF deficits (planning, organization), high emotional arousal, and sensory sensitivities all make a person function poorly and can easily be misattributed by other people to "character flaws." Individuals with ASD have heard remarks throughout their lives such as "He [she] doesn't keep his [her] room clean because he [she] is just plain lazy." As a result of such misattributions, many have learned to hide their problems from people in order to avoid criticism—but through strategies that are maladaptive. Andrew's case, which is mentioned again under "Organization and Time Management Skills" below, serves as a good example of this point.

Because there can be a tendency to try to hide deficits, talking openly with the therapist about these issues makes some patients feel very uneasy. The therapist can assure the reluctant patient that this type of self-assessment is something that most typical adults do naturally. As far as tasks of daily living, a typical healthy adult who knows he or she is not good at something (e.g., balancing the checkbook, cooking, fixing leaky pipes) will find somebody else to do it for him or her, either getting a family member or friend to do it, or hiring someone to do it. Occupational choices are also affected by a typical adult's realistic assessments about his or her own deficits. Part of the effort of choosing a profession, for example, involves ruling out things that a person knows he or she *would not* be good at doing. Like so many things that typical people do without much conscious thought, people with ASD need to go through this process with explicit guidance. Normalizing the need to go through this self-examination will often increase the patient's willingness to find ways to compensate for his or her deficits.

To facilitate this process, I wrote a self-help book for adults with ASD, *Living Well on the Spectrum: How to Use Your Strengths to Meet the Challenges of Asperger Syndrome/ High-Functioning Autism* (Gaus, 2011). It can serve as a companion to the sessions when self-acceptance and stress management goals are being addressed, including the skill areas targeted in this section. The coping skills training from which patients with ASD most commonly benefit are *organization and time management, problem solving, relaxation,* and *assertive communication.* All can be seen as strategies for compensation in that they help individuals manage their deficits more effectively. Most of the therapy approaches discussed here have a long history of demonstrated efficacy with typical adults. Because they are so thoroughly presented by their original sources, they are not described in detail here. Descriptions are given of any special considerations or modifications the therapist may make for adults with ASD, but references to more comprehensive instructions for the techniques are provided for readers who are less familiar with them. There are some cognitive strategies (reappraisal, self-instruction) and mindfulness-based CBT strategies (emotion identification/acceptance, mindfulness exercises) that, though often considered part of coping and stress management, are addressed in Chapters 7 and 8, when the treatment of comorbid mental health problems is described.

Organization and Time Management Skills

It is not uncommon for people with ASD to have problems organizing spaces (e.g., living space, work space, carrying cases/bags). Related to this are problems often seen with creating or following a schedule. Chronic lateness is a complaint for some patients, whereas for others, a sense of "never getting anything done" contributes to stress. The EF deficits described in Chapter 2 likely contribute to some patients' poor awareness of how they are spending their time, or to their unrealistic ideas about what can be completed in an hour or a day. The following list includes examples of strategies that can help patients manage space and time more effectively. These can be practiced by using a variety of materials and media, including smartphone applications.

- Use an organizational checklist to clean out and organize small spaces.
- Make environmental modifications so spaces are "friendly" to sensory or EF profile.
- Build in times for discarding unneeded items during the weekly routine.
- Use a blank daily schedule template to take baseline data on how time is being spent.
- Make a "to-do" list and put items in priority order.
- Set small realistic goals for each day or week.
- Use visual cues to help remind self about tasks.

The self-help book *The Smart but Scattered Guide to Success: How to Use Your Brain's Executive Skills to Keep Up, Stay Calm, and Get Organized at Work and at Home* (Dawson & Guare, 2016) is a guide for any adult wanting to improve EF skills and has many more strategies like the ones listed above. Autism-specific tools can be found in Gaus (2011).

One of the interventions that was built into Andrew's treatment plan was time management training. Among his other problems, he had great difficulty completing the tasks for which he was responsible, mostly related to housekeeping. His parents reported that they were often frustrated with him when he lived in their house, as he always had a cluttered room. He never seemed to complete tasks they would ask him to do in the family home. They viewed him as a procrastinator, and when they got angry with him, they would call him lazy. Now that he was living in his own apartment, his whole place was "a cluttered mess." Andrew told me that he felt overwhelmed by the tasks, and although he always intended to do them, he had no idea of how to start. He had learned to "yay say" his parents, always promising to do things they asked him to, while thinking that he did not know how to get started. He was afraid to discuss this problem with them, and his lack of communication with them only heightened their frustration with what they viewed as procrastination. The discussion he had with me revealed that he believed he did not have enough time to do all of the things he needed to do. This outlook was puzzling because he worked fewer than 40 hours a week and had very few commitments outside of work. After exploring this area more, it seemed that he was distorting time in several ways. One was that he thought he had less time than he really did. The other was that he estimated the amount of time some tasks would take as being longer than they really would. In addition, he seemed unable to choose a task to do at any given moment. If he had some time available, he would ponder all the tasks he could possibly think about, all at once, and get so overwhelmed by this process that he would choose none. Finally, he did not know how to break down a big task into smaller steps.

To address this problem, Andrew was first asked to log his time for 1 week. He was given a blank activity schedule sheet (from Persons et al., 2000) that shows a week with each day broken down into 1-hour blocks. He was asked to fill in each hour, noting the activity he was doing at that time. He was instructed not to try to modify how he spent his time because the purpose was to get a picture of how he *typically* spent his time. After he completed this assignment, he was able to use the visual representation to more accurately assess his availability. Then he was asked to make a list of all of the things on which he felt he was behind. When asked to put them in priority order, he had difficulty. He paused and thought about each one but reported that he did not know how to choose which one should go first because they were all important. An entire session was spent teaching Andrew a prioritization system by categorizing each item as one of the following:

- *"Urgent*—I must do this ASAP" (neglecting it would cause imminent threat to my health, safety, or financial standing).
- *"Important*—I would like to do this soon" (nonurgent things that would make me feel good or involve a commitment I have made to someone else).
- *"Can wait*—I would like this to be done sometime in the next 6–12 months" (I would enjoy seeing this done, but no harm will be done if I do not do it soon).

After the list was categorized, Andrew was shown how to make a to-do list. As mentioned, he had a tendency to think of *all* the things he had to do all the time. Even after he had made his prioritization list, he seemed to have difficulty mentally filtering out the items that were less important from those that were more important. Therefore, when he made his to-do list for the upcoming week, he was directed to also make a not-to-do list, where all of the things that he had not chosen for the week would be written. He was told that he was not allowed to do the things on the not-to-do list. A self-instructional strategy was suggested; he was told that if he found his mind wandering to the things on the not-to-do list, he was to say to himself, "Andrew, you are not allowed to do those things this week. Don't use time and energy focusing on not-to-do items. You need your energy for what is on this week's list. Look at your to-do list *only*." This strategy was meant to alleviate some of the pressure he seemed to be putting on himself to complete too many things in too little time. Finally, he was shown how to take a large task (e.g., cleaning out the basement) and make it into a list of smaller tasks that did not all need to be done on the same day or in the same week (e.g., pick up garbage from basement floor, sort recycling items, sort items for donation, designate different storage areas for different types of things, buy or repair shelving units). Andrew reported an improvement in his task management after practicing these strategies over several weeks.

Problem-Solving Skills

Because of the difficulties experienced by these patients in regulating their emotions and sensory experiences, they are easily overwhelmed by problems that may seem minor to other people. They have difficulty drawing inferences from information (Rumsey & Hamburger, 1988) and are also subject to repeat errors despite feedback that they are incorrect responses (Hoffman & Prior, 1982). In one study of problem-solving ability in adolescents with ASD, subjects were presented with novel problem scenarios. Compared with typical controls, they showed poorer memory for pertinent facts in the scenario, less generation of appropriate solutions, and difficulty choosing optimal solutions (Channon, Charman, Heap, Crawford, & Rios, 2001). Teaching them a traditional problem-solving formula, based on the work of D'Zurilla and colleagues (e.g., D'Zurilla, 1986; D'Zurilla & Goldfried, 1971), can give them one tool for modulating the intense emotional reaction they may have to an unexpected problem by learning to (1) define the problem more objectively, (2) practice generating and choosing viable options, and (3) evaluate their own performance of solutions. The process involved in filling out a worksheet, such as the one shown in Figure 6.3, can help some patients decrease their arousal level in the face of an overwhelming problem. The therapist may need to take more time teaching these skills than might be necessary with a typical adult. In Gaus (2011), a modification of the traditional problem-solving model is presented in which some steps are broken down into smaller separate steps to appeal to the learning style of people with ASD. As shown in Figure 6.3, Step 3 was added to allow the patient an opportunity to consider some ASD-specific issues that might be interfering with solution generation. Steps 5 and 6 represent components of what would be a single step in the traditional model, but warrants separation for this population to reduce the risk of becoming overwhelmed. A multimodal schematic diagram that can be used to present the model to patients is shown in Figure 6.4. Once the patient has learned how to fill out a sheet (while in a calm state, of course), it can later become a self-soothing activity in the face of a significant dilemma. As one patient put it, there is comfort to be found in "having something to do" with the thoughts and feelings that are "wreaking havoc in the mind." Reading the sheet and writing in answers is incompatible with other maladaptive reactions that many adults with ASD have reported in the face of extreme stress (e.g., nonfunctional rumination, screaming, punching walls, banging head on objects), and the structure that is provided by the problem-solving formula is appealing to people with ASD.

Figure 6.5 contains an example of a problem that was effectively managed by Rachel, a 36-year-old woman with ASD who was introduced in Chapter 1. Three full sessions were spent on this exercise, which was based on the Gaus (2011) adapted problem-solving worksheet. In the first, she described a conflict that had arisen between her work schedule at a new job and her physical therapy appointments, which she needed to help in the healing of a shoulder injury. She had not taken any active steps to solve the problem but was becoming increasingly angry and frustrated each day. Her anger was directed toward others in her life and was beginning to affect her interactions with her boss. The worksheet was introduced and problem identification was completed. The second session was spent finishing the sheet, and the third was spent following up. The overlap with other therapy components is apparent in Figure 6.5, in that assertiveness skills, reappraisal, self-monitoring, and self-reinforcement were involved. This

(Text resumes on page 182.)

Go through these steps in order by answering each question. Try to focus on one step at a time and be sure to complete all eight steps without skipping any.

1. **Problem identification:** *What is bothering me in this situation?*

   _____

   _____

2. **Goal selection:** *How do I wish it could be different?*

   _____

   _____

3. **Identification of obstacles:** *What is getting in my way?*

   _____

   _____

   _____

4. **Generation of alternatives:** *What are the possible solutions for the obstacles?*

   _____

   _____

   _____

   _____

   _____

5. **Consideration of consequences:** *What are the pros and cons of each solution?*

   _____

   _____

   _____

   _____

   _____

   _____

6. **Decision making:** *Which solution(s) should I try first?*

   _____

   _____

   _____

7. **Implementation:** *Now I will try the solution(s) and track my progress.*

   _____

   _____

   _____

8. **Evaluation:** *Did it meet my goal, or do I need to try a different solution?*

   _____

   _____

   _____

FIGURE 6.3. Problem-solving worksheet.

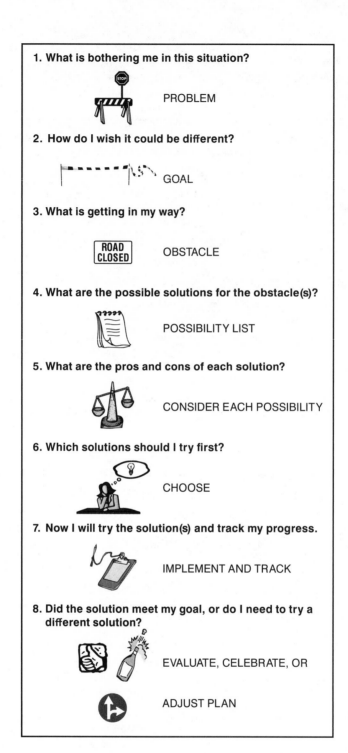

1. What is bothering me in this situation?

PROBLEM

2. How do I wish it could be different?

GOAL

3. What is getting in my way?

ROAD CLOSED   OBSTACLE

4. What are the possible solutions for the obstacle(s)?

POSSIBILITY LIST

5. What are the pros and cons of each solution?

CONSIDER EACH POSSIBILITY

6. Which solutions should I try first?

CHOOSE

7. Now I will try the solution(s) and track my progress.

IMPLEMENT AND TRACK

8. Did the solution meet my goal, or do I need to try a different solution?

EVALUATE, CELEBRATE, OR

ADJUST PLAN

FIGURE 6.4. Problem-solving steps. From Gaus (2011). Copyright © 2011 The Guilford Press. Reprinted by permission.

1. **Problem identification:** *What is bothering me in this situation?*

   I have to go to physical therapy three times a week. The physical therapy office gave me appointment times that are during my work hours. I asked my boss if I could come in late a few days a week and she said no.

2. **Goal selection:** *How do I wish it could be different?*

   I want to be able to make my physical therapy appointments.

3. **Identification of obstacles:** *What is getting in my way?*

   My anxiety about others getting mad at me is getting in the way. My lack of experience voicing my needs (being assertive) leads me to run out of ideas of what to say. Then I assume I have to put up with what others decide for me, even if it is not the best for me.

4. **Generation of alternatives:** *What are the possible solutions for the obstacles?*

   a. Ask the physical therapist to change the time.

   b. Avoid physical therapy for a few weeks.

   c. Try to sneak into work late, hoping the boss will not notice.

   d. Talk to the boss again, explain more about the situation.

   e. Talk to the boss again and offer to work late on the days I come in late.

   f. Approach the boss in a demanding fashion and tell her she is being insensitive.

   g. Quit my job.

5. **Consideration of consequences:** *What are the pros and cons of each solution?*

   a. The office sounded firm about these times. It is not likely to work.

   b. I may go backward in my healing.

   c. It will cause more anxiety and stress trying to avoid being caught.

   d. This may work because I had not gone into detail with her.

   e. She would like the idea of my making up the time.

   f. She would become angry, and the problem would not be solved.

   g. I like my job, and it would be a great loss.

6. **Decision making:** *Which solution(s) should I try first?*

   Considering all of the possibilities, there are three things I could try. I am going to start with the one most likely to work. Alternatives (d) and (e), in combination, stand the best chance. If not that, I will try (a).

7. **Implementation:** *Now I will try the solution(s) and track my progress.*

   I made an appointment with my boss and explained the situation again, offering to work late on the days I come in late. She said that she would allow it, but did not want it to go on indefinitely. She still seemed annoyed, but she agreed.

8. **Evaluation:** *Did it meet my goal, or do I need to try a different solution?*

   At first I felt like I had failed, because she was annoyed with me. Then I realized that I met my goal. I can go to my appointments. I will speak to my physical therapist again and find out how long it will go on so I can bring that information back to my boss. I am proud of myself for handling this problem directly.

FIGURE 6.5. Rachel's problem-solving example.

overlap is consistent with D'Zurilla's (1988) suggestion that problem-solving training, when used with other treatment methods, should not be applied as a separate treatment procedure but integrated with the overall treatment plan.

Relaxation Skills

People with ASD have difficulty modulating affect and reading their own internal cues of distress—intervention for which is presented in Chapter 8. Nevertheless, teaching relaxation skills can be a valuable component of the treatment plan as a proactive method for patients to use to lower chronically elevated arousal. Groden and her colleagues have been providing strategies for relaxation to people with autism and related conditions for nearly 40 years, since the classic book on teaching these skills to people with developmental disabilities was published in 1978 (Cautela & Groden). Now in its second edition (Groden, Weidenman, & Diller, 2016), this book continues to serve as a valuable resource because it presents both pictures and step-by-step instructions for delivering a variety of relaxation inductions to people at a wide range of functioning levels. I find that relaxation can be taught to people with ASD in much the same way as it would be to any adult population, so therapists who are well versed in behavior therapy and CBT will find that they can proceed with very few modifications. Therapists who are new to this approach may refer to Bernstein and Borkovec (1973) or Goldfried (1971, 1977) for an overview of the historical theoretical underpinnings and practical application of relaxation training.

Some people erroneously equate mindfulness and meditation practices with relaxation strategies. Though the regular practice of mindfulness can result in an overall more relaxed state for many people, that is not the goal. Those strategies are not described in this chapter, as they will be detailed more in Chapter 8.

To summarize this section, strategies for building coping skills in patients with ASD were presented, including organization and time management, problem solving, and relaxation. In contrast to the previous section on social skills, this section focused on the self-management skills that have less of a social component but are crucial for managing the tasks of daily living and minimizing stress.

Chapter Summary and Conclusions

This chapter presented intervention guidelines for teaching adults with ASD the major skills that their typical adult peers have attained more naturally. The failure to acquire these skills by adulthood is what defines ASD as a developmental disability. However, this chapter introduced a *habilitation* model that assumes that many of these skills can be learned, even though the individual has already reached adulthood. The strategies presented here could benefit any person with ASD, even if there is no mental health problem present. The next chapter describes methods for treating the comorbid mental health issues that are usually present in psychotherapy cases, using a traditional cognitive therapy model as the basis.

CHAPTER 7

Intervention

Addressing Comorbid Mental Health Problems

This chapter presents strategies for treating the comorbid mental health problems that are so often seen in psychotherapy patients with ASD. Up to this point in the book, it has been emphasized that individuals with ASD have idiosyncratic ways of processing information and communicating that warrant special considerations by psychotherapists. This chapter, in a seeming contrast to that point, promotes the idea that people with ASD should be offered the same CBT interventions that would be offered to any adult who is struggling with anxiety, depression, or chronic stress. Previous chapters discussed how the core problems of ASD result in different patient presentations than those of typical adults. This chapter "switches gears" to highlight how these patients can benefit from treatment in much the same way as typical adults, once the therapist accounts for their atypical developmental histories.

I have found that the traditional cognitive theory of emotional disorders (Beck, 1976) can be used to explain the anxiety and mood problems that are seen in adults with ASD. In Chapter 2, this point was illustrated with Figures 2.4 and 2.5, which noted the developmental processes involved. If one assumes this formulation, CBT can be applied with very few modifications. The presence of an ASD, although warranting thoughtful approaches to assessment and the need to build a working relationship, should not "sidetrack" the cognitive-behavioral therapist away from using the tools that have a strong evidence base for the treatment of adults who do not have ASD (Butler et al., 2006; Hofmann et al., 2012) and some promising results for adults with ASD (Spain et al., 2015). The therapist can avoid this trap by using the individualized case formulation approach that was described in Chapter 4. Each new patient in an outpatient psychotherapy setting, whether having ASD or not, can be viewed as a person with a mental health problem whose symptoms have developed out of a unique combination of factors and who should be offered evidence-based interventions to reduce his or her symptoms.

For example, take two patients who come in for treatment who are both diagnosed with major depressive disorder after the initial assessment. One has ASD and the other does not. Both should be offered a traditional CBT package to address their depression because its efficacy has been demonstrated in adult populations. The only difference is that the patient with ASD may need additional components in his or her treatment plan, *along with* the traditional CBT, in order to *build skills* that the typical depressed patient would already possess, or to *optimize the effectiveness* of the traditional CBT. These skills were presented in Chapter 6.

This chapter describes how some of the essential techniques of CBT can be applied with adults who have anxiety or depression co-occurring with ASD. The literature presenting the theories, techniques, and empirical evidence supporting CBT is vast and spans over 50 years. Because of space limitations, this chapter does not provide a comprehensive description of every protocol that could be used with adults who have ASD. It is also not necessary, if the assumption that adults with ASD should be offered the same interventions that would be offered to anyone is accepted. The purpose of this chapter is therefore not to review the CBT literature but to stimulate readers to think about adult cases of ASD in a way that would lead them to consider drawing from that literature while planning treatment. Readers who are not familiar with the fundamentals of CBT, as per Beck's cognitive theory, are referred to Beck (1995) and Persons and colleagues (2000), which both provide excellent and easy-to-understand introductions for the newcomer. The terminology used in this chapter is drawn largely from those two sources. The assumptions behind all of the interventions described in this chapter are as follows:

- *Schemas* are cognitive structures containing deeply held, broad *core beliefs* that allow a person to make meaning of events. People generally have a set of adaptive schemas along with a set of maladaptive ones. Psychopathology is a response to life events that have activated maladaptive schemas.
- *Intermediate beliefs* are the attitudes, assumptions, and rules about how people, including the self, should behave and be evaluated. These are the vehicles through which the core beliefs are expressed from day to day and can be dysfunctional when a maladaptive schema has been activated.
- *Automatic thoughts* are the more immediate thoughts that occur in the face of a specific situation and reflect the individual's interpretation of what is happening. Automatic thoughts are driven by associated core and intermediate beliefs and are dysfunctional when a maladaptive schema has been activated.

According to Beck (1995), the intervention should begin with modifying dysfunctional automatic thoughts, the bottom of the list just presented, and work upward. Automatic thoughts are the easiest to access and modify, whereas the core beliefs within schemas are the most difficult to modify and are addressed later in treatment. This chapter is organized in that order to describe CBT implementation for adults with ASD. *Introducing the cognitive model* to the patient is discussed first, followed by strategies for identifying and responding to *dysfunctional automatic thoughts*, then *intermediate beliefs*, and finally *schemas*.

Introducing the Cognitive Model to the Patient

At the end of Chapter 5, which was about orienting the patient to treatment, there was brief mention of the need to educate the patient on the cognitive model. Using the diagram from Persons and colleagues (2000), presented in Figure 2.3, is often helpful in terms of presenting the rationale for treatment. Often preliminary steps must be taken before it can be presented in this fashion, however. One of the useful tools for beginning this process is the *thought record*. Teaching the patient to use it will not only lead to important data collection but also to training the individual on the theory behind the interventions that will be implemented.

Using the Thought Record to Define Automatic Thoughts

Introducing the *thought record*, also referred to in the literature as the dysfunctional thought record (DTR; Beck, 1995), early in treatment is a useful way to explain the assumptions and rationale of CBT to the patient. Slightly different versions can be found in CBT texts, but all ask patients to keep a log of upsetting situations, including the date and a description of the event, and to write down the associated thoughts and emotions that they experienced at the same time.

Some patients with ASD may need extra instructions and practice if they do not immediately know what the therapist means by the term *thought*. Most have an intellectual understanding of the word but may have difficulty accessing their own thoughts while describing an account of a disturbing situation, or understanding that they are examining their own thoughts from an observer's point of view. They also may be intimidated by the worksheet itself. The therapist can assess for these potential obstacles by asking the patient to come up with an example within the session, based on something that caused distress within the previous week. A discussion that took place with Bob in the third session is used to illustrate this aspect. As mentioned when Bob's case was introduced in Chapter 1, he was very hostile toward me in the earlier sessions, which is evident in this example.

THERAPIST: This week I am going to ask you to start logging your thoughts and feelings each time you hear some upsetting news on TV or on the radio.

PATIENT: I already told you what I thought. Why do I have to write it down? Didn't you keep notes on what I said?

THERAPIST: I do keep notes, but they are to help me with the job I have to do in our work together. Those notes will not help you in the job you have to do in our work together. The notes that are going to help you the most are the ones you take yourself.

PATIENT: This is bullshit. I'm sick. Can't you see that? I won't remember to write anything down. You should be able to see that.

THERAPIST: I can see that you are sick. And you are suffering quite a lot. And what I am asking you to do *is hard*. I wish there were a way I could make your symptoms disappear without having to ask you to do something hard. But I can't. I need you to be the observer of what happens during the week, and the log I am asking you to keep will help me to help you.

PATIENT: Well, who said I am not a hard worker? I can work hard. Are you saying I can't handle something hard? I can do hard things. But why can't I just tell you my answers every week? A log sounds complicated.

THERAPIST: I do think you can handle it, but I am going to make sure you get all the instructions you need before you are sent off on your own to do it. Let's take a look at how the log works. (*Draws a chart on poster paper with three columns, labeling them "Date," "Situation," and "Thoughts." The other columns included on a typical thought record—such as "Behaviors," "Emotions," and "Responses"—are left off deliberately to avoid overwhelming the patient.*) Can you tell me the last time you got some upsetting news from the media?

PATIENT: Last night.

THERAPIST: OK. So, I will show you how the sheet would be used. I am going to write yesterday's date in the first column, under "Date." What did you see or hear on the news?

PATIENT: On TV, they were talking about how bad security is at airports. They were saying that it's still bad, even now. I mean, does that make any sense to you? What are they trying to do, scare everyone? How do they expect people to function after they hear that?

THERAPIST: OK, so I am going to write that under "Situation." I will paraphrase what you said: "Watching a news story about inadequate airport security." Does that cover it?

PATIENT: I guess. Yeah.

THERAPIST: OK, now, can you tell me what thoughts went through your mind as you were watching that news story?

PATIENT: I just told you! Jesus.

THERAPIST: You did give me some of your reactions, about them trying to scare everyone and how it could get in the way of people functioning, but it sounded like you were asking me what I thought—they were questions. Also, I was not sure those were thoughts you are having right now, in this moment, or whether you were thinking them when you watched the news program last night.

PATIENT: I don't know what you mean. Thoughts are thoughts.

THERAPIST: Yes, and they are all relevant. But on the log, we just need to capture what was on your mind right at the time of the situation we are recording, or immediately after it—almost like we were running a tape recorder in your head while this was going on so we can record the thoughts you're having in the moment.

PATIENT: I don't know. I can't really tell the difference—I can only think of what I am thinking now.

THERAPIST: Well, to tell you the truth, we are at a disadvantage today because we are trying to get this down a whole day after it really happened. This will be easier for you when you are doing it right after something happens—closer to the moment. But let's see if we can come up with a way to tell the difference between now and then. We'll start with now. What are you thinking now about this story?

PATIENT: The news reporters are trying to scare everyone. It's outrageous.

THERAPIST: OK. Good. Now, do you think that thought was in your mind as you watched the news last night?

PATIENT: No. I was thinking more about the security people, that they are failing at their jobs. They are supposed to protect us. And they are failing. And there's nothing to stop another terrorist attack. I mean, who is going to stop it? Don't you worry about this? How can you do your job while this is going on? I don't see how anybody can concentrate on anything but this!

THERAPIST: All right. It sounds like you were able to name different thoughts you were having last night. I will write in the "Thoughts" column "The security people are failing at their jobs. They are supposed to protect us. They are failing. There's nothing to stop another attack." Does that about cover the thoughts you were having last night?

PATIENT: Yes. I think that's it.

THERAPIST: OK. You managed that very well. Like I said, this was extra hard because we were trying to do it after the fact. And you were still able to do it, with that extra challenge. So, I think you will find it a little easier when you are doing it at the moment. So, I am going to print out a sheet for you that looks just like the one I drew up here, and I am going to ask you to copy what I wrote up here, and that will be your sample for the week. Then, as these types of incidents happen, you will log them in the same way, starting right underneath the sample. Do you have any questions about it?

PATIENT: No. I get it now.

I dealt with three obstacles as I introduced the exercise. One was Bob's hostility, which I hypothesized was his tactic for avoiding a task by which he was intimidated. The second is that he was having difficulty with the metacognitive task of trying to think about thoughts retrospectively. Third, the activity increased his anxiety, as evidenced by his repeated questions to me that were very similar to the ritualistic questioning he engaged in at home with his parents. In response, I had to give him clearer instructions about the worksheet without giving him the impression that I doubted his ability because his own self-doubt was the suspected root of his intimidation and resultant hostility. I also chose not to answer some of the questions he was asking, so as not to reinforce the ritualistic behavior that was part of his presenting problem. Instead I stayed focused on the task and only responded to his questions about the activity at hand. I gave him a partial thought record as homework—that is, it was missing columns for "Emotions," "Behaviors," and "Responses" because it was my judgment that he would not have been able to handle that much new information in this session. As it turned out, he was very compliant with the homework and brought the record to the next session with three different entries added. These are shown in Figure 7.1.

In each of the following 2 weeks, another column was added, first "Emotions" and then "Behaviors," and only after ensuring proficiency was achieved with the previous task. Figure 7.2 shows a sample entry from a complete record he had brought in later in the process. "Responses" were not filled in yet because the record was being used at this point as a tool for eliciting information, not for intervening. Once he was able to use a full record, enough data was collected to present the visual model of his symptoms, shown in Figure 7.3. This graphic aid was used to explain to Bob how his obsessions and compulsions were being maintained and also introduce the idea of his core beliefs/schemas, which had been extracted from patterns noted in the thought records. Once he understood that his beliefs contributed to his anxiety—his thoughts about the need to be protected and his compulsive questioning—we could then explore how the cycle was perpetuating anxiety in the long run. This explanation made it easier for him to accept

Date	Situation	Thoughts
11/29	Watching a news story about inadequate airport security	The security people are failing at their jobs. They are supposed to protect us. They are failing. There's nothing to stop another attack.
12/1	Saw a website about terrorist groups	What's to stop a terrorist from getting on a plane in Afghanistan, Pakistan, or Iraq and flying a plane into another American building. Security is horrible at the airports. What if the pilots become terrorists? Why isn't anyone stopping this?
12/3	Heard someone say something on the radio about nuclear weapons	I wonder if Iraq has to do more testing before they launch a missile. What if we missed the testing? We could have missed it. We fell asleep on 9/11, we could sure miss this. No one seems to be doing anything about this. How come no one is doing their jobs?
12/6	Saw something on TV about Saddam Hussein	What if he flees his country, then launches nuclear missiles from another part of the world? He does not care about his own people, anyway. I heard he gassed some of them. I want to know who is watching him. Who is going to stop him?

FIGURE 7.1. Partial thought record as initial homework assignment for Bob.

the rationale for the exposure and response prevention approaches that I planned to implement with him.

It is not uncommon for patients with ASD to have some difficulty initially grasping the idea of monitoring and recording thoughts. Some are reluctant to accept the idea because they confuse the concept of internal dialogue or self-talk with "voices" that psychotic people hear. They are afraid that if they begin to examine their self-talk, it means that they are "hearing voices" and that the therapist might diagnose them as having schizophrenia. The therapist may have to spend some time normalizing self-talk and differentiating it from the break from reality that occurs in psychosis. For other patients, the concept is too abstract, and they do not initially understand what the therapist is asking of them. Two strategies can be used to enhance the learning, each one working with different patients. One is to use *visual aids* and the other is to use illustrative *metaphors*.

Date	Situation	Thoughts	Emotions	Behaviors	Responses
12/22	Saw a story about how other American buildings could be good targets for terrorists. My parents were not home.	Why aren't they beefing up security if they know this? They're not doing their jobs. How can they tell us about this and then do nothing about it?	Scared, angry	Called my brother to ask him if he heard the story and what he thinks about it.	

FIGURE 7.2. More complete thought record entry for Bob. From Persons, Davidson, and Tompkins (2000). Copyright © 2000 the American Psychological Association. Adapted by permission.

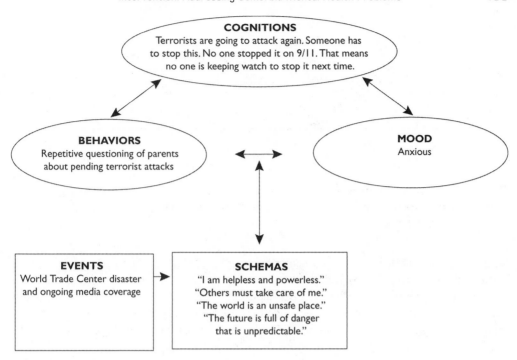

FIGURE 7.3. Beck's cognitive theory explaining Bob's obsessions and compulsions. From Persons, Davidson, and Tompkins (2000). Copyright © 2000 the American Psychological Association. Adapted by permission.

Visual Aids

As mentioned earlier, I keep a dry-erase board or a large pad of poster paper on hand. To accommodate patients who prefer electronically displayed images, PowerPoint slides or other images can be put up on a computer monitor and sent to the patient's smartphone. Regardless of media the therapist chooses to use, diagrams and drawings are often helpful with many in this population, and when presenting the thought record and cognitive model to some patients with ASD, pictures can help make abstract concepts more concrete for them. For others, text-based reminders are helpful for the patient to look back at between sessions, so encouraging the patient to take notes, either on paper on a smartphone, can facilitate learning for those who prefer visual to verbal aids. Visual aids such as the ones shown in Figure 7.4 can be used to help those who are having difficulty with metacognition, or thinking about thoughts. These are the classic cartoon symbols that are suggested by Gray (1994) for teaching people with ASD that thoughts are a type of speech, the only difference being that we do not say them out loud.

Metaphors

Other patients enjoy and learn from using metaphors when talking about abstract concepts. One was used with Bob, above, when I suggested that he imagine a tape recorder running in his head, recording thoughts as they occur. Another is to suggest to the patient that there is a narrator or news commentator on duty all day inside his or her

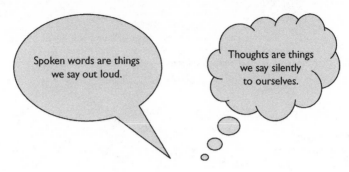

FIGURE 7.4. Cartoon symbols used to define thoughts. From Gray (1994). Copyright © 1994 Jenison Public Schools. Adapted by permission of Future Horizons, Inc.

head, who is constantly making comments and remarks about what is happening. One patient came up with his own metaphor once he began to understand this concept. He said he had a "board of directors" in his head who were dialoguing throughout the day on what was happening in his life. Once he described this image, it was easy for the therapist to ask him to write down what "the members of the board" were saying.

Identifying and Responding to Dysfunctional Automatic Thoughts

After the patient understands what automatic thoughts are and that they can be monitored and recorded, the therapist can begin to help him or her evaluate them. The idea that thoughts can be *dysfunctional* is another concept that may be difficult for some patients with ASD to accept at first. The thought record can help with that process. After the patient has practiced filling it out repeated times, the therapist can begin asking the key questions involved in an evaluation of the thoughts. As a starting point, I often assign the book *Feeling Good* (Burns, 2009) to patients to introduce them to the rationale behind cognitive restructuring, which is learning to reconceptualize or reframe problem situations. Another helpful book for patients with ASD is *Exploring Depression, and Beating the Blues* (Attwood & Garnett, 2016), which provides ASD-friendly strategies to teach cognitive restructuring. Even if books are not assigned (e.g., some patients may have obstacles that would interfere with reading it), at the very least the patient is introduced to the concept of *cognitive distortions*.

Identifying and Responding to Cognitive Distortions

To begin the process of evaluating dysfunctional automatic thoughts, I always present a list of common cognitive distortions to the patient, as illustrated in Table 7.1, which is based on Beck (1995), Burns (1999), and Persons and colleagues (2000). I find the list a useful starting point with this population for several reasons.

- The list format in which the material is presented seems to appeal to the *rule-driven learning style* that so many patients with ASD have.

- The "multiple-choice" nature of the material allows patients to rely on *recognition* of their own patterns without having to *access* the language to describe them. They can read the items, rule out what does not fit them, and choose what does fit. This method alleviates the difficulty that is inherent in the alexithymic (problems accessing language to describe mental states) tendencies of these patients. I have observed that they tend to be good at recognizing themselves; they choose errors on the list that are consistent with what I have observed in them through other means.
- When they see these errors on a list in a published book, it *normalizes their experience* for them, and they often ask, "You mean other people have these problems, too?"
- The terms that are used on the list can become part of a *common language* between the patient and the therapist.

TABLE 7.1. Common Cognitive Distortions

- *All-or-nothing thinking:* There are only two categories for everything. You see things in terms of "black or white," "good or bad," "smart or stupid," "beautiful or ugly," etc. It is hard for you to see things on a continuum or in "shades of gray."

- *Catastrophizing:* You exaggerate the possible negative outcomes of an incident. A minor problem is assumed to have catastrophic implications. For example, "I lost my car keys, so that means I will develop Alzheimer's" or "My boss reminded me of an upcoming deadline, which means he is getting ready to fire me."

- *"Should" statements:* You have a set of strict rules about how you or other people are supposed to act or handle things and exaggerate the consequences if a rule is violated. For example, "I should be able to keep my room organized at all times or else I am irresponsible" or "Bank tellers should always be polite or else they should be fired."

- *Personalization:* You overestimate your role in the actions of other people, including strangers. You assume you are the reason for others' behavior without considering alternative explanations. For example, "My professor did not call on me when I had my hand up because she thinks I am an idiot" or "A store clerk gave me the wrong change because he knows I am a sucker."

- *Labeling:* You engage in negative "name calling" by assigning unfavorable labels to yourself or other people without having evidence for your conclusion. "I am a *loser* because I couldn't get a date" or "He is a *selfish bastard* because he would not help me with my project."

- *Mental filter/disqualifying the positive:* You have a filter in your mind that only allows negative information in; you pay attention only to the negative details about yourself or others and "filter out," ignore, or disqualify positive information. For example, you focus on one mistake you made at work as a sign of failure, but you ignore the positive feedback you recently got from your boss.

- *Mind reading:* You assume that you know what other people are thinking or what their intentions are, even if you have no evidence for it. For example, "She mentioned her vacation because she knows I don't have enough money to take a trip and she wanted to hurt my feelings."

- *Emotional reasoning:* You let your feelings guide your reasoning. You use the logic, "If I feel it, it is true." For example, "I am afraid to fly, so it must be dangerous."

- *Overgeneralization:* You make global statements and conclusions about singular events. For example, "I could not get the lawnmower started today—I am terrible with mechanical things" or "My daughter did not do her chores this week. She is never going to be a responsible person."

Note. Data from Burns (1999); Beck (1995); and Persons, Davidson, and Tompkins (2000).

Cognitive Distortions in ASD

It has been well documented through neuropsychological research that people with ASD are subject to cognitive rigidity. The findings reviewed in Chapter 2 suggested that they have difficulty shifting attention and mind-sets and also have a tendency not to look at the "big picture" or gist of a collection of information or stimuli (i.e., central coherence). Unfortunately, their information-processing style provides a "hot breeding ground" for the types of cognitive distortions listed in Table 7.1. I have found that people with ASD are vulnerable to any of the cognitive distortions, and like the general adult population, each patient makes his or her own unique combination of errors. However, the one that is found in every patient with ASD I have met is *all-or-nothing* thinking.

Because of neuropsychological dysfunction, people with ASD generally have great difficulty thinking about things on a continuum; there are no "shades of gray." Information is placed in dichotomous mental categories and held there in an inflexible way. Just a few examples of these categories are found in the way people are evaluated; they are seen as either good or bad, nice or mean, and smart or stupid. Task or work performance is seen as either perfect or terrible, a total success or a total failure, and superior or inferior. Not only do these patients have difficulty quantifying things in gradients but they also seem to have a very low tolerance for uncertainty. They tend to become highly anxious in situations where an absolute answer is not immediately available.

In Bob's case, for example, he was having more difficulty than the average American citizen assimilating the new idea that terrorists could attack on American soil. He could not easily modify his previous dichotomous thinking on this issue, which was "Terrorist attacks *do* occur other places, but they *do not* occur in my country." This was connected to "I *will not be killed* if I live in a country where there are no terrorist attacks, but I *will be killed* in a country where terrorist attacks occur." Last, "Authority figures should protect me from harm and I am safe if they are *doing their jobs,* but if anything bad happens, it is because *they are not doing their jobs* and so I am not safe." As mentioned, every American was faced with this challenge and found it painful, but most people were able to assimilate the information in a way that allowed them to continue functioning. Bob's dichotomous thinking style was a major contributing factor to the anxiety that was so disabling to him at the point of intake.

Eliciting Automatic Thoughts and Identifying Cognitive Distortions

The thought record is, as mentioned, one way to identify patterns of dysfunctional automatic thoughts and distortions. Some patients, even after demonstrating competence in using the thought record, will lose their ability if they are highly distressed and emotionally aroused by an event. An alternative method, a *visual downward arrow* technique for helping the patient identify dysfunctional automatic thoughts, is proposed here for those situations.

VISUAL DOWNWARD ARROW

The downward arrow technique is a strategy in which a patient is asked to take one automatic thought and try to trace the "chain" of automatic, more superficial thoughts that lead to the deeper core belief that is driving it. It was introduced as a self-help worksheet by Burns (1980), and it directs patients to think about the process as "peeling successive layers of skin off an onion to expose the ones beneath" (p. 264). Beck (1995) later described how a therapist can use a downward arrow interviewing technique to help patients do the same thing in session. A case example, Seth, is used to demonstrate how a modified downward arrow strategy can help a patient whose emotional arousal is interfering with the identification of key automatic thoughts and beliefs.

Seth is another patient who was introduced in Chapter 1. As a quick review, Seth is a 44-year-old single Jewish unemployed man who was referred by his vocational counselor in order to address occupational concerns. He lives with a roommate in an apartment and receives weekly visits from a staff member of an assisted living program for adults with developmental disabilities. He is a part-time college student, pursuing an associate's degree in computer science. After a comprehensive assessment, his diagnoses (DSM-5; American Psychiatric Association, 2013) were:

- Autism spectrum disorder (Asperger's disorder)
  - *requiring support for deficits with social communication (Level 1)*
  - *requiring support for restricted, repetitive behaviors (Level 1)*
  - *without accompanying intellectual impairment*
  - *without accompanying language impairment*
- Generalized anxiety disorder

Despite the fact that he had learned to use the thought record, Seth arrived in one session in a state of agitation and arousal, unable to articulate what was upsetting him beyond the repeated phrase, "I will be homeless soon." He was unable to report what was upsetting him, and he had not used the thought record to record the incident. It took a whole session for him to become calm enough to have the following discussion, which took place within the last 5 minutes of the session.

PATIENT: This morning my roommate asked me to clean up some crumbs I left while preparing a snack late at night.

THERAPIST: And that is why you will be homeless?

PATIENT: That's right. Any day now.

THERAPIST: How does your roommate's request make you homeless?

PATIENT: I just know it. I will be homeless. I can see it coming.

THERAPIST: Could you try to get some of your thoughts about this down on a thought record this week?

PATIENT: OK.

THERAPIST: This is a good example of how some of your automatic thoughts are causing you to be anxious, but I don't think you had time today to really name all of the thoughts you are having. I suspect there are a lot that are leading you to believe you will be homeless, but we don't have any more time to work on it today.

PATIENT: OK. I'll try to write them down.

Seth returned the following week, but he had not used the thought record to document the incident with his roommate. Seth tended to be compliant with homework in the past, so I assumed that this task was too difficult for him at this time; his emotional arousal seemed to be interfering with his ability to examine his thoughts more objectively. In this session, he continued to repeat that his roommate's request for him to clean up crumbs was an absolute indicator that he would be homeless soon, but he was unable to link the roommate's feedback to homelessness in any logical way. Various verbal probes were unsuccessful. I decided to use a version of the downward arrow questioning technique, but do so by incorporating visual aids. First I drew the diagram in Figure 7.5 on poster paper. Knowing that Seth was a computer science major and enjoyed programming, I chose to use flowchart symbols to illustrate the thinking process. It was presented in this way:

> "OK. Look at this flowchart. Let's make believe we are trying to find a bug in a computer program. We will start by drawing the two components we already know about. They are here: 'My roommate asked me to clean up crumbs from the counter,' *therefore* 'I will be homeless soon.'"

After that, I drew another picture, shown in Figure 7.6, and said the following:

THERAPIST: Now, I made another flowchart here. You can see that I took the same two components we were just looking at and put them on this sheet, but notice that there are a whole bunch of steps in between them. These steps suggest that there are a whole bunch of thoughts you are having, one right after the other, to lead from this point (*pointing to the first thought*) to this point (*pointing to the last thought*). The connection is really not as direct as you first thought. Do you think that is possible?

PATIENT: I guess so. It just happens so fast. I can't help it.

THERAPIST: You're right. It does happen fast. When you went from getting feedback from your roommate to being homeless, you were traveling a hundred miles an hour, so everything that happened in between was a blur. We are just going to slow it down now, looking at that road you traveled in slow motion, frame by frame. Now we are going to fill in the steps in between. Think about each one as an "if–then" statement that you use in computer programming. We will go very slowly, and I will give you plenty of time to think about each one. OK?

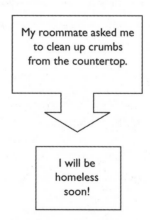

FIGURE 7.5. Introducing Seth to the thought flowchart.

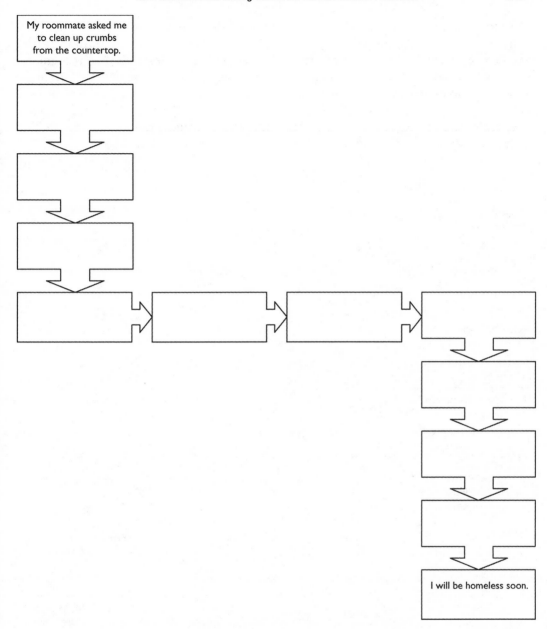

FIGURE 7.6. Seth's thought flowchart at the beginning.

I had several objectives in this exercise. The first was to help Seth slow down his automatic thoughts so that he could become more aware of the content of each one. This idea was influenced by a worksheet I had seen in Brownell's (2000) cognitive-behavioral weight management program, called "The Behavior Chain." Patients who are strug-gling with episodes of overeating are asked to write down, on a picture of a chain, the series of behaviors, thoughts, and feelings that lead up to the incidents. I believed that Seth needed to go through this process with his thoughts, rather than overt behaviors, and that a visual prompting system would help him to do it more effectively than a purely verbal one. The second objective was to help him use the logical thinking that he demonstrated in other areas of his life (e.g., computer programming) to recognize the erroneous assumption he was making in this situation by linking feedback from a roommate to becoming homeless. Finally, in line with the traditional *downward arrow* objective, I wanted to uncover the core belief that was operating behind these automatic thoughts. The following dialogue is what led to the outcome presented in Figure 7.7, where all of the steps of the flowchart are filled in with automatic thoughts.

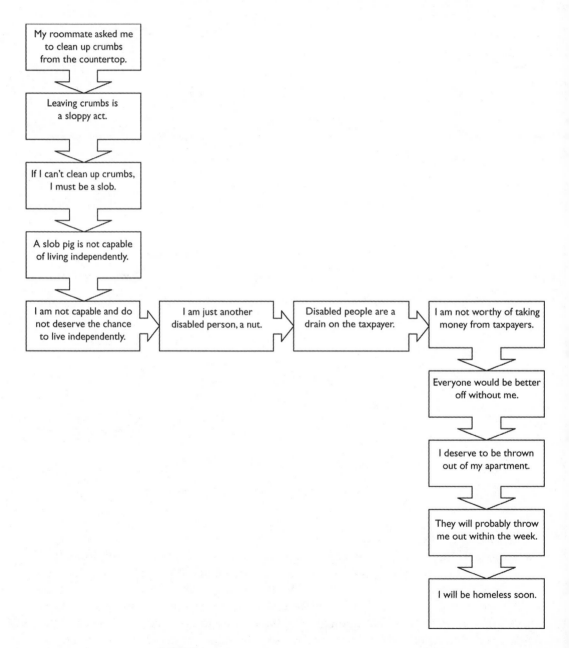

FIGURE 7.7. Seth's completed thought flowchart.

THERAPIST: Start with the first step, again, "My roommate asked me to clean up crumbs." Now I am going to say it a little differently, and you pick up where I leave off. Remember, don't say, "I will be homeless" at this point because that is way over here (*pointing to the last step*). We are trying to find all of the if–then statements that led up to that because it really wasn't a direct connection the way you first experienced it. Ready? "My roommate asked me to clean up crumbs and that means. . . ."

PATIENT: Well, leaving crumbs is a sloppy act.

THERAPIST: OK. I am writing "Leaving crumbs is a sloppy act." And that means . . .

PATIENT: If I can't clean up some crumbs, I must be a slob.

THERAPIST: "If I can't clean up some crumbs, I must be a slob," which means . . .

PATIENT: A slob pig is not capable of living independently.

THERAPIST: "A slob pig is not capable of living independently," therefore . . .

PATIENT: I am not capable and do not deserve the chance to live independently.

THERAPIST: OK, I am writing that. And that means . . .

PATIENT: I am just another disabled person, a nut.

THERAPIST: Therefore . . .

PATIENT: Disabled people are a drain on the taxpayer.

THERAPIST: So . . .

PATIENT: I am not worthy of taking money from the taxpayers . . .

THERAPIST: Which means . . .

PATIENT: Everyone would be better off without me.

THERAPIST: And that means . . .

PATIENT: I deserve to be thrown out of my apartment.

THERAPIST: Therefore . . .

PATIENT: They will probably throw me out within the week.

THERAPIST: And so . . .

PATIENT: I will be homeless soon (*chuckles*).

THERAPIST: OK. That was great. You really caught on fast to this. Now we have a map that shows how you got from the incident with your roommate to the idea that you would be homeless. There was a total of (*counts the boxes on the diagram*) 10 thoughts you had that linked the incident to your final conclusion. What is your reaction to this diagram, now that it is all filled in?

PATIENT: I'm surprised. I didn't know I had so many thoughts. And some of them sound silly to me now. I mean, it seems ridiculous now that I see it on paper, the way I was thinking.

The session continued with a discussion about which boxes he was already beginning to challenge himself by labeling them as "silly" and "ridiculous." He was asked to identify the cognitive distortions he was exhibiting, and he correctly named *all-or-nothing thinking, catastrophizing,* and *jumping to conclusions.* He was also asked to choose which statements were supported by evidence, and which were not. As a precaution, I followed up on the statement "Everyone would be better off without me" and ruled out suicidal ideation. Finally, he was asked to pick which statement seemed to be the weakest, and to come up with an alternative statement to replace it. Though the topic was not addressed in this session, two schemas about himself were implicit in the entries on the flowchart, and these schemas ended up being major themes that we addressed in later sessions. They were "I am incapable" and "I am undeserving of good things." It is unlikely that any of this information would have been accessible to Seth or me without the stimulation provided by this visual strategy.

Recognizing and Modifying Intermediate Beliefs

As mentioned, the automatic thoughts are the more superficial things that people say to themselves in the moment as events are occurring; they are the words being uttered by the internal "narrator" or "commentator" who is making remarks about everything that is happening while a person is awake. The cognitive model assumes that these thoughts are generated by more broadly held attitudes, assumptions, and rules—called intermediate beliefs—about how people should behave and be evaluated. These are the links between the deeper and more broadly held core beliefs, which make up schemas, and the superficial automatic thoughts.

Intermediate Beliefs and ASD: Rules

People with ASD often have a relatively large collection of intermediate beliefs, particularly the type that are formulated as *rules*. I hypothesize that the development of an elaborate set of rules is a coping strategy. On some level, these individuals have been aware since early childhood that they do not understand a lot of the things that are going on around them, especially in the social domain. The difficulty they have inferring information that is not concretely tangible leaves them with a sense of being lost or disoriented in new situations. They therefore "latch on" to any set of rules that are tangible, and if none is available, they will create their own. Rules allow them to navigate situations that are otherwise overwhelming or frightening to them. However, because of the problems they have with drawing inferences and getting the "big picture" or gist of a situation, they rely on *atypical* means of creating these rules. These atypical means make them more vulnerable to maladaptive or erroneous intermediate beliefs.

Dr. Temple Grandin, a scientist, author, and lecturer who has ASD, describes this process from a firsthand account in her book *Thinking in Pictures* (Grandin, 1995). She also gives an example of *atypical rule development* when she speaks on the topic of autism. She shows photographs of two very different-looking dogs and describes how, when she was a young child, she could not understand what unified all of the creatures that people were calling *dogs*. After observing many types of dogs, she was finally able to link them together in terms of the shape of their noses. She noted that, without exception, all animals that people labeled *dogs* had the exact same nose pattern, no matter what their body shape, size, color, or coat type. She also noticed that other animals, such as cats, horses, cows, and sheep, did not have that nose pattern. Therefore, the rule she developed was "All animals with this particular nose pad are called dogs." She ends the story by humorously noting, "I would have been in big trouble if I had seen any bears at that time, as I later learned that they have that same nose pad" (Grandin, 2003).

Grandin's example shows how learning a simple labeling process is laborious for a person with ASD, whereas it comes so naturally and without conscious thought to a typically developing child. Yet, as illustrated in her example, the high intelligence that is common with some forms of ASD allows these individuals to apply logic to link together the pieces of information they have gathered to arrive at some kind of guiding principle. Social cognition, which is far more complicated than labeling static images of animals, requires a person to gather information from many different sources, some of which are invisible and most of which are constantly shifting and changing. Unfortunately, given the information-processing deficits found in people with ASD, they end up arriving at many erroneous and maladaptive guiding principles as they try to make sense of their own role in their social environment.

Psychotherapy patients with ASD must learn to articulate their rules, evaluate them, and replace the maladaptive ones with more useful ones. It is important for the therapist to recognize that a heavy reliance on rules is a crucial and adaptive compensatory strategy for patients with ASD, and they should not be discouraged from using it. The goal of the therapy is to teach them how to *evaluate* their rules in a more effective way so that they can better recognize ones that are not working for them and replace them with ones that will.

The following two examples illustrate the process of helping patients with ASD verbalize, evaluate, and replace maladaptive intermediate beliefs, which tend to be dominated by rules. The first presents the use of a modified activity schedule with Bob, and the second illustrates a dysfunctional beliefs worksheet with Seth.

Intervening with Maladaptive Rules

Using an Activity Schedule as a Behavioral Experiment

Bob's case has been described throughout this book, and an example from his thought record was presented earlier in this chapter. One of his treatment goals was to increase his self-reliance and independence, and this example shows how an activity schedule was used to address some of his maladaptive intermediate beliefs regarding self-care.

As mentioned, Bob's treatment initially focused on decreasing his obsessive–compulsive symptoms surrounding his fear of terrorism after 9/11. Although it is not described here, exposure and response prevention was implemented, and the target symptoms significantly improved across the first 6 months of treatment. After that point, however, he continued to show depressive symptoms, including neglect of self-care. Because the acute fear of terrorism had dissipated, I could more easily explore his anxiety about his diabetes. It was hypothesized that his depression was secondary to the belief that he was helpless in the face of his medical problems. Despite the fact that he had been diagnosed with the illness 8 years before, he had never successfully adapted, either emotionally or behaviorally, to the new role his doctors and parents were advising him to play.

Bob reported that he was continually distressed by thoughts about the negative health consequences he might face, such as losing his eyesight or having his feet amputated, if his diabetes was poorly controlled over the years to come. However, he expressed puzzlement over the fact that these thoughts did not motivate him to follow a proper diet or exercise regularly. Although he had a strong desire to change his eating and exercise habits, he felt thwarted to do so by a frustrating struggle with a series of rules he had developed over the years since his diagnosis. He referred to them as "mental habits" and recognized that they were irrational. However, he did not believe he could change them. After examining data on Bob's automatic thoughts, the following list of rules, or intermediate beliefs, was created:

- *I must follow a strict diet that has none of my favorite foods included.*
- *If I don't follow a strict diet, it means I am not capable of caring about my health.*
- *Eating is my only source of pleasure; I have to binge just before I start my diet because it may be my last time to enjoy food.*
- *If I can't even eat right, there is no sense in exercising; it will just be canceled out by my binges.*
- *If I can't even take care of my health, then there is no sense in doing anything else to improve my life; going to day treatment is a waste of time.*
- *I must start my diet on a Tuesday so I won't mess it up with weekend binges; because there are some Monday holidays, Tuesdays are always safe.*
- *If I mess up and eat something bad, it cancels out any healthy eating I have done. I have blown the diet, which proves I am not capable of taking care of my health.*
- *Once I blow it, I shouldn't bother starting again until Tuesday.*
- *If I don't get myself into gear soon, I'm going to go blind or lose my feet.*

Bob was first asked to examine the advantages and disadvantages of holding these beliefs. In sum, he believed most of the beliefs on the list motivated him to take care of his health and were therefore advantages. The disadvantages were that they made him feel very anxious because they placed pressure on him, and some of the rules actually contradicted one another, leaving him confused and more anxious. After listing the disadvantages, he was able to recognize that the advantage he had described was erroneous. The rules were, in reality, *not* motivating him to practice healthy eating at all, but were probably driving him to binge and avoid healthier habits. After acknowledging that these beliefs were based on faulty assumptions and were not helping him toward his goal of a healthy lifestyle, he expressed frustration because he still did not know how to challenge those beliefs when they appeared as automatic thoughts from day to day. He stated that he did not believe that he was capable of changing "the rules" even though he now knew they were dysfunctional.

A behavioral experiment was initiated involving a custom-made activity schedule form. The objective was to help Bob write new replacement rules and to collect data to support the validity of the new rules. Before designing the activity schedule and with the therapist's guidance, Bob came up with a list of three more functional rules that addressed the main themes seen in his list of maladaptive rules. Though he did not believe them very strongly, he agreed to test out the following new ideas:

- *I can practice healthy eating habits on any day and can include some foods I like. Each day is a separate time frame in which I can make eating choices. Each day counts as 1 day. One healthy eating day stands alone and one unhealthy eating day stands alone. An unhealthy eating day does not cancel out previous healthy eating days. I can try to <u>slowly increase</u> the number of healthy eating days I have each month.*
- *I can work on more than one thing to improve my life, even if I am not doing any of them*

perfectly. I can go to day treatment <u>more often</u> than before, even if my health is not perfect. I can exercise <u>more often</u> than I was before, even if my eating is not perfect.

* *I have other sources of pleasure in my life besides eating. They include bowling, tennis, and movies. I can do those things <u>more often</u>.*

The language used in these rules, such as "slowly increase" and "more often," was designed to address Bob's dichotomous thinking. These rules were then translated into the following measurable goals:

* *I will attend two leisure activities outside of my house per week (e.g., bowling, tennis, movies).*
* *I will increase the number of days of healthy eating each month.*
* *I will increase the number of days I exercise each week until I reach four times/week for 20 minutes.*
* *I will attend my day treatment program more often each month.*

A monthly activity schedule was designed that allowed Bob to monitor and record his progress on each of these goals. A monthlong sheet was chosen over the traditional weekly activity schedule sheet because it was thought that Bob would benefit from seeing gradual changes occur across a longer time frame. Figure 7.8 shows a blank copy of the form.

During the first month Bob used the form, we discussed it every week. He reported that the structure it provided was appealing to him. He looked forward to putting a checkmark in a box when he knew he had completed an activity and, interestingly, he also looked forward to putting an X in a box when he knew he had not achieved a particular goal for a day. He admitted that the X symbol took on a punitive meaning and that he actually took pleasure in "giving an X" to himself. Because of the risk he was at for distorting his interpretation of it, I made sure to probe each week about how Bob was using the data coding system. Sure enough, by the second week, he had begun to give himself Xs when they were not warranted. For example, he'd put an X in the exercise box on a day he had indeed exercised. He reported that he had eaten poorly that day, so he did not think he deserved "credit" for the exercise he'd done because the unhealthy eating had probably canceled out the positive effects of the exercise. I asked him to explore the advantages and disadvantages of keeping inaccurate data. He could not name any advantage and quickly recognized that he had drifted into following one of his old, maladaptive rules. I also emphasized the need to look at each little box on the sheet as a separate entity, reflecting only what had happened for *that* goal on *that* day. Ironically, I encouraged his dichotomous thinking style in order to facilitate accurate data by saying, "*This* little box on *this* day is asking you a 'yes or no' question—either you exercised or you didn't. Which is it?"

Figure 7.9 shows the activity schedule for Bob's first month of data collection. After converting each goal's data into percentages, Bob expressed surprise that he had achieved anything at all. Even his most difficult goal, practicing healthy eating, showed a 10% success rate. He acknowledged that without this data sheet, he would have "given a zero" to himself if asked to rate his own progress. After several months of data collection, he could see a trend of improvement in his lifestyle behaviors, and this improvement supported the validity of the new rules he had written.

Month _____ Year _____

Please answer the four questions each night before you go to bed.

Daily Data Collection

Date	1	2	3	4	5	6	7	8	9	10	11	12	13	14	15	16	17	18	19	20	21	22	23	24	25	26	27	28	29	30	31
Did you attend a leisure activity outside the house today?																															
Did you practice healthy eating today?																															
Did you exercise for 20 minutes today?																															
Did you attend day treatment for the full scheduled time?																															

Key: ☑ = completed task

 ☒ = did not complete

 N/A = not required on this day

Month-End Evaluation of Goals

Goals	Month-End Tally	Percentage of Success
1. Attend two leisure activities outside per week, or 8 days/month.	/8	
2. Increase the number of days per month of healthy eating, or more days than previous month.	/30 or /31	
3. Exercise for 20 minutes 4x/week, or 16 days/month.	/16	
4. Attend day treatment program on all scheduled days, or 12 days/month.	/12	

FIGURE 7.8. Monthly activity schedule.

From Valerie L. Gaus (2019). Copyright © The Guilford Press. Permission to photocopy this figure is granted to purchasers of this book for personal use or use with individual clients (see copyright page for details). Purchasers can download enlarged versions of this figure (see the box at the end of the table of contents).

202

Month April   Year 2007

Please answer the four questions each night before you go to bed.

Daily Data Collection

Date	1	2	3	4	5	6	7	8	9	10	11	12	13	14	15	16	17	18	19	20	21	22	23	24	25	26	27	28	29	30	31
Did you attend a leisure activity outside the house today?	✗	✗	✗	✓	✗	✗	✓	✗	✗	✗	✗	✗	✗	✓	✗	✗	✗	✗	✗	✗	✗	✗	✗	✗	✗	✗	✗	✓	✗	✗	
Did you practice healthy eating today?	✗	✗	✗	✗	✗	✗	✗	✓	✓	✗	✗	✗	✗	✗	✗	✗	✓	✗	✗	✗	✗	✗	✗	✗	✗	✗	✗	✗	✗	✗	
Did you exercise for 20 minutes today?	✗	✗	✗	✗	✗	✗	✓	✓	✓	✓	✓	✗	✗	✗	✗	✗	✓	✗	✗	✗	✗	✗	✗	✗	✗	✗	✓	✗	✗	✗	
Did you attend day treatment for the full scheduled time?	NA	NA	✗	✓	NA	✓	NA	NA	NA	✗	✗	NA	✗	NA	NA	NA	✗	✓	NA	✗	NA	NA	NA	✗	✗	NA	✗	NA	NA	NA	

Key: ☑ = completed task

  ☒ = did not complete

  N/A = not required on this day

Month-End Evaluation of Goals

Goals	Month-End Tally	Percentage of Success
1. Attend two leisure activities outside per week, or 8 days/month.	4/8	50%
2. Increase the number of days per month of healthy eating, or more days than previous month.	3/30 or /31	10%
3. Exercise for 20 minutes 4x/week, or 16 days/month.	7/16	44%
4. Attend day treatment program on all scheduled days, or 12 days/month.	3/12	25%

FIGURE 7.9. Bob's completed monthly activity schedule.

203

Creating a Dysfunctional Beliefs Worksheet: Challenging "One-Liners"

Another example of maladaptive intermediate beliefs phrased in the form of rules can be found in Seth. As mentioned, he was diagnosed with generalized anxiety disorder (GAD) along with ASD, and he was the subject of the *thought flowchart* presented earlier in this chapter. Two of Seth's core beliefs about himself—"I am incapable" and "I am undeserving of good things"—were reflected in some of the automatic thoughts elicited on the thought flowchart worksheet.

When these beliefs were explored more with him, Seth was able to connect some of them to the ideas that were conveyed to him by his parents while he was growing up. He reported that he had a very vivid auditory memory for the things his mother and father would say to him as they were trying to teach him various lessons; he could virtually hear each parent saying his or her favorite phrases in his head, in the exact voice and tone used decades before. Even though his parents were alive and active in his present life, they were not saying these things to him anymore. Nevertheless, he tended to apply them as rules in a very literal way in his daily life, and they were contributing to the anxiety that was one of his presenting problems. As they were being examined in session, Seth began calling them "one-liners." As an exercise, he was asked to list all the one-liners that were most active for him in the present. They were:

- *Don't take what doesn't belong to you.*
- *Don't you lose money.*
- *You go after breakfast.*
- *Boys play with boys and girls play with girls.*
- *Don't leave your seat until you are finished with your work.*
- *Pick up your feet when you walk.*
- *Don't open an umbrella in the house.*
- *Don't ever walk around nude.*
- *No fun until the work is done.*
- *If you don't go to the bathroom every day, you will get <u>cancer</u>, like your uncle.*
- *Look at him! Why can't you do things like him? He is better than you are.*

Many of these phrases are stereotypical things that some parents said to their children during the era Seth grew up in (1950s and 1960s), and after Seth finished writing them down, he laughed as he read them out loud. When asked why he was laughing, he said, "I guess these don't make sense anymore." It was explained to Seth that children understand things in very concrete ways, and parents often oversimplify things to help children understand new concepts. When children grow up, they reshape the rules as their life changes and their responsibilities grow, and they learn to apply the rules more flexibly. If the rules are kept in their child form, then they would be too rigid for an adult to follow because an adult's life is more complicated in many ways. For example, the admonition "No fun until the work is done" may be a way to teach a child to prioritize and begin to take responsibility for small amounts of work. If this rule were taken literally by an adult, however, that person would never have fun because an adult is never really completely finished with *all* of his or her chores and responsibilities.

In order to reinforce the differentiation between the function served by the one-liners at one point in his life versus the function they serve in the present, an exercise was assigned. A three-column worksheet was created: In the first column, all of the one-liners were listed; the second column was entitled "Function for children," and the third was "Consequences if applied too literally in adulthood." Seth was asked to think about each rule, and imagine why a parent would say it to a child or how it might be functional for helping a child understand certain concepts. Then he was asked to list the dysfunction it would create if it were applied too literally by an adult, at an age where the concrete nature of the rule no longer fit. The finished worksheet is presented in Figure 7.10. This process strengthened Seth's belief that the one-liners were no longer rational

One-liner	Function for children	Consequences if applied too literally in adulthood
Don't take what doesn't belong to you.	Teaches kids not to steal—prevents criminal behavior	Impairs functioning by preventing you from even touching anything
Don't you lose money.	Teaches kids that money is to be valued—prevents wasting	Afraid to take risks—deprive self of pleasure
You go after breakfast.	Enhances good toileting practices—routine	View self very negatively if a day is missed—look at self as failure or something is wrong (e.g., cancer)—impairs functioning
Boys play with boys and girls play with girls.	Teaches identity and promotes social skills—may prevent sexual improprieties in older children	Limits choices for friends—impairs building friendships—limits choices for professionals—promotes bias and prejudice
Don't leave your seat until you are finished with your work.	Teaches children to maintain attention to a task—to complete a job	May prevent taking necessary breaks
Pick up your feet when you walk.	Teaches children not to shuffle and wear out shoes and make noise	Walk awkwardly as if marching in a parade or in military
Don't open an umbrella in the house.	Superstition and safety	May prevent air drying a wet umbrella
Don't ever walk around nude.	Teaches appropriate appearance in public	May interfere with ability to perform essential ADLs or respond to emergencies
No fun until the work is done.	Teaches children priorities and responsibilities	May never have pleasure as an adult—that can lead to depression, inability to function, and possible hospitalization
If you don't go to the bathroom every day, you will get CANCER like your uncle.	Encourages children to stay regular for health reasons (old wives' tale)	Scheduling problems, heightens fears about medical conditions
Look at him! Why can't you do things like him? He is better than you are.	Trying to teach child through example	Constantly compare self to others—seek out ways to put others above self—damages self-esteem

FIGURE 7.10. Seth's one-liner worksheet.

or functional for him, and this realization made it easier for him to "write new rules" for himself in later sessions, as his core beliefs about himself were further modified.

Modifying Schemas

Schemas are the most difficult cognitive constructs to modify. They are made up of the beliefs that, developmentally, came first in a patient's life and have the longest reinforcement histories—but are addressed last in treatment. Only after patients gain some experience with the process of identifying and modifying automatic thoughts and intermediate beliefs can they begin to challenge the deeper and broader core beliefs. A helpful metaphor that I use with patients is to imagine that the task in CBT is to tear down an old shed that is not useful anymore. The shed is a wooden structure covered in shingles, and it sits on a cement foundation. One would have to remove the components starting from the top and working down. First comes the roof and exterior walls (automatic thoughts), then the framing and floorboards (intermediate beliefs), and finally the cement foundation (schemas). Developmentally, when the shed was built, the concrete foundation was laid first, the framing was based on that foundation, and the exterior laid over that frame. Because the foundation had to hold everything else up, it is deeply rooted, solid, and hard to break apart.

The cognitive rigidity in ASD that has been mentioned so often in this book makes it even more difficult than it would be with typical adult patients to modify the core beliefs that comprise schemas. Even with typical adults, Persons and colleagues (2000) suggest that it is not feasible to modify all of a patient's maladaptive schemas, and that only one or two core beliefs about the self or others can be targeted in therapy. This idea applies to patients with ASD, as well.

Common Core Beliefs in ASD

Beck (1995) presents a list of the most common maladaptive core beliefs that theoretically underlie psychopathology, and categorizes them as either beliefs about being *helpless* or beliefs about being *unlovable*. This list is presented in Table 7.2.

Patients with ASD usually have at least one core belief from each category that will become a focus in therapy. The most common of these beliefs I have encountered in adults with ASD are about being . . .

- Helpless
- Powerless
- Inadequate
- Defective
- Incompetent
- A failure
- Unattractive
- Unwanted
- Bad
- Unworthy
- Different
- Bound to be alone

The themes of helplessness, incompetence, defectiveness, and unworthiness were apparent in the cases of Bob and Seth, used earlier in the sections on automatic thoughts and intermediate beliefs. Those cases are revisited here, as well as the cases of Andrew and Rose, to illustrate the application of techniques for modifying schemas. Included below are descriptions of *continuum techniques* and the *core belief worksheet*.

TABLE 7.2. Categories of Core Beliefs about Self

Helpless core beliefs

I am helpless.	I am inadequate.
I am powerless.	I am ineffective.
I am out of control.	I am incompetent.
I am weak.	I am a failure.
I am vulnerable.	I am disrespected.
I am needy.	I am defective (i.e., I do not measure up to others).
I am trapped.	I am not good enough (in terms of achievement).

Unlovable core beliefs

I am unlovable.	I am unworthy.
I am unlikable.	I am different.
I am undesirable.	I am defective (i.e., so others will not love me).
I am unattractive.	I am not good enough (to be loved by others).
I am unwanted.	I am bound to be rejected.
I am uncared for.	I am bound to be abandoned.
I am bad.	I am bound to be alone.

Note. From J. S. Beck (1995). Copyright 1995 by Judith S. Beck, PhD. Reprinted by permission.

Continuum Techniques

The dichotomous thinking to which people with ASD are prone warrants the use of techniques that have been developed for typical adults who exhibit polarized thinking. Continuum methods are CBT strategies designed to help patients develop a new mental representation of an idea that was previously seen in all-or-nothing terms (Beck, 1995; Padesky, 1994; Persons et al., 2000). It works by having a patient take a negative statement (usually about the self) that is global and break it down into more specific criteria. The specific criteria are then turned into some type of rating scale that allows the person to evaluate him- or herself along a continuum. Those ratings are then used to challenge the original global statement, which usually reflects a maladaptive core belief. The cases of Andrew and Bob are used to illustrate.

Andrew's case was used in Chapter 6 to illustrate perspective-taking skills and time management. Again, he is a 32-year-old man who has a degree in culinary arts, works as a manager in a gourmet food shop, and engages in model railroad building as a hobby. His presenting problems were depressive symptoms and lack of satisfying relationships. After his assessment, his diagnoses (DSM-5) were:

- Autism spectrum disorder (Asperger's disorder)
  - *requiring support for deficits with social communication (Level 1)*
  - *requiring support for restricted, repetitive behaviors (Level 1)*
  - *without accompanying intellectual impairment*
  - *without accompanying language impairment*
- Persistent depressive disorder (dysthymia), early onset
- Avoidant personality disorder

Andrew's core beliefs about himself were "I am a failure" and "I am unwanted." Although he was chronically dysphoric (hence the dysthymia diagnosis), his mood would become more depressed and irritable around times he perceived to be life's "mile markers"—mainly his birthday and New Year's Day. In one late December session, he came in reporting a high level of anger, mostly toward himself. He stated that as the new year approached, he could only think about how he is failing to move forward in his life. Despite some progress that had been made in therapy, in this session, he appeared to be regressing in that he was repeating many of the maladaptive automatic thoughts that had been addressed many months before. They all had the theme of "I am a failure."

I chose to use a cognitive continuum intervention to address the activation of Andrew's core belief of failure, which had been triggered by the impending new year. One of the statements Andrew made in the session was chosen for this exercise: "The decade is half over already, and I have not succeeded. I have not accomplished anything." The cognitive continuum intervention is illustrated in the following dialogue:

THERAPIST: Let's turn that statement into a rating. Imagine a scale from 1 to 10 (*draws a horizontal line on poster paper*): 1 represents absolutely no success (*writes on one end*), whereas 10 represents total success (*writes on the other end*); 5 would be somewhere in between (*fills in the rest of the numbers between 1 and 10*).

PATIENT: OK.

THERAPIST: Now, tell me how you would rate your overall success this year, compared to 5 years ago, since you seemed to focus on the decade being half over.

PATIENT: I'd give myself a 1—no success.

THERAPIST: OK. Now, on the bottom of this paper I'm going to make a list. Tell me all of the things in your life that you think define success. Is success just one thing? Or are there a few things in your life that you would like to be more successful in?

PATIENT: Having a good job. Having enough money to support myself. Having a girlfriend. Having friends. Driving a decent car.

THERAPIST: (*after writing the list*) Anything else?

PATIENT: No, that's about it.

THERAPIST: OK. I'm going to make two columns next to your five criteria for success. One represents where you were 5 years ago, and the other one represents now. Start with your job. How would you rate yourself, using this 10-point scale, on where you were with the job situation 5 years ago?

PATIENT: Oh, God. It was a 1. I didn't have a job at all.

THERAPIST: OK. I will write that here. Moving over to the other column, how would you rate yourself now compared to then?

PATIENT: Umm. Well, I don't really like my job right now, but at least I have been able to stick with it for 3 years. And I did get promoted this past year. I guess I would have to give myself a 5.

THERAPIST: OK. Now let's do the same thing for the next criterion on your list, having enough money to support yourself. Where were you 5 years ago?

PATIENT: Another disaster. I had no money. I was living with my parents. A 1.

THERAPIST: And now?

PATIENT: My parents still give me money, but at least I am in my own place, and I am paying for most of it myself. That would be a 5, too.

THERAPIST: Next is having a girlfriend. Five years ago?

PATIENT: A 1, of course. And a 1 now, too. It's never gonna happen.

THERAPIST: OK, 1 for then. Let me ask you something before I write a 1 for now. I know you don't have a girlfriend now. But do you think you are any closer to it than you were back then? For instance, you have worked hard practicing some of the skills you learned here, and you have been successful in striking up an acquaintance with that one female coworker. I don't necessarily mean she will become your girlfriend, but I mean you have learned some things that are making you more comfortable talking to women. If you consider that, do you still think you are in exactly the same place you were 5 years ago on this issue?

PATIENT: I guess not. But chatting a few times with my coworker still seems pretty lame. I will have to give myself a 3 on that.

THERAPIST: What about friends?

PATIENT: Five years ago, it was about a 2. I always kept in touch with my one friend from high school. And now, it would be about a 6, I guess. I go out with some guys from work sometimes. And I hang out with my brother's friends. And I like some of the guys in my model railroad club. So that has gotten better, I guess.

THERAPIST: Last is your car.

PATIENT: (*Laughs.*) That is pretty clear-cut. My parents bought me a new car 5 years ago. It's not the greatest, but at least it was new. I would have to say 5 for then. Now it's an old, not-so-great car. Now it gets a 1!

Andrew was then asked to calculate his average success score for 5 years ago, which turned out to be 2, and for the current year, which was 4. A graph was made as a final step in this exercise, so that Andrew could see visually how his success rate really had gone up according to his more detailed analysis. This process provided data that were inconsistent with his core belief of "I am a failure."

In Bob's case, the monthly activity schedule that was presented earlier also served as a cognitive continuum exercise. At the end of each month, as mentioned, the percentages of success on each of his goals were calculated. These data were plotted on a graph that was also reviewed each month with him. Bob's core belief, "I cannot take care of myself," was challenged whenever this data graph was reviewed. He was "forced" to attribute even small increments in his percentage rates to his own effort.

Core Belief Worksheet

Another strategy for modifying schemas (core beliefs) is the core belief worksheet developed by Beck (1995). It is meant to help a patient reinforce cognitive changes that have taken place in earlier sessions. In some ways, it can be considered a relapse prevention exercise, in that the changes in automatic thoughts and intermediate beliefs that are learned in therapy are not likely to "stick" if they are not reinforced repeatedly. Only through that reinforcement process can underlying schemas truly change.

The worksheet requires the patient to list a maladaptive core belief on the top of the sheet, then rate, on a scale of 0–100%, how much it is believed right now, the most it was believed over the past week, and the least it was believed over the past week. Then the patient records the new, more adaptive belief and rates how much it is believed right now. The rest of the sheet comprises two columns for the patient to use, over the course of a week, to log evidence that contradicts the old belief and supports the new one, and also to log evidence that supports the old belief but is reframed in a new way.

The case of Rose is used to illustrate how this exercise was implemented, with some modifications. Rose was introduced in Chapter 1 as a 41-year-old single Irish American Catholic woman who was referred to therapy by her case manager because of a recent increase in angry outbursts and anxiety. Rose also has a long history of socially inappropriate behavior that has interfered with her occupational functioning. She lives with five other people in a group home for adults with developmental disabilities. Her intellectual functioning was borderline to low average, and she was capable of living and working more independently than she was, but her significant inflexibility and impulse control problems were interfering. After her intake sessions, she was diagnosed (DSM-5) as follows:

- Autism spectrum disorder
  - *requiring support for deficits with social communication (Level 1)*
  - *requiring substantial support for restricted, repetitive behaviors (Level 2)*
  - *with mild intellectual impairment*
  - *without accompanying language impairment*
- Attention-deficit/hyperactivity disorder, combined presentation
- Persistent depressive disorder (dysthymia), early onset

The goals for Rose were to decrease the frequency of angry outbursts (involving screaming, shoving, or punching peers and support staff), increase impulse control, and increase her understanding and acceptance of her disability.

Rose's core beliefs about herself were "I am defective," "I am not good enough," and "I am bound to be rejected." Her automatic thoughts and intermediate beliefs were dominated by all-or-nothing thinking, and she had a strong tendency to place herself and other people into narrowly defined categories. All people were labeled as good or bad according to only two sets of criteria. They were either *disabled* (bad) or *normal* (good). She believed that her lifelong learning problems had come from a disability (making her bad), but that the social rejection she had faced in her life was due to people mistakenly and unfairly labeling her as "retarded." Her intellectual functioning level was higher than most of the peers she had been placed with since elementary school up through the present. Her family was supportive and inclusive of her in all holidays and celebrations, which gave her many opportunities through her life to mingle and socialize with typical people. These individuals were tolerant of her behavioral differences, so her comfort level and identification with "normal" people was strong. She fantasized about moving out of her group home and into her own apartment, at which point she could find a regular job and then better fit in and be accepted. Her need to access adult disability services only highlighted her status as a disabled person, which made her feel angry.

In the first several months of treatment, psychoeducation about ASD was provided to Rose, and she was eager to learn what it was and how it would affect her. During this period, she was engaged in a day service program that focused on prevocational services for adults with developmental disabilities. She continually expressed shame about being "put with retarded people," however. She often reported feeling "sorry for" people with more severe disabilities, but also angry that others might think she is "retarded." Rose described how she always knew that she had "learning disabilities," and in some ways, she was relieved to find out that the ASD diagnosis explained a lot of the obstacles she had faced in her life. However, she also felt a desperate need to be "normal," and labeling herself as "disabled" seemed to go against that goal.

Rose's treatment plan had several components, but only one is described here. The goal of increasing her understanding and acceptance of her disability was a priority because her beliefs about the meaning of having a disability were contributing to her anger problems. The core belief "I am defective" was embedded in her attitudes about disability (intermediate beliefs) and her automatic thoughts (all-or-nothing thinking about disabled people). For example, an attitude she held was "If you are disabled, it means you are retarded." This attitude drove the automatic thought she had whenever she observed obvious impairments in her peers at home and at her day program, which was "Look at that poor person who can't control herself. I hope I don't look like that."

One of the exercises that was done with Rose was a modified core belief worksheet. In order to challenge the belief "I am defective," Rose had to first gather evidence for and against some of the attitudes she held about disabled people (which were really intermediate beliefs). Rose learned best when ideas were broken down into concrete steps, so this worksheet was designed to appeal to that style. As a homework assignment one week, she was asked to write down all of the characteristics she believed disabled people held. She came back to the next session with a list.

Disabled people are:

* *Stupid*
* *Ill-mannered*
* *Crazy*
* *Angry*
* *Poor*
* *Useless*

Next, she was asked to rate how much she believed each one. Then she was asked to produce evidence that supported the statement as well as *two forms* of evidence to contradict it. Not only was she asked to think of people who were disabled who did not possess the negative trait named but also to name some nondisabled people who *did* possess the trait. Finally, the worksheet required her to rate the strength of her belief after she examined the evidence. Although each individual belief about disability was really an intermediate belief, it was hypothesized that the core belief listed at the top of the sheet was being challenged through each of these steps, and that Rose would learn best if the process was broken down in this way. Figure 7.11 presents the worksheet after her first use of it. Her all-or-nothing thinking style led her to rate the strength of each belief as 100% before examining evidence. This worksheet was assigned to her on a weekly basis thereafter, so that she could gather ongoing evidence in her day-to-day

Old Core Belief: <u>I am defective because I am disabled.</u>

New Belief: <u>I have a disability, but I am not defective.</u>

Statement about disability	How strongly do you believe this now?	Evidence to support that disabled people have this trait	Evidence to support that some disabled people do not have this trait	Evidence to support that some nondisabled people do have this trait	How strongly do you believe the statement after examining the evidence?
Disabled people are stupid.	0–100% <u>100</u>	The people in my house and program are disabled, and they also look retarded.	My cousin's daughter is in a wheelchair, and she is very smart.	My uncle Joe is not disabled, but he is very stupid.	0–100%? <u>50</u>
Disabled people are ill-mannered.	0–100% <u>100</u>	I am disabled, and I am rude sometimes.	My cousin's daughter is in a wheelchair, and she is also very polite and nice.	My cousin Gretchen is not disabled, and she is very rude all of the time.	0–100% <u>40</u>
Disabled people are crazy.	0–100% <u>100</u>	The people in my house and program who yell look like they are disabled and crazy.	Christopher Reeve was disabled, but he was not crazy.	My sister is kind of crazy, but she is not disabled.	0–100% <u>50</u>
Disabled people are angry.	0–100% <u>100</u>	I am disabled, and I am very angry.	The guy who runs the Asperger support group is disabled, but he is always in a good mood.	I saw a very normal, nicely dressed man screaming at the gas station guy. He was very angry.	0–100% <u>70</u>
Disabled people are poor.	0–100% <u>100</u>	All the people in my program look like they have no money. We all have to follow a tight budget.	I read an article about famous people with dyslexia who are disabled and rich!	Both of my uncles are poor, but they're not disabled.	0–100% <u>30</u>
Disabled people are useless.	0–100% <u>100</u>	We are all put in a silly day program instead of real jobs because we are useless.	Christopher Reeve was disabled, but he was not useless. He helped thousands of people.	Lots of people who are not disabled do not want to work because they are lazy.	0–100% <u>20</u>

FIGURE 7.11. Rose's belief worksheet.

212

life and repeatedly rate the strength of each belief. The ratings gradually decreased as she gathered more evidence.

Chapter Summary and Conclusions

In summary, this chapter described how traditional CBT strategies can be applied to the mental health problems seen in patients with ASD. With only a few special considerations and modifications, CBT can be offered to adults with ASD to alleviate symptoms of anxiety and depression. The cognitive model is relevant to this population of adults, who are vulnerable to maladaptive schema development, an overreliance on dysfunctional rules, and all-or-nothing thinking. Several case examples were used to illustrate how tools such as the thought record, activity schedule, downward arrow, cognitive continuum, and core belief worksheet can be used with these patients. The next chapter covers mindfulness-based CBT approaches, sometimes called "contextual" or "third-wave" CBT, which are showing promise in helping adults with ASD with both their core symptoms as well as comorbid mental health problems.

CHAPTER 8

Intervention

Addressing Emotion Regulation Problems Using Mindfulness-Based Strategies

People with ASD have problems with the regulation of emotion, as evidenced by several studies reviewed in Chapter 2. Given the wide variety of mental health disorders that are characterized by problems with emotion regulation (ER), many interventions have been designed to help people enhance their awareness of internal states (emotions, cognitions, and physical sensations) in order to better manage automatic, intense emotional responses and to decrease impulsive reactivity to triggering stimuli. Many of these treatment approaches incorporate "mindfulness"- and "acceptance"-based strategies. As with the previous intervention chapters, this is not meant to be a comprehensive set of instructions on how to implement these treatment approaches because these are detailed in manuals elsewhere. Instead, this chapter outlines the rationale for considering the inclusion of mindfulness and acceptance strategies in the CBT treatment plans of adult patients with ASD who show significant problems with ER. An overview of the presenting problems that warrant the consideration of these strategies is provided along with recommended resources that allow interested readers more in-depth study. Several techniques are described, using case examples for illustration.

ER and ASD

The field of psychopathology research in the general population has incorporated the study of ER and its role from a transdiagnostic perspective in the development and maintenance of mental health problems (Kring & Sloan, 2010). Researchers in the ASD field have recently followed suit, as questions are being asked about the role ER impairment plays in both the severity of ASD symptoms as well as the development of comorbid mental health problems, such as anxiety and depressive disorders. ER is a complex, multifaceted process that can be impaired in several ways across different patients. This can best be understood in the context of a working model of effective ER. To consolidate the concepts presented in Chapter 2, we can broadly define ER as a two-stage process, with each stage involving several subtasks. In the first stage of effective ER, a person must be able to *perceive*, fairly accurately, an internal event that would be considered an emotion. This includes recognizing that something is happening (e.g., "I am experiencing an emotion . . ."), labeling it correctly (e.g., " . . . and it is called anger [or fear, sadness, joy, etc.]"), then assessing the level of arousal or intensity of the emotion (e.g., " . . . and it is very intense"). The second stage begins when a person decides that the emotion warrants modification (e.g., "I need to get this arousal level down") and then uses strategies to *regulate* or change the emotional experience and/or alter the level of arousal (see Gross & Thompson, 2007, for a detailed model of what these strategies are and how they are employed in nonclinical samples of typical people). This requires a person to possess the necessary skills (assuming he or she has acquired them through the course of development); be able to access those strategies when needed; and finally, to apply them flexibly. If successful, the person will be able to adapt to the event and continue with the usual activities of daily living and optimal functioning. For the purposes of illustration, this description exaggerated the amount of conscious decision making that a person would do in a real scenario, as typical people are likely performing these operations in a more fluid and less conscious fashion.

When people struggle with ER problems, impairments can be at one or several points in the process described above. A patient's presenting problem might be related to problems with perceiving emotions in him- or herself, deficiencies in skills needed to regulate emotional arousal, or difficulties accessing and applying acquired skills flexibly and in the appropriate context. As outlined in Chapter 2, there is a growing body of evidence that people with ASD are more likely than typical people to have problems at all stages of the ER process. They are more likely to have difficulty with the *perception of* internal states, also called alexithymia (Berthoz & Hill, 2005; Maisel et al., 2016; Samson, Huber, & Gross, 2012). This deficit in the fund or accessibility of words to describe subjective mental states has been shown to be associated with autism symptom severity (Maisel et al., 2016), but it is still unclear whether it is a core feature of ASD, a separate but common comorbidity (e.g., Shah et al., 2016), and/or a direct consequence of ASD symptoms. Regardless, this ability can be considered a prerequisite for later stages of effective ER. It is not surprising, then, that people with ASD have also been shown to have difficulty demonstrating adaptive *regulation* strategies. They are more likely to report nonacceptance of negative thoughts and emotions (Maisel et al., 2016; Swain et al., 2015), intolerance of uncertainty (Maisel et al., 2016), and less flexibility in applying regulation strategies, as evidenced by a preference for using emotional suppression more often than cognitive reappraisal (Samson et al., 2012).

When a therapist determines that an adult patient with ASD is struggling with one or several stages of ER, and hypothesizes that those impairments are contributing to the presenting problems, skill-building goals in this arena can be incorporated in the treatment plan. While Chapter 6 focused on targeting core ASD problems and Chapter 7 focused on targeting comorbid mental health problems, the assumption in this chapter is that addressing ER problems can help a patient with either. Depending on the other factors outlined in the patient's case formulation, building ER skills can improve the ASD problems in social functioning and restrictive, repetitive behaviors. This will reduce stress in a patient who may not even meet criteria for a comorbid mental health problem, thereby enhancing quality of life and reducing risk for the development of behavioral or psychiatric disorders. For those adults who do have anxiety and depressive disorders along with ASD, teaching ER strategies can be effective components in the treatment of those problems.

The next section outlines treatment approaches that have been established for teaching ER skills to people without ASD, but who have other mental health problems. Some of these *mindfulness-* and *acceptance-*based treatments have also shown promise for patients with ASD.

Mindfulness-Based Interventions in CBT

For the past 20 years, the evolution of CBT has led to the inclusion of strategies that teach patients mindfulness practices for better ER. Mindfulness-based CBT approaches are not meant to replace traditional CBT, but to add components that allow a therapist to choose from a wider variety of strategies and have more flexibility when teaching patients skills to manage overwhelming negative thoughts and emotions. At the risk of oversimplifying with a brief definition, mindfulness practices are strategies that help a person pay attention to experiences in the present moment in an accepting way and without judgment (Kabat-Zinn, 1990). These are ancient practices that have religious origins (e.g., in Buddhism), the value of which was recognized by several modern scientists and practitioners, who extracted elements for secular application in primary health care (e.g., Kabat-Zinn, 1982) and mental health care (Hayes & Wilson, 1994; Linehan, 1993a, 1993b; Teasdale, Segal, & Williams, 1995) settings.

Like CBT was an outgrowth from traditional behavior therapy, mindfulness-based therapies represent an outgrowth from traditional CBT. Through this expansion process in our field, authors have nicknamed these new approaches as "third-wave" or "third-generation" therapies. Those terms assume that the genesis of *behavior therapy* was the *first wave* of applying behavioral and learning principals to alleviate clinical problems. With a commitment to using objective observations of problem behavior, behavior therapy interventions are based on behavior analysis and identifying the function of target behaviors in the context of antecedents and consequences. This understanding comes from both an individualized assessment of the patient (e.g., Gelfand & Hartmann, 1984), as well as the evidence provided by psychological research (e.g., Ross, 1981), and the goal is to provide a patient with relief by using these principles. The commitment to using evidence-based approaches, fueled by compassion for human beings who are suffering, represented the elegance and appeal of this movement. When the field shifted toward considering private events (thoughts and emotions) as contributing factors along with overt behaviors, environmental-setting events, and consequences, the term *cognitive* was added to the behavior therapy name, giving rise to the *cognitive-behavioral therapy* term used throughout this book. This shift is what some would call the *second wave* of behavior therapy. Interventions were added that were meant to modify thoughts (e.g., cognitive restructuring, reappraisal), as well as behaviors and environmental factors, with the goals of alleviating distress and decreasing maladaptive behavior. The practices of using objective measures, conducting individualized assessments to understand the function of behavior, and relying on psychological research to design treatment plans remained as fundamental principles. In that sense, the second wave was adding to existing concepts, without changing the core assumptions or removing previously established practices. Similarly, in the 1990s, when some CBT researchers and intervention developers began incorporating new approaches that were based on mindfulness practices, the core principles of behavior therapy and CBT remained intact. All previously established methods for intervening on thoughts and behaviors are still used, but *third-wave mindfulness-based CBT* represents a shift toward also using strategies that do not necessarily alter the *content* of patients' thoughts, but rather teaches them methods for observing thoughts and changing the way they relate to the thoughts (e.g., acceptance) instead of trying to change them.

Of course, with any growth spurt comes growing pains. There have been ongoing debates about whether the inclusion of mindfulness and acceptance strategies in the family of interventions included in CBT is really a "new wave" that warrants differentiation from more traditional forms of CBT (e.g., Hofmann, Sawyer, & Fang, 2010). When considering these approaches for use with patients who have neurodevelopmental disorders, including autism, Leoni, Corti, and Cavagnola (2015) suggest that the utility of mindfulness-based treatments lies in the very same behavioral elements that constituted the first wave of behavior therapy. One might even go so far as to suggest that the third wave is more conceptually related to the first wave than the second wave. For example, acceptance and commitment therapy (ACT; Hayes & Wilson, 1994), one of the approaches that is often associated with the third wave, has its basis in behavior analysis, not CBT per se.

Because these theoretical debates will likely continue for years to come and could fill a whole volume, I have adopted the most neutral and descriptive language possible in this book, for the sole purpose of giving the reader enough information to be able to explore these interventions for some patients. I do not use the terms *third wave, new wave,* or *third generation* from this point on; the word *wave* has been used so many times in the last several paragraphs, it could make one's head spin, so it is time to wave (last time) good-bye to that. Instead, the term *mindfulness-based CBT* is used to refer to any CBT treatment plan that includes elements of traditional behavior and cognitive therapy, as well as more recently researched approaches that teach patients how to focus on events in the immediate present and to accept certain phenomena that are not readily changeable.

As illustrated throughout this book, adults with ASD benefit from individualized treatment plans, each based on a patient-specific case formulation. It has been noted by many in the CBT treatment literature for typical (non-ASD) patients that it is rare for therapists to implement a "pure" treatment package—that is, CBT protocols that are well established through multiple randomized controlled trials (RCTs) are not carried out as written when patients have multiple diagnoses in outpatient settings (Frank & Davidson, 2014; Persons, 2008; Persons et al., 2000). Considering both the nomothetic evidence base and idiographic hypotheses about an individual person (Persons et al., 2000) is the spirit in which I suggest including mindfulness-based strategies for some patients. I briefly describe the mindfulness-based treatment packages that have received the most attention in the CBT literature over the past 20 years as the nomothetic basis of this chapter, before illustrating idiographic-based applications for adults with ASD. They are ACT, dialectical behavior therapy (DBT), and mindfulness-based stress reduction (MBSR).

Acceptance and Commitment Therapy

ACT was developed and first described in an article by Hayes and Wilson (1994) and elaborated in a book by Hayes, Strosahl, and Wilson (1999). This approach assumes that human suffering is caused or worsened by attempts to avoid the experience of pain, and that the ability to use language gives people many complicated ways to practice that avoidance. At the core of ACT's transdiagnostic model of mental health, psychopathology risk is related to psychological inflexibility. The more inflexible a person is, the more likely to suffer and struggle with mental health problems. Thereby, interventions have been designed to increase psychological flexibility, which is defined as a multifaceted concept, with each domain offering a point of intervention. ACT strategies aim to help patients learn to (1) accept painful thoughts and emotions, (2) stay in contact with the present moment, (3) clarify personal values, (4) commit to action based on values, (5) view self as context, and (6) defuse from negative thoughts. The first two objectives are accomplished through mindfulness practices. The third and fourth objectives are accomplished through values clarification and action planning exercises. The last two objectives are accomplished by teaching clients "defusion" strategies, or to notice their thoughts and judgments about events and themselves and observe them from a distance, without taking them literally (or to be fused with them). While this practice shares some qualities with traditional CBT-based cognitive restructuring, in ACT, there is no emphasis on changing the content of the thoughts or debating with oneself about the evidence for the thought. Reappraisal is encouraged, but with the idea of choosing what to do about a negative thought. Rather than argue with it, push it away, or try to replace it with a different thought, there is also a choice to notice it and just let it be while attending to other aspects of the present moment at the same time.

Therapists are encouraged to attend training seminars, access supervision, and pursue self-study activities to develop their skills in applying ACT. There is no required certification one must receive before offering ACT to patients, but there are many options for ongoing development and improvement in skills. I, like many of my colleagues, began to consider ACT strategies after attending several intensive workshops and then pursuing peer supervision options in my region. While I would not call myself an ACT expert, my basic CBT practice is now informed by the ACT model, and some of the tools I acquired from workshops and readings in ACT have become standards in my CBT toolkit. Examples of those are illustrated later in this chapter.

Applications of ACT for Mental Health Problems in the General Population

ACT was designed as a set of methods to help people change the behavior of their choosing and to more effectively cope with painful experiences, but does not target a specific diagnosis or disorder. Nevertheless, clinical researchers have tested its efficacy for specific disorders since its inception, and the most recent review and meta-analysis of that research was provided by Öst (2014). Though ASD is not mentioned in any of the articles that met criteria for inclusion in this review, the treatment of the disorders that are commonly seen as comorbid conditions in adult ASD were analyzed. The author evaluated the degree of empirical support for many disorders by using American Psychological Association guidelines for classifying evidence-based treatment (as described by Chambless et al., 1998; Silverman & Hinshaw, 2008). I include here only the ones that have been mentioned earlier in his book as comorbidities of patients with ASD. While not *well established* for any disorder, ACT was deemed *possibly efficacious* for depression, psychosis, obsessive–compulsive disorder (OCD), anxiety, substance use disorders, chronic pain, and work-related stress, and *experimental* for borderline personality disorders (BPD) and trichotillomania. Studies that allowed comparison with traditional CBT protocols led to the conclusion that ACT is as effective (with slightly higher effect sizes being nonsignificant) as traditional CBT. This is consistent with the suggestion that mindfulness-based interventions offer CBT therapists additional treatment components that allow more flexibility in applying an existing and well-established evidence-based family of treatments.

Applications of ACT for People with ASD

The ER difficulties that are well documented in ASD provide the rationale for using ACT for some patients. Several clinical researchers have called for the use of interventions to improve ER in people with ASD by targeting some of the very same characteristics that the ACT model directly addresses: cognitive inflexibility (Samson et al., 2012; White et al., 2014), nonacceptance of emotion (Maisel et al., 2016), and intolerance of uncertainty (Maisel et al., 2016; South & Rodgers, 2017). Though these authors do not mention ACT specifically, the elements associated with ER impairment and mental health problems are found in the ACT treatment approaches. While no RCT has been conducted to date for ACT with patients with ASD, it has been applied and described anecdotally by some (e.g., Nichols, Sheehan, & Zito, 2017). The only published research to date was a quasi-experimental pilot study in which ACT skills were taught through a 6-week group program to a sample of cognitively able adolescents and young adults with ASD, conducted in their school setting (Pahnke, Lundgren, Hursti, & Hirvikoski, 2013). The program did not target any particular comorbid diagnosis, but aimed to increase the participants' ability to cope with the stress of living with ASD. Students were taught strategies for acceptance of thoughts/feelings/sensations, values identification, using values for goal-directed behavior, increased flexibility in perspectives on self and on problem solving, defusion (decreasing literal meaning of thoughts), and mindfulness practices for stress management. Pre- and postassessment on measures of stress, hyperactivity, emotional distress, and prosocial behavior revealed significant improvement in all areas, and these results held up at a 2-month follow-up assessment. Much more research is needed before we can say ACT is a well-established evidence-based approach for ASD, but we do have a solid rationale for teaching these skills to improve ER in our patients.

Anecdotally speaking, in my practice, I have found that adults with ASD respond more quickly to reappraisal strategies that involve acceptance of a thought as opposed to changing a thought. Because people with ASD can be very rigid in holding on to an idea, it is sometimes easier to teach people to accept the presence of the thought and work with it, rather than try to convince them to challenge the rationality of the thought and to replace it. For example, if a patient were to tell me that he is angry because a fellow passenger on a city bus deliberately bumped into him, I can take the cognitive restructuring route and encourage him to examine the evidence for this thought and then try to modify the thought so that it is less distressing (e.g., exploring the possibility that the passenger lost his balance or was distracted). This can be difficult and time-consuming with a person with cognitive rigidity and a very literal understanding of language. However, if I encourage him to accept the thought as is, but relate to it differently (defusion) by asking him to say, "I am *having the thought* that the passenger deliberately bumped into me" instead of "That passenger deliberately bumped into me," we save ourselves the trouble of debating about what is really going on with the other passenger (and since he lives in a very crowded city, there is some chance that the person did bump him on purpose). It also frees us up to explore strategies of observing, describing, and sitting with the painful emotions that come along with the idea that a stranger would be aggressive toward him, such as the anxiety or anger that would be natural in this situation. This objective would be consistent with the need to address the nonacceptance of emotion that has been mentioned several times as a hypothesized factor related to the ER difficulties observed in people with ASD, such as rigid use of the maladaptive strategy of emotion suppression.

Dialectical Behavior Therapy

DBT was first described in an article by Linehan, Armstrong, Suarez, Allmon, and Heard (1991) and elaborated in a book and accompanying manual by Linehan (1993a, 1993b). This structured treatment package was carefully designed to help patients with suicidal and self-injurious behavior, many of whom met criteria for BPD. Because these patients were not adequately helped by existing behavior therapy methods at the time, Linehan tailored this approach to address each hypothesized obstacle to treatment success. DBT is based on a biosocial theory (Linehan, 1993a) that assumes BPD at its core is a problem of ER impairment—the severe emotional distress and disruptive, unsafe maladaptive behavior are largely driven by deficits in ER. Effective ER fails to develop when a person with biologically based emotional vulnerability (e.g., easily aroused, slow to recover from high arousal) is raised in an invalidating environment, where caregivers communicate that the individual's responses and reported experiences are not valid (e.g., incorrect, inappropriate, unacceptable). When there is a paucity of opportunities to learn effective ER from the direction and role modeling of supportive adults, any child is at risk for diminished ER capacity, but this problem is exacerbated when the child is born with a biologically based vulnerability to emotional arousal.

DBT is rooted in learning theory and principles of behavior analysis, but it is distinguishable from traditional behavior therapy, not only because of the biosocial theoretical assumptions described above but also because of the dialectical philosophy that both therapists and patients are asked to assume while doing this work. Adopting a dialectical worldview involves accepting that two seemingly opposing ideas or statements can both be true at the same time. For example, part of the therapeutic alliance that is so essential in DBT includes the acceptance of the patient as is (validation) while at the same time facilitating change (building skills). Teaching the patient to apply a dialectical philosophy while facing life's challenges is one of the goals of DBT, as it addresses the rigid dichotomous thinking so often observed in BPD. Linehan recognized in the early stages of developing DBT that mindfulness practice is a "core skill" that lays the foundation to help patients to learn ER. Without abandoning her behavior analysis principles, she integrated mindfulness and acceptance strategies to create a comprehensive, holistic protocol requiring both acceptance and change.

The intervention has five functions and is delivered across several modes. The functions of DBT are to (1) enhance the patient's *capabilities*, (2) improve the patient's *motivation*, (3) ensure new capabilities are *generalized* from the therapy setting to the patient's everyday life, (4) enhance the *therapist's* capabilities and motivation to treat patients effectively, and (5) structure the *environment* to support both the patient's and therapist's capabilities. These objectives are carried out through multiple therapeutic and training activities. At the outset of a course of DBT treatment, patients and therapists are asked to commit to the following:

- Twelve months of participation in a weekly skills training group, where a qualified therapist will teach essential skills for improved *mindfulness, interpersonal effectiveness, ER,* and *distress tolerance.*
- Weekly individual therapy with a qualified therapist (who is typically not the same person as the skills training group leader) for individualized attention to reinforce practice of the new skills and address factors that interfere with practice.
- Coaching between sessions via telephone to support the practice of newly learned skills in real-life situations.
- Weekly team consultation meetings among therapists to ensure adherence to the model and the provision of necessary emotional support for the stress inherent in treating patients with frequent crises.
- Ongoing environmental modifications, individualized to each case, that further increase the likelihood of generalization and reduce the risk of crisis escalation and dropout (e.g., include family in the treatment, reduce the size of the therapist's caseload).

To be implemented as designed, standard DBT can be offered only by teams of practitioners who have been intensively trained and work together. For example, there can be no fewer than two therapists involved in one patient's treatment (skills trainer plus individual therapist), and ideally there are more in the weekly team meeting to provide support and interventions for the therapists themselves, who are treating patients who are often high risk and have complex needs. In the 25 years that have passed since Linehan's (1993b) first manual was published, however, its utility for other problems has been established. In Linehan's (2015) recent updated treatment manual, the founder reviews that literature, describes modifications, and encourages the use of DBT beyond the treatment of BPD. Some of those points are covered in the next section.

Applications of DBT for Mental Health Problems in the General Population

Standard DBT is the package that was described above, and it has the strongest evidence base for the treatment of BPD, but also has support for treating eating disorders, substance use disorders comorbid with BPD, other Cluster B personality disorders, and depressive disorders in older adults (see Linehan, 2015; Miller & Rathus, 2000, for reviews). In addition, it has been successful with age-appropriate modifications of therapy materials for the treatment of suicidal adolescents (Miller, Rathus, & Linehan, 2007; Miller, Rathus, Linehan, Wetzler, & Leigh, 1997; Rathus & Miller, 2015) and adolescents with bipolar disorder (Van Dijk, Jeffrey, & Katz, 2013).

With the expansion of the applications of DBT has come the recognition that the skills training component of the standard package has great utility as a stand-alone treatment for a variety of mental health problems. This involves teaching the skills training modules, typically in a group therapy setting, without concurrent individual therapy. While not yet tested in people with ASD, there is growing empirical support, as reviewed by Linehan (2015), for its effectiveness in treating some of the comorbid conditions mentioned in this book, such as depression, eating disorders, problem drinking, and attention-deficit/hyperactivity disorder (ADHD).

Applications of DBT for People with ASD

The idea of offering DBT to people with ASD is in its infancy. There has been no RCT of DBT for ASD published to date. Nevertheless, several clinical researchers have proposed it, using existing research on the ER impairments associated with ASD along with apparent applicability of the DBT skills training curriculum for such problems. Hartmann and colleagues (2012) provide a detailed rationale for offering DBT to people with ASD. They outline the obvious overlap between BPD and ASD in terms of ER impairment, but also point out distinctions between the two patient populations, and suggest modifications in standard DBT to address those. For example, people with BPD often have intact basic social skills and can engage in successful reciprocal conversations and make use of non-verbal communication when not in crisis; their interpersonal skills are most impaired if they have conflict with someone or become emotionally aroused. People with ASD, on the other hand, are lacking those basic social "building blocks" and those deficits are more pervasive. Therefore, the authors suggest, DBT for ASD would need to be adapted to interweave the teaching of basic social skills into all four of the skills training modules. Interestingly, these authors also point out that in some domains, people with ASD may be *more* skilled than people with BPD. For example, people with ASD may be more likely to withdraw to themselves when stressed than people with BPD. While this can be viewed as maladaptive at times, in the context of DBT, this natural ability can be reinforced and built upon as a crisis survival strategy, such as the "STOP" skill or the self-soothing skill in the distress tolerance module of DBT.

Brown (2016) has created a DBT adaptation for teaching ER skills to people with developmental disabilities. The main objective for creating this package was to address the learning needs of a variety of people with intellectual disability (ID; not ASD per se). Nevertheless, the concrete breakdown of the concepts along with the use of visual symbols could be very helpful for people with ASD who do not have ID. It is designed to be offered as a stand-alone skills training intervention. Brown is an intensively trained DBT therapist and based her program on the principles of DBT, but because the layout of the curriculum is different from what is found in standard DBT, she refers to it as a "DBT-informed" program.

Because I believe DBT skills training has so much promise to help people with ASD, I was excited to see the topic addressed at the 21st annual meeting of the International Society for the Improvement and Teaching of Dialectical Behavior Therapy (ISITDBT) in 2016. A clinical workshop was included in the program that presented an adapted DBT approach that is specifically designed for people with ASD without ID. The presenters are intensively trained DBT therapists who are actively treating people with ASD with this model (Walsh-Bender & Kappenberg, 2016). For many of the same reasons outlined above, the rationale for using this approach is rooted in the biosocial theory that drove the original development of DBT. People with ASD have a biologically based vulnerability to emotional sensitivity and reactivity. Because of their obvious behavioral differences, they are more likely than typical children to experience invalidating environments. Even loving and dedicated parents can be perplexed by unusual behaviors, teachers less likely to understand their needs, and peers more likely to reject and ridicule them. Without any modification necessary, Linehan's (1993a) biosocial theory would predict ER impairment in adulthood for people with ASD.

Anecdotally speaking, several colleagues of mine who are actively providing DBT on fully functioning DBT teams have commented on the increasing frequency with which they end up with patients with ASD on their caseloads. Most of the time, the clients are referred for DBT because of concerns about high-risk behavior or severe ER problems (e.g., as seen in suicidal adolescents), not because they have ASD. In many cases, the individual has not been diagnosed with ASD, or it is not mentioned at intake as the main reason for seeking DBT. Though I am only beginning my own training in DBT (just finished a skills training course at the time of this writing), I have been fortunate enough to develop a collaborative relationship with a DBT team in my region. For some of their patients who have ASD, they consult with me about ASD issues. Conversely, when I have a patient with ASD whose ER problems and impulsive behavior are too severe to be adequately treated in my sole-practitioner setting, I refer to the DBT team, where they assess the need for standard DBT or stand-alone DBT skills training. A transfer of care or collaborative treatment effort will be planned, based on the patient's need.

In conclusion, DBT holds a lot of promise to help people with the ER problems that come with ASD. Though modifications are needed to adapt to the specific needs of this population, the appeal of DBT is that it saves us from having to "reinvent the wheel" to treat problems that are so like those found in other disorders with severe ER impairment. At the same time, I strongly advise those CBT therapists who have not been trained in DBT to do intensive coursework and seek supervision from an experienced DBT practitioner before using these approaches with patients who have significant ER impairments.

Mindfulness-Based Stress Reduction

MBSR was first described by Kabat-Zinn (1982) as an approach for treating chronic pain in a primary care medical setting. Kabat-Zinn is both a scientist, with a PhD in molecular biology from MIT, and a practitioner of meditation and yoga in his personal life. Early in his career he saw the value of integrating ideas that came from the seemingly disparate arenas of learning (science and religion) to help people who were suffering with the physical pain associated with chronic medical conditions. With a scientific interest in using mind–body interventions in medicine, his approach is firmly rooted in the field of behavioral medicine, with most MBSR programs being offered in medical facilities.

MBSR is an 8-week group program that can be offered to anyone and is not meant to treat a single diagnosis; a healthy adult with no diagnosis would benefit, for example, by learning skills to manage normal daily stressors and to enhance quality of life. It is presented more like a class than a therapy group. Instructors are people who have gone through extensive training to implement the structured curriculum, which includes secular practice of mindfulness skills, beginner yoga skills, psychoeducation about stress, and some cognitive strategies for increasing one's awareness of thoughts.

Segal, Williams, and Teasdale (2001) introduced mindfulness-based cognitive therapy (MBCT) as an adaptation of Kabat-Zinn's course to be delivered in mental health treatment settings. The outline (8-week curriculum) and modality (group program) of

MBSR were maintained, but some content was modified to specifically target the symptoms of chronic depression, and is presented more like a psychotherapy treatment program. The design is based on the hypothesis that by integrating mindfulness practices with traditional CBT, therapists can help patients with a history of recurrent depressive episodes to lower their risk of relapse. Teasdale and colleagues used the term *attentional control* to describe to their behaviorally oriented colleagues what the function of mindfulness strategies is, as patients are taught not to try to control thoughts and emotions but instead to control the way they pay attention to those events.

Both MBSR and MBCT are considered part of a family of approaches now called mindfulness-based programs (MBPs) by Kabat-Zinn and his colleagues (Crane et al., 2016). Both are based on the same fundamental principles and are taught by instructors who have committed to their own personal practice of daily meditation. There are some practical differences of interest to CBT therapists who may want to pursue advanced training in one of these programs, or who want to refer a patient to the program best suited for the presenting problem. MBSR instructor training can be commenced by people with a wide variety of educational backgrounds and disciplines, requires six intensive courses, several silent retreats, and independent study before certification can be sought. For MBCT, on the other hand, instructor training is usually open only to people who already have a background in a professional mental health discipline (psychology, social work, psychiatric nursing, psychiatry). There are fewer hours of classroom-based courses, but more independent study and supervision requirements. In both programs, a professional can expect to spend 2–3 years of preparing before receiving teacher certification. Whether a therapist plans to pursue advanced training or not, taking the 8-week MBSR course as a participant can be a useful way to become oriented to the approach.

Applications of MBPs in the General Population

MBSR has been most effective in helping people manage their physical pain and to reduce stress, anxiety, and depression related to medical illness, including cardiovascular disease, breast cancer, and psoriasis (for reviews, see Grossman, Niemann, Schmidt, & Walach, 2004; Khoury et al., 2013). It has also been shown to help healthy adults to cope more effectively with stress and improve quality of life (see Chiesa & Seretti, 2009, for a review). Neuroimaging studies have provided preliminary evidence that MBSR is associated with beneficial neural changes in both healthy people as well as clinical samples, showing that this nonmedical intervention can actually change how the brain functions (see Hatchard et al., 2017, for a review). Because MBSR is not meant to be a psychotherapy intervention, it does not have an evidence base as a stand-alone treatment for mental health disorders. One study compared it to CBT group therapy for social anxiety disorder (SAD). While MBSR was as effective as CBT in improving mood, daily functioning, and quality of life, CBT was more effective in reducing symptoms of SAD (Koszycki, Benger, Shlik, & Bradwejn, 2007).

MBCT, in contrast to MBSR, is tailored to be a mental health intervention, with a specific focus on depression. Even so, it is not meant to be the first-line treatment for depression, as it targets the factors pertinent to relapse prevention in patients who have recurrent episodes. One RCT showed that MBCT is most effective in preventing recurrence of depression in patients who had had at least three previous depressive episodes

(Teasdale et al., 2000). It has also shown promise in reducing anxiety and associated depressive symptoms in patients with GAD (Evans et al., 2008).

Applications of MBPs for People with ASD

There has been only one study in which MBSR has been applied with adults with ASD. Sizoo and Kuiper (2017) compared MBSR to CBT in targeting anxiety symptoms, depression scores, ASD symptoms, rumination, and global mood. Both approaches were similarly effective in improving all of the target variables. The few other studies of MBPs in ASD have explored MBCT. The MBCT protocol of Segal and colleagues (2001) was modified for adults with ASD (by changing some of the language and exercises to be less ambiguous and by adding an extra session to the standard program) and named "mindfulness-based therapy for autism spectrum disorders" (MBT-AS) by Spek and colleagues (2013) and tested in an RCT. The aim was to reduce symptoms of depression and anxiety, with the hypothesis that reduced rumination tendencies would be the mechanism of change. Rumination is defined as a tendency to think repetitively about the causes, situational factors, and consequences of one's own emotional experiences, and can be conceptualized as a form of nonacceptance of emotion. Because the thinking styles of people with ASD make them prone to rumination (nonacceptance of emotion) and MBPs result in reduced rumination in the general population, MBT-AS was expected to be helpful to these adult subjects. Results indicated that the treatment group showed significant reduction in depression, anxiety, and rumination compared to the wait-list control, and increased positive affect after the 9-week group program. There was a potential mediation effect for rumination changes in relation to changes in anxiety and depression levels. In another study of MBT-AS, the investigators repeated the treatment with five groups of adults with ASD, finding similar success in improving depressive and anxiety symptoms, associated with decreased rumination (Kiep, Spek, & Hoeben, 2015). These effects were maintained as measured at a 9-week postintervention follow-up. In another preliminary study of feasibility and efficacy, Conner and White (2018) implemented a similar protocol with nine adults with ASD diagnosis. Unique to this study was the treatment delivery modality, which was through individual psychotherapy sessions, a departure from the group modality used in other studies. The modified MBCT intervention targeted the ER impairments that are common for people with ASD. Seven of the nine participants reported improvement in at least one of the ER domains of impulse control, access to ER strategies, and emotional acceptance. This study also provided evidence for the feasibility of offering a modified MBCT intervention to adults with ASD.

In sum, MBPs are viable approaches to target ER problems and enhance quality of life for adults with ASD. They are not meant to be used as stand-alone treatment protocols for specific mental health disorders, but have great potential to serve as an adjunct to a course of individual psychotherapy. In my own practice, I rely on a stress reduction center in my region, where MBSR courses are offered on a regular basis (and where I took the course myself). For some patients, whose treatment plans warrant ER skill building, I refer them to an MBSR course for a more intensive learning experience than what I can provide. In those cases, individual sessions with me continue, where I can give the patient guidance on using the new skills to address the specific presenting problems.

Improving Identification of One's Own Emotions

As mentioned earlier, ER is a multistage process, with the recognition of internal states coming first, followed by attempts to regulate those experiences. Clinical focus on ER problems and improving them starts with targeting impairments in the ability to recognize one's own emotions, or alexithymia. Some authors include alexithymia under the umbrella of ER, while others describe it as a separate but related concept. I prefer the former conceptual framework, as the recognition of emotion represents the very first moment in the whole ER process; later-stage skills cannot be fully learned or demonstrated without the prerequisite perceptual processes functioning properly. Despite a continuum model, I organized the sections ahead into two separate categories. Strategies for improving the perception and identification of emotional experiences are covered in this section, while strategies for applying actions (behavioral or mental) to regulate these experiences are covered in the following section.

Strategies for teaching emotion recognition and identification have been designed by professionals from a variety of disciplines and theoretical orientations. The common objectives of most tools for psychoeducation about emotion are to (1) increase *general knowledge* about human emotion, (2) improve *emotion vocabulary* and the ability to *connect emotion words to subjective experiences* of emotion, and (3) improve the ability to detect and self-assess the *intensity* of emotions and to be aware of ongoing changes in arousal levels.

The tools a therapist chooses depends on the learning style of the patient. Some patients respond more to multimodal tools that combine words, pictures, colors, and action-oriented exercises involving movement. Others respond better to conventional text-based reading materials and written worksheets. In my own work with adults, it has been challenging to find tools that are age appropriate. If you browse the multitude of education and therapy tool catalogues that are available, you will see many games and toys that are designed to teach children emotion identification and self-awareness of emotion, but many of those are not appealing to adult patients. Examples of the ones I have found are described below, with notation about which of the three objectives listed above are addressed and what modalities are utilized. This information is also summarized in Table 8.1.

DBT ER Skills Training Module

The skills training manual that is used in standard DBT (Linehan, 2015) includes a module for the teaching of ER skills. The lessons start out with a focus on understanding what emotions are and why we need them. Also included are richly detailed handouts that are useful for improving emotion vocabulary. Definitions and synonyms are provided for the basic emotions *anger, disgust, envy, fear, happiness, jealousy, love,* and *sadness*. The information is provided with text-based handouts and worksheets. The *DBT Skills Training Manual for Adolescents* (Rathus & Miller, 2015) has a similar ER training module, but in modifying the materials for younger people, the authors added illustrations and nonverbal symbols that are very useful for some adults with ASD. These worksheets can be used to meet an emotion psychoeducation goal in a CBT treatment plan, even if the therapist is not delivering a DBT intervention.

TABLE 8.1. Tools for Psychoeducation about Emotion

Name of program or tool	Provides general knowledge about human emotions	Targets emotion vocabulary, recognition, and labeling of own emotions	Targets self-assessment of the intensity level of own emotions	Text-based presentation of materials	Multimodal presentation of materials
DBT Emotion Regulation Skills Training Module (Linehan, 2015)	✓	✓		✓	
DBT Emotion Regulation Skills Training Module for Adolescents (Rathus & Miller, 2015)	✓	✓		✓	✓
"The Role of Your Emotions" chapter in *Living Well on the Spectrum* (Gaus, 2011)	✓	✓		✓	✓
Alexithymia Reduction Treatment (Levant, Halter, Hayden, & Williams, 2009)		✓		✓	
The Incredible 5-Point Scale (Buron & Curtis, 2012)			✓	✓	✓
Feelings Rating Scale from the Emotion Regulation Skills System (Brown, 2016)			✓	✓	✓
Exploring Feelings for Anxiety (Attwood, 2004a) and Anger (Attwood, 2004b)		✓	✓	✓	✓
Bodily Map of Emotions (Nummenmaa, Glerean, Hari, & Hietanen, 2014)		✓			✓
Talk Blocks for Work (Innovative Interactions, 2000)		✓			✓

Living Well on the Spectrum

In the self-help workbook that I wrote for adults with ASD (Gaus, 2011), there is information and worksheets designed to help the reader with the first two objectives listed above. In a chapter called "The Role of Your Emotional Differences," readers are given basic scientific information about human emotion, including the definition and function of feeling states. Figures 8.1 and 8.2 are examples of how the material is presented, combining text with pictures. Also included is material designed to improve emotion vocabulary and to build connections between the specific emotion words of *joy, anger, sadness,* and *fear* and the associated arousal states. The illustration in Figure 8.3 is used to help the readers of that book understand those concepts.

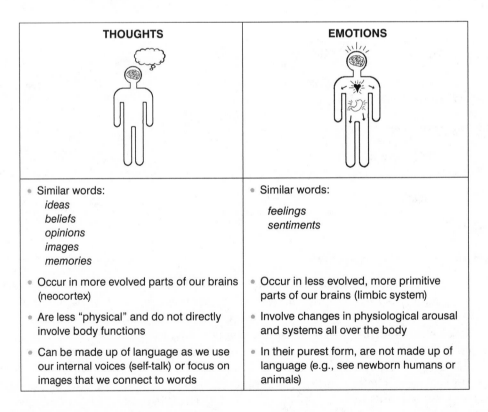

Notes

✓ Scientists who study human emotion have a long way to go before giving us all the facts. The following three assumptions came from some of their findings:

✓ <u>Emotions</u> and <u>thoughts</u> are different from each other.

✓ There are basic human emotions that can be described by these four words:

    1. Joy
    2. Sadness
    3. Anger
    4. Fear

✓ Each basic emotion serves an important function to help us survive.

FIGURE 8.1. Emotions: Why humans have them. From Gaus (2011). Copyright © 2011 The Guilford Press. Reprinted by permission.

THOUGHTS	EMOTIONS

• Similar words:
  ideas
  beliefs
  opinions
  images
  memories
	• Similar words:
	
	  feelings
	  sentiments

• Occur in more evolved parts of our brains (neocortex)	• Occur in less evolved, more primitive parts of our brains (limbic system)
• Are less "physical" and do not directly involve body functions	• Involve changes in physiological arousal and systems all over the body
• Can be made up of language as we use our internal voices (self-talk) or focus on images that we connect to words	• In their purest form, are not made up of language (e.g., see newborn humans or animals)

FIGURE 8.2. Differences between thoughts and emotions. From Gaus (2011). Copyright © 2011 The Guilford Press. Reprinted by permission.

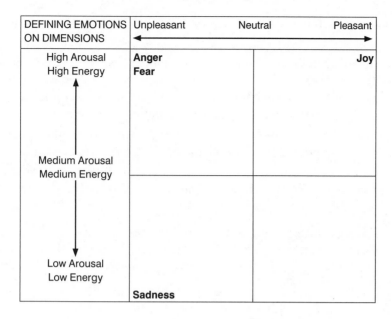

DEFINING EMOTIONS ON DIMENSIONS	Unpleasant Neutral Pleasant	
High Arousal High Energy	**Anger** **Fear**	**Joy**
Medium Arousal Medium Energy		
Low Arousal Low Energy	**Sadness**	

FIGURE 8.3. Defining emotions on dimensions. From Gaus (2011). Copyright © 2011 The Guilford Press. Reprinted by permission.

The dialogue below took place in a session when some of this material was being introduced to Carl, the man mentioned in Chapter 1, who came in for help with adjustment problems related to aging. His treatment plan called for emotion education. One of the maladaptive behaviors that his supporters were concerned about was his frequent use of 911 and ambulance trips to the local emergency room, most of which resulted in a discharge and medical reports ruling out the need for treatment. One hypothesis was that he had difficulty differentiating between symptoms of medical problems and the signs of being anxious or frustrated. Here the therapist is proposing the idea of working on this.

THERAPIST: So you said you felt "funny" when you called for an ambulance over the weekend. Was it more like you were coming down with a physical illness, or more like you were upset . . . emotionally upset?

PATIENT: Hmm. Hard to tell.

THERAPIST: Yes, it can be hard to tell. When people are emotionally upset, there are changes inside the body that feel the same as some types of medical symptoms.

PATIENT: Yeah. I like to have the ER doctor figure that out. That's why I'd rather just go to the ER. Better to be safe than sorry.

THERAPIST: I agree—it is better to be safe than sorry when it comes to medical problems. And you certainly have had your share of medical problems.

PATIENT: You got that right.

THERAPIST: You mentioned last week that each ambulance ride ends up costing you a lot of money because a big portion of it isn't covered by your insurance.

PATIENT: I know. I wish I didn't have to use it so much.

THERAPIST: Well, like you said, you are trying to be cautious. I know you and your visiting nurse will keep working on the protocol for calling 911. While you work with her over the next few weeks on that, you and I can be doing some work here to help you catch the signs of emotional upsets. I can give you some information and tips on how to be a better detector of your own emotions.

PATIENT: Well, I think I am pretty happy most of the time. Like, I'm usually thinking about things that are fun for me. Like the next museum trip I have planned.

THERAPIST: And that is exactly why you are doing so well living by yourself and being independent—you are optimistic and enthusiastic about staying active.

PATIENT: Yeah—I like to have fun!

THERAPIST: That's the spirit! Everybody has some moments when they are not feeling so happy, though. It is normal to sometimes feel frustrated or nervous or sad.

PATIENT: I just push those ideas away.

THERAPIST: That's a natural response to unpleasant things in life. Yet, we can sometimes cope more effectively with difficult moments when we are more aware of what is happening inside of us as well as outside of us. There are lots of things that happen on the inside of us. Look at this diagram about thoughts and feelings.

PATIENT: Aren't thoughts and feelings the same things?

THERAPIST: Not exactly. They both happen on the inside, but there are some differences that you will see here. (*Gives the patient handouts containing the diagrams shown in Figures 8.1 and 8.2.*)

Before the therapist could move into teaching Carl methods for coping with stress and regulating his emotions, Carl would need, as prerequisites, a basic working knowledge about emotions and strategies for observing them in himself. The above excerpt was from the first of many sessions spent on this topic.

Alexithymia Reduction Treatment

The alexithymia reduction treatment (ART) manual (Levant, Halter, Hayden, & Williams, 2009) provides a 6-week psychoeducational group intervention that is not designed for any particular diagnosis, but targets alexithymic tendencies in men. Lessons and homework assignments include worksheets to develop a better emotion vocabulary and to keep an emotional response log to increase self-awareness of these phenomena. The information is presented in text-based worksheets. Though it was designed for men, the emotion education tools it provides would be useful for any adult patient who needs to build these skills.

Exploring Feelings Manuals

In Attwood's *Exploring Feelings* manuals, a CBT group treatment is detailed to treat anger (2004b) and anxiety problems (2004c) in youth with ASD. Though it is not geared toward adults, the "affective education" exercises provided in both manuals are excellent for teaching emotion concepts to adult patients, as well. There are both text-based and experiential exercises to enhance emotion vocabulary, and to teach self-assessment of intensity. For example, to teach the idea that emotions can vary in intensity, an exercise called the "Rope Game" is used. Participants are asked to get out of their seats and stand at particular points on a rope that has been placed on the floor to represent the level of intensity experienced of a given emotion. This example of multimodal presentation of material—in this case, movement and visual symbols—can be very helpful to some patients.

The Incredible 5-Point Scale

In what has become a classic book in the world of special education, now in its second edition, Buron and Curtis (2012) provide a set of tools designed to improve social cognition and ER in students with ASD. The authors are teachers who were aiming to help students in school-based settings, but the approach is useful for psychoeducation about emotion in adult therapy settings, as well. The curriculum teaches students how to use a 5-point rating system to assess and rate the varying intensity of stress, emotional experiences, and behaviors. Every worksheet is based on the same model, which is presented as a color-coded scale, with 1 being the least intense, and 5 being the most. The value of the tool lies in the flexibility it offers to individuals, teachers, and therapists. Figure 8.4 is an example of the worksheet that a patient could use to evaluate stress. In this black and white diagram, the color words were inserted next to each level to describe the illustrations as they appear in the original materials. For patients who have not yet developed a strong emotion vocabulary, the word *stress* can be a generic term for emotional arousal, and this worksheet can be used to begin practicing the self-assessment of varying intensity. Blank templates of the scale can be used to fill in specific situations in the user's life. Using a patient's special interests can be a powerful way to enhance the tool. Figure 8.5 illustrates how a worksheet was individualized for Carl, using his special interest in the art of Fabergé. Because he already had a working knowledge of the emotion of happiness, that was the feeling that was chosen to introduce the idea of rating varying levels of emotional experience. His expression of joy and excitement over the works of Fabergé was so frequent and observable, it seemed like the most logical subject for this exercise. The worksheet was introduced to him, with the instructions to find pictures of his favorite pieces of art to bring in and paste on the sheet. The activity took place over several sessions, and laid the groundwork for subsequent work that would be done around negative emotions.

The Feelings Rating Scale from the Emotion Regulation Skills System

The Emotion Regulation Skills System for Cognitively Challenged Clients (Brown, 2016) is a DBT-informed program that includes a rating scale that uses both words and nonverbal visual symbols to help patients learn to self-assess emotional intensity. The scale goes from 0 to 5 and includes verbal descriptions, cartoon drawings, and graphics that suggest increasing intensity. The 0, for example, has the words *no feeling* next to it, with a cartoon of someone in a bed sleeping; the 1 has the words *tiny feeling* next to it, with a cartoon of a mildly concerned face; and so on. The font size of the numbers also increases in size to suggest growing intensity, such as:

0 1 2 3 4 5

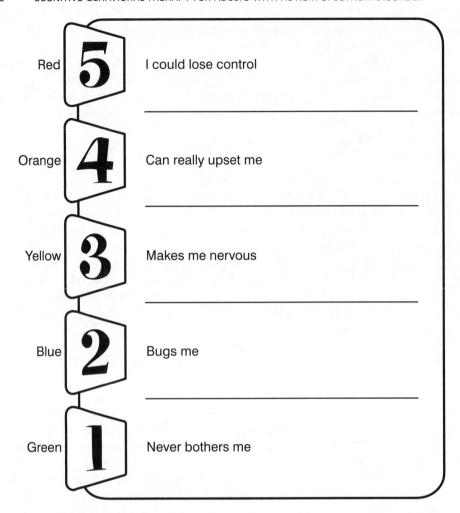

FIGURE 8.4. The Incredible 5-Point Scale for rating stress. From Buron and Dunn (2012). Copyright © 2012 AAPC Publishing. Adapted by permission.

Even if a therapist is not using the program in its entirety, the rating scale is useful to teach patients to pay attention to varying emotional arousal levels within themselves because of the multimodal presentation of the concept.

The Bodily Map of Emotions

For those patients who enjoy learning about the scientific aspects of psychology, the Bodily Map of Emotions (Nummenmaa, Glerean, Hari, & Hietanen, 2014) diagram can be an appealing way to introduce some general knowledge about human emotions, as well as to increase emotion vocabulary. The one-page tool came from a study done with healthy adults in which subjects were asked to color—using a mouse and specially designed computer graphics program—a blank silhouette of a body, to self-report their reactions to various emotion stimuli. When presented with a variety of emotion stimuli

stimuli (words, stories, movies, facial expressions), subjects "painted" the body to indicate where they felt increasing (warm colors) or decreasing (cool colors) activation while exposed to each stimulus. The resulting body maps show regions whose activation was reported to increase or decrease when feeling each of 14 emotions: anger, fear, disgust, happiness, sadness, surprise, neutral, anxiety, love, depression, contempt, pride, shame, and envy. The findings were consistent across conditions in 701 adults, with representation from both Western European and Eastern Asian cultures. The diagram can be used as a handout and is available for downloading as a full-color PowerPoint slide through the original open-access article at the National Academy of Sciences (*www. pnas.org/content/111/2/646*). It introduces the idea to adult patients that human beings experience a variety of emotions and that those phenomena are felt throughout the body, while being careful to explain that these are not exact replicas of solid objects, the way a topographical map of a mountain range would be, for example. Because they

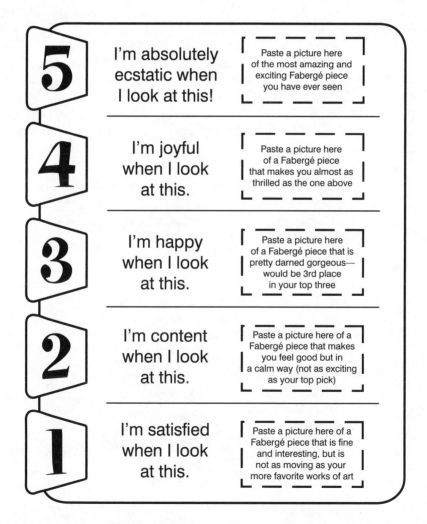

FIGURE 8.5. Carl's Incredible 5-Point Scale for rating happiness. From Buron and Dunn (2012). Copyright © 2012 by AAPC Publishing. Adapted by permission.

are pictorial representations of the averaged data derived from the subjective experiences of many people, each map may not look the same for each individual person (e.g., the way disgust appears on the map may not be exactly the way every person feels it). Discussing this diagram can pave the way toward helping the patient to pay attention to the internal sensations associated with different emotions, as well as the emotion vocabulary that is detailed in the figure.

Talk Blocks

Another approach for teaching emotion vocabulary and connection to subjective states can be found in Talk Blocks for Work (Innovative Interactions, 2000). Capitalizing on the strong visualization skills that many adults with ASD have, the Talk Blocks serve as a visual multiple-choice cue set to help the patient recognize and differentiate his or her feelings and needs in stressful situations. The appeal of this tool is the age-appropriate focus found in a multimodal presentation, which is a rare combination of features. Designed for adults to use for workplace dilemmas, this is a set of six blocks, each with a picture and phrase on each of the six sides. Three blocks are red, to symbolize feelings, and three blocks are blue, to symbolize needs. Each subset of blocks, therefore, gives the patient 18 choices to help him or her access the words that best describe subjective experiences. Table 8.2 shows the lists for each of the block subsets.

As the patient expresses distress over a conflict or dilemma, the therapist can present the Talk Blocks. While showing the patient that there is a picture and phrase on each

TABLE 8.2. Words and Phrases Presented on Talk Blocks

Red feeling blocks	Blue need blocks
I FEEL . . .	*I NEED . . .*
Angry	*To be listened to*
Appreciated	*No interruptions*
Exhausted	*Time alone*
Happy	*More information*
Pressured	*Nourishment*
Undervalued	*To talk*
Anxious	*More support*
Bored	*To assert myself*
Motivated	*To set some limits*
Focused	*To take a break*
Impatient	*Solutions*
Productive	*To listen*
Frustrated	*To have fun*
Irritable	*To laugh*
Overwhelmed	*To be patient*
Excited	*To calm down*
Successful	*To stop and think*
Disappointed	*To take a deep breath*

Note. From Innovative Interactions, LLC (2000). Copyright 2000 by Innovative Interactions, LLC. Reprinted by permission.

side, the therapist first hands the patient the red ones and says, "Which of these words best describes how you feel? You can pick more than one if you want." Many patients appear to have a "lightbulb" experience as they select the block that matches how they feel. They exclaim something like "Oh, this is it! 'Overwhelmed.' That is how I feel" but they had not been able to come up with the word on their own. After choosing the feeling word(s), the patient is handed the blue blocks and the therapist says, "OK, you feel overwhelmed at work. Now, what do you think you need to help you with that feeling? In other words, which of the phrases on these blue blocks best describes something that you think would help you feel less overwhelmed?" Finally, the patient is asked to string together the words and phrases chosen into a sentence. Figure 8.6 shows the blocks the way they would appear for the following:

I FEEL anxious, therefore I NEED more information.
I FEEL overwhelmed, therefore I NEED to take a break.

Not all of the feeling words are "pure" emotions, but serve the purpose of building a connection between subjective states, whether they be emotions or beliefs and words, and the fact that those states can prompt a need for change. Many adults with ASD have strong verbal skills and rich vocabularies but are missing the *connection* between words and subjective states. An example of this can be seen in this unexpected event with one of my patients. At the beginning of one session, a patient with ASD and superior

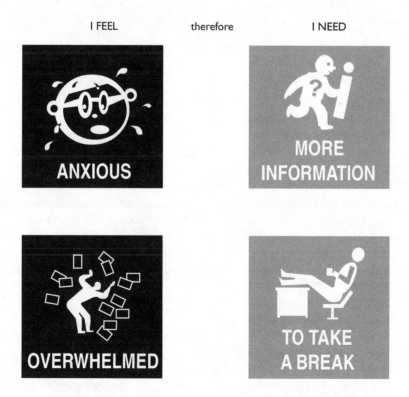

FIGURE 8.6. Examples of Talk Block sentences. From Innovative Interactions, LLC (2000). Copyright © 2000 Innovative Interactions, LLC. Reprinted by permission.

intellectual ability noticed the Talk Blocks sitting on my desk and asked about them. I had not planned to use them with him, but I showed them to him and explained their purpose. He seemed amused as he spent a few minutes looking through them and putting sentences together in what appeared to be a playful way, but he did not seriously connect them to anything in his life. The session turned to the regular agenda and the blocks were put away. The following week, the blocks were not out, and I had forgotten about this patient's interest in them. He asked to see them again, saying that he wanted to tell a story about something that had happened to him at his job. As I went to look for the blocks, he said, "Oh, never mind. Don't get them. I remember them." He proceeded to name off almost all of the 36 words that were on the six blocks! I was shocked by this display of uncanny visual memory (which is not uncommon among people on the autism spectrum), as he had only spent a few minutes looking at them the prior week. Needless to say, the blocks were incorporated into his plan because he responded so positively to them. Interestingly, he did end up needing a lot of practice before he could associate these words that he had memorized so easily with actual subjective states he was experiencing in his life.

The Talk Blocks have recently gone out of production, but are still available through third-party sellers. This approach can be applied through the use of homemade materials, even if a therapist does not have access to the blocks. The patient is taught several things by practicing this exercise repeatedly through a variety of real-life scenarios. One is to increase emotion vocabulary while also improving the ability to make connections between subjective states and words. Another is the idea that a feeling can actually prompt one to change something in the environment in order to relieve distress, which is the foundation of ER. This concept provides an excellent segue into the next section on ER skills to help patients with acceptance of emotion and tolerance of distress.

Improving ER Skills

This section provides examples of how mindfulness and acceptance-based interventions can be used to teach adult patients with ASD more adaptive strategies for regulating negative emotions. The research on ER in people with ASD reviewed earlier suggests problems with nonacceptance of emotion, intolerance of uncertainty, and inflexibility in applying ER skills. By viewing these problems as points of intervention in a treatment plan, the therapy goals become (1) increase acceptance of emotions, (2) increase tolerance of uncertainty, and (3) increase flexibility in applying acquired ER skills. Case examples are used to illustrate how methods described in earlier sections can be applied for specific ER problems in adult patients with ASD.

Increasing Acceptance of Emotion

It is common for people with ASD to struggle with the acceptance of internal events that are negative. This may be partly due to the lack of knowledge about emotions and emotion vocabulary mentioned in the previous section. Because nonacceptance of emotion and rumination are associated with some symptoms of ASD as well as comorbid mental health problems, techniques that have been designed to target that can be offered to patients with ASD. Assuming a patient has received sufficient psychoeducation about emotion, work on accepting those events in oneself can begin.

Rachel was introduced in Chapter 1 as a 36-year-old woman, newly diagnosed with ASD after years of multiple misdiagnoses. Her treatment plan involved several goals that included acceptance, as she had sought therapy to help herself adjust to the new knowledge she had gained about her own diagnosis of ASD. This dialogue is from a session in which emotion psychoeducation had been the focus, with this excerpt showing when the topic switched from emotion identification to acceptance of emotion.

PATIENT: Well, I understand all of those emotion words and what they mean. I majored in English! But I am not a very emotional person. Not at all.

THERAPIST: What do you mean?

PATIENT: I don't have many emotions. Really. Just anger. Yeah, I am either fine, or angry. And when I'm angry, everyone knows it! But most of the time, I am logical.

THERAPIST: Do you mean you don't experience emotions like sadness or fear?

PATIENT: Logic takes over if those things appear. You see, I am very practical. Those emotions are not practical.

THERAPIST: Given that material we reviewed about the function of emotions for human beings, can you think of some ways sadness or fear might be practical at times— may even have some survival value?

PATIENT: Yes, I suppose. But it's never really gotten me anywhere. If I think I am getting sad or scared, it annoys me and I just shut it off . . . use my logic to solve problems.

THERAPIST: So you get annoyed about being sad or scared? Like getting upset about being upset?

PATIENT: Yes. Like I said, anger is the easiest for me. So, it's easier to be angry than sad or scared.

THERAPIST: Have I mentioned yet the idea of "secondary emotion"?

PATIENT: I don't think so.

THERAPIST: It's a term psychologists use to describe when we have an emotional reaction to having an emotional reaction.

PATIENT: (*Laughs.*) That is kind of a mind-bender!

THERAPIST: Yes! It is! We humans do that sometimes and it tends to backfire by making us even more upset.

PATIENT: Hmm. Actually, that makes sense. I never thought about that before. My logic tells me we are on to something here. (*Laughs again.*)

After this discussion, Rachel was given some material from *The Illustrated Happiness Trap* (Harris & Aisbett, 2013), a book I often use to introduce patients to the concepts around accepting emotions and making the choice not to engage in suppression strategies. Based on the concepts of ACT, this easy-to-read book, that has cartoons to illustrate the concepts, is a useful tool for teaching acceptance-of-emotion strategies. In a subsequent session, Rachel was given some handouts about the mindfulness practice of "staying" in one's "wise mind" mode (Linehan, 2015). Using the illustrated handout found in the adolescent adaptation (Rathus & Miller, 2015), Rachel was taught about the benefits of accessing her "wise mind" by paying attention to both her "reasonable mind" and her "emotional mind" to be most effective in solving her problems. Like many patients with ASD, Rachel found relief in the idea that she would not have to give up her logical side in order to accept more openly her emotional experiences, as the "wise mind" relies on both.

Increasing Tolerance of Uncertainty

Facing uncertainty is an experience that most human beings find stressful. Having the ability to tolerate uncertain circumstances is an essential ER skill. Impairment in this ability is associated with ASD and some of the comorbid conditions common to these adult patients. Strategies to improve this skill are essential in the treatment plans of many of these adult patients.

Seth was introduced in Chapter 1 and described further in Chapter 7 (the "thought flowchart") as a 44-year-old man with maladaptive stress responses and occupational problems. With a comorbid diagnosis of GAD, intolerance of uncertainty was central to his struggles. Some of his maladaptive behavior served the function of providing him a sense of certainty and control, although at a high price. For example, he had a history of abruptly ending friendships after minor, normal misunderstandings. His reasoning was that he would rather end it himself than wait for the day that the friend might end it. The dialogue below illustrates how this tendency appeared within the therapy relationship. I take time off approximately three times each year, for about 1 week each time. Each time a vacation was impending, the discussion of the schedule would take place approximately 6 weeks ahead of time. After several years of working with Seth, I became frustrated with the fact that the conversation would go in an almost identical fashion, every time, as follows:

THERAPIST: I want to go over the schedule with you for the near future. I am going to be away the week of August 20th, so we will not be able to meet that week.

PATIENT: (*low groan, grimacing expression, hands splaying in the air*) Well . . . well . . . well, let's skip the whole month! We have to skip the whole month! No sessions in August at all. That's it. Skip the month.

THERAPIST: I will only be gone for 1 week. We can meet the other 3 weeks in August. I will be here.

PATIENT: No! It's easier to just skip the month. No sessions. That's it!

THERAPIST: Seth, you don't have to come to meet me the other weeks that I am here in August. That is up to you. I do want you to know that I am available, and will hold the time slots open for you for the time being. You can decide when we get closer to the date, but I am available on the other weeks if you want to come in.

PATIENT: It's just easier to skip it. I don't want to have to worry about something else throwing off the schedule. You might get stuck out of town or sick or something. It's easier to just cut it now!

THERAPIST: Every week, one of us could get stuck or sick or something. Every week we make an appointment for the next week, *with* the possibility that one of us could get stuck or sick. What makes the likelihood higher that it will happen when I am on vacation?

PATIENT: (*appearing calmer*) It's not. OK, just pencil me in on the other dates. I feel better when there is a routine. I don't like the routine to change. That's all.

Even though we managed to get through the scheduling issues each time I had a vacation planned, the resolution did not ever generalize to the next time. He would always respond in the same exact way, as if we had never resolved the issue before. In hindsight, I realize I should have integrated this issue into our treatment plan, but I had mistakenly chalked it up to a nuisance factor around scheduling with this patient, as his complex problems had me thinking we had "bigger fish to fry." I had simply come to accept that this was a ritual that I would have to tolerate, until one day, he shifted my thinking. Here is the dialogue from that session:

THERAPIST: So, I want to go over the schedule for the near future. I am going to be away for the week of June 5th. So, I will not be able to meet that week (*bracing herself for the usual "skip the whole month" routine*).

PATIENT: (*long silence, then a sigh*) Why don't you just retire?!?

THERAPIST: (*loud laugh*) What? (*more loud laughing*)

PATIENT: (*loud laughing*) That's an interesting idea I gave you, eh? (*more loud laughing*)

This was not my proudest moment as a therapist because my laughter was an involuntary outburst, triggered by his unexpected deviation from the ritual. I was grateful for his laughter, which was a sign to me that he was not offended by my response. Ironically, it was his spontaneous change in the routine that allowed me to view this pattern from a different perspective than the one I had for several years.

Seth and I were able to use this experience constructively to increase his tolerance of uncertainty, in part thanks to the ACT technique of "defusion." One assumption of ACT is that people can become "fused" with their thoughts, resulting in repetitive patterns of maladaptive thought and behavior that have been conditioned and underlie many mental health problems. In simple terms, thoughts are stories we are telling ourselves using language. Fusion refers to believing these stories as if each one is literally true, and is central to the chronic worrying that is observed in GAD. Defusion, on the other hand, is the process of observing the story, without taking the words literally. It is a reappraisal strategy that is aimed at an internal event (a thought), and involves placing one degree of separation between what the story is saying and what you literally believe. Without planning it, Seth's remark about retirement and then our shared laughter was enough to defuse both of us from the "skip the whole month" story. With that, I was freed up to be able to offer more ACT-based defusion strategies to address the function of his maladaptive attempts to create certainty within relationships (e.g., impulsively ending friendships). His insistent remarks about canceling all therapy sessions within each month of a vacation had the same function as terminating friendships in which some minor misunderstandings had occurred—to avoid the seemingly intolerable distress associated with uncertainty. In subsequent sessions, I asked him to list phrases that expressed his intrusive worries, including:

- *My therapist will not ever return from her trip.*
- *My friend will end the friendship because of our misunderstanding.*
- *I cannot bear the uncertainty of waiting for bad news.*

I asked Seth to rewrite each phrase with the additional opening words of "I am having the thought that . . ." The newly phrased sentences were:

- *I am having the thought that* my therapist will not ever return from her trip.
- *I am having the thought that* my friend will end the friendship because of our misunderstanding.
- *I am having the thought that* I cannot bear the uncertainty of waiting for bad news.

After many repetitions of each phrase, Seth was eventually able to articulate an understanding that his thoughts did not necessarily reflect reality. After this, he was able to more effectively reappraise similar thoughts when they arose in his life. He sometimes used the phrase "My worst fear is that this will happen, but that is not the same as it actually happening." Other times he might say, "My mind says this, but it doesn't make it true." As he became more practiced in phrasing his worries that way, his willingness to refrain from impulsive attempts to make things more certain also increased, as he realized he could tolerate the uncertainty and continue to engage in his activities of daily living, even when he was having a worry thought.

As a side note, the routine he developed after this for every vacation-planning discussion is to simply say, with a smile, "Why don't you just retire?" followed by a long laugh and a look to me to laugh with him. This shared joke has become a ritual, as well, but a more healthy and adaptive way for Seth to cope with his discomfort, as he no longer insists that we "skip the whole month." In addition, through humor he is communicating his understanding that his attempts to control uncertainty are at best, ineffective, and at most, something to laugh about, representing successful defusion. The thoughts still come, but he feels less controlled by them.

Increasing Flexibility in Applying ER Skills

Many adults with ASD come to therapy already having acquired some effective coping skills, self-taught through life experiences, acquired from therapeutic supports, or a combination of both. For some the difficulty is in applying these skills flexibly to more effectively regulate emotional experiences. For example, a strategy that is effective for a person in one situation (stepping outside for a brief moment of fresh air to cope with the pressure of working in a crowded noisy office) may not be applied in another situation if the latter is not recognized by the individual as similar enough to the former to apply that skill (when feeling overwhelmed by a crowded noisy family reunion, failing to recognize the likelihood that a brief break out in the fresh air may be helpful). Or an effective skill (listening to relaxing music near bedtime on a stereo system) may need to be only slightly modified to use it across more situations (when away from home), but the individual with ASD may not recognize the possibility of modifying it (bring a portable listening device) or may not immediately be able to design a modification for it (unsure how to search for suitable listening devices).

Mindfulness practices, by definition, improve an individual's ability to control attentional processes. By learning to pay attention more fully, in the present, to both external and internal stimuli, people can become more flexible in how they direct their focus. This allows for more immediate recognition of opportunities for reappraisal, an early-stage regulation process that is more adaptive than suppression, which is a late-stage regulation strategy that is less adaptive and associated with more cognitive and behavioral rigidity (Gross & John, 2003). There is no reason to assume people with ASD cannot learn to gain better control over their attentional processes and then enjoy the benefits of these added skills. In fact, my clinical observations of adults with ASD have led me to believe that they often have better control over their attentional processes than typical people in some situations.

Because of their lifetime struggles with unique sensory experiences, adults with ASD have a highly developed ability to narrow their focus on one part of the environment or a specific sensory experience in order to modulate the effects of being in an overstimulating environment. This survival skill has been important for adults who have achieved independent living and working, keeping up the appearance of "normalcy" for long stretches of each day. For example, one patient who worked in a crowded accounting office reported that the job was difficult when he first started it because he could not tune out the voices of coworkers as they did their work. He could hear up to 20 people talking at once, even though they were each at their desks speaking at a volume that is appropriate in a work environment. Because the job was important to him and he believed that his coworkers were simply doing their jobs, he adapted by focusing his attention on a very low humming sound that his computer would produce almost continuously. He could still hear the voices and he was not trying to drown them out, but became very practiced at attending to the humming. He described it as a "steadying" sound that allowed him to do his work even though he could still hear everything in the office. He had never received mindfulness training, nor had he been given any help with this issue. He came up with this strategy himself, relying on his natural ability to control his attention. Nevertheless, this was taxing to him, as the effort to keep this up all day long would leave him exhausted by the time he finished his shift.

While adults with ASD possess some characteristics that may give them a propensity to learn mindfulness skills, they need help building a wider repertoire of these strategies. For patients who report unique sensory experiences, like the office worker described above, introducing mindfulness strategies that utilize multiple senses can be helpful because they offer adults with ASD more ways to generalize existing ER skills. One source can be found in the *DBT Skills Training Manual, Second Edition* (Linehan, 2015), from the mindfulness exercises for learning the "observing" skill that focuses on "coming back to your senses." Patients are given a wide variety of methods for observing experiences in the present using vision, sound, smell, taste, touch, and breathing sensations. The senses can also be used to expand awareness by focusing on one sensory experience, then add another and another within a single exercise. For example, a very simple way to introduce the idea is illustrated in the dialogue below:

THERAPIST: OK, let's take a moment to observe some things in this room right now. First, please name four things you can see, right now, from where you are sitting.

PATIENT: The lamp, the tissues, the plant, your shoes.

THERAPIST: Good! Now name three things you can hear.

PATIENT: The clock ticking, the sound machine outside the door, birds outside.

THERPAPIST: Terrific. Now, name two things you can feel, through touch—things that are contacting your skin.

PATIENT: My socks, and, hmm, the chair arm on my elbow.

THERAPIST: Great! Now, name one thing you can smell.

PATIENT: Leather.

THERAPIST: You got it. You just paid attention to some things that were there all along, but by focusing your attention on them in this way, you are expanding your awareness, in the present, which is essential for mindfulness practice.

This is a simple exercise that can be done in any order the therapist sees fit (e.g., change the order or senses or the number of things to name in each step). The purpose is to give a task that illustrates the concept and is relatively easy to do, thereby giving the patient an immediate success experience.

Sensory-based mindfulness strategies were used to help Edwin—a 27-year-old man with ASD and a history of major depressive disorder with recurrent episodes—increase his participation in a previously enjoyed activity. Edwin had been an avid reader before his first major depressive episode. As his depressive symptoms improved through the course of treatment, he wanted to return to reading fiction books as a hobby. He became frustrated when he tried, however, because he could not concentrate as well as in the past. Intrusive self-critical thoughts challenged his ability to focus even further. A schedule was implemented in which he would read for 15 minutes a day for 1 week, with the idea that the time segments could be lengthened gradually in the subsequent weeks. After he tried this plan for 1 week, he came into session reporting disappointment in himself and skepticism about the plan. He had adhered to the schedule, but had processed very little of the book, as most of each 15-minute segment was spent "fighting off" distractions and trying to "clear my mind" of negative thoughts.

Referring to some acceptance strategies with which he was already familiar, it was agreed that "fighting off" distractions was not likely to be effective. Instead, it was agreed that staying engaged in the book even though distractions and critical thoughts were present would be the goal. The use of sensory-based strategies was suggested to facilitate that engagement because they do not rely on language. Edwin was instructed to pay attention to the nonverbal aspects of the book page whenever he felt "hijacked" by intrusive thoughts. Because reading is such a language-based activity, and his intrusive thoughts were also language based and competing with the content of the book, it was hypothesized that expanding his awareness to nonverbal aspects of the activity would allow him to stay engaged. He was asked to pay attention to the following features of the book whenever he was feeling distracted or having difficulty concentrating:

- The visual aspects of texture on the paper of the pages
- The feel of the texture of the paper on his fingers
- The color and shade of the paper
- The shape of each letter formed by the font
- The contrast between the ink color and the paper color
- The smell of the paper and ink

For the next week, the schedule was implemented again, only now the goal was clarified to be to stay engaged with the book in any variety of ways for 15 minutes each day. Though it was counterintuitive, this reading activity did not require him to absorb the content of the book in order to be successful. After 1 week of this homework, he came back in and reported that he was able to complete the exercise every day. He did get distracted and did have some intrusive thoughts, but using the sensory strategies helped him to stay with the book because, as he put it, shifting to the nonverbal aspects of the book seemed to decrease the "voice volume" of the intrusive thoughts. By the fifth day, he was able to read some passages and absorb some of the story in his book. This illustrates one example of using mindfulness-based strategies to increase flexibility of thoughts and behaviors.

In sum, mindfulness skills offer patients methods by which to increase flexibility. By using some strategies that the patient is already using on his or her own, then expanding on them, flexibility is being reinforced. Because mindfulness skills are best taught by therapists or instructors who have had a lot of formal training in these practices, not all therapists reading this will feel equipped to provide this to their patients themselves. In cases where a therapist recognizes the need for a patient without having the skill set to teach mindfulness, the patient can be referred to an MBSR class or a DBT skills group for an adjunctive service to the individual work that can continue at the same time.

Clarifying Values

One of the essential elements of mindfulness-based CBT involves clarifying and referring to the patient's personal values. Both ACT and DBT have treatment components that are targeted toward helping patients clarify their values and to make active choices that will allow them to live in accordance with them. A clear sense of one's values has a positive reciprocal relationship with the ability to practice mindfulness and acceptance strategies. Helping patients clarify the principles that are most important to them and which they want to use as guides through their lives is empowering to them, and serves as the basis for behavioral activation strategies in the therapy. Values clarification work can be introduced at any point in the sequence of skill-building interventions. In ACT, the ideas are introduced in the later stages of treatment and in DBT within the later part of the ER skills training module, though both approaches are meant to be flexible and can be applied in any order, depending on an individual's needs. For adults with ASD, I have introduced it at various points, depending on how it fits into the individualized case formulation. More often I find myself introducing it in the early part of treatment, as the patient's personal values are used when explaining the rationale for other interventions later in the course of therapy.

There are many ways values clarification can be implemented. Worksheets and exercises can be found in DBT and ACT books, including Ciarrochi and Bailey (2008), Harris and Aisbett (2013), Hayes and Smith (2005), Linehan (2015), and Rathus and Miller (2015). Open-access resources for this purpose can be found on the Association for Contextual Behavioral Science (ACBS) website (*https://contextualscience.org/acbs*), many of which are available to everyone, as well as a wider range of tools for members of ACBS. The case example below illustrates the use of my favorite method for integrating the patient's values into the treatment, which is a card-sorting exercise.

Values Card Sort

The Values Card Sort was created by Ciarrochi and Bailey (2008) and appears in their ACT-based manual as part of an assessment device called the Survey of Guiding Principles (SGP). An exercise using this tool was implemented with Edwin, the 27-year-old man mentioned in the previous section, who came in with a diagnosis of ASD and depression. As a part of his orientation to treatment, the exercise was used to help with establishing goals for therapy. Ciarrochi and Bailey's card deck was used, along with a modification of the rating sheet by Whiting (2012), downloaded through the ACBS website (*https://contextualscience.org/the_survey_of_guiding_principles_questionnaire_and*).

The following dialogue illustrates how the exercise was introduced to Edwin:

THERAPIST: This exercise is to help you clarify your personal values. By values, I mean those principles you really want to live by—that guide you and give your life meaning—those things that you can't imagine your life *not* having. And when I say things, I don't mean tangibles or material things. I mean what you want to stand for and how you want to relate to the world and people around you. At the risk of sounding corny, your values are your strongest wishes about *who* you want to be, *how* you want to live, but not what you *have* in terms of material things. What gives your life meaning is defined by your values.

PATIENT: So, you mean goals.

THERAPIST: Goals can be formed from values, but values are more like directions—metaphorically speaking—like heading east or heading north. A goal is an obtainable outcome that when complete, is no longer necessary. Goals can be designed and carried out in the service of a value, but values are ongoing. A value is used the way you would use a compass—it is always there, directing you, and does not stop operating after you arrive at a particular destination. So, my value could be "I want to always head east," and one goal could be "I want to see a landmark east of here—the Montauk lighthouse—the eastern-most tip of Long Island." Once I arrive in Montauk and visit the lighthouse, my goal is complete, but my value is still alive, allowing me to make another goal to continuously live in accordance with my value. In my metaphor, I would need to make a new goal to continue east, whether it be get in a boat, a plane, or a wet suit.

PATIENT: (*Laughs.*) OK. So, in this exercise, you're going to give me some values. Then we can set goals from them.

THERAPIST: At the end of this exercise, you will surely have a list of values. But I will not be giving them to you. Through the exercise, you will see that you already have them. You had them before you walked in today; in fact, you have had them for most of your life. Today's exercise is meant to help you focus on them and get them into clear view. Though our values are always with us, we don't always pay attention to them. So, this exercise was designed by psychologists who do a lot of research about how people develop and use their values in living satisfying and meaningful lives.

PATIENT: OK. That sounds interesting.

THERAPIST: So, I am going to hand you a deck of cards. On each card is printed a value that a person may or may not have. (*Randomly selects two cards from the deck and shows the patient; see Figure 8.7 for illustrations of sample cards.*) See, this one says, "Helping others." That is a value that researchers have found to be very important

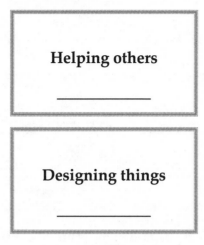

FIGURE 8.7. Examples from the Values Card Sort deck. From Ciarrochi and Bailey (2008). Copyright © 2008 Ciarrochi and Bailey. Reprinted by permission.

to some people, and less important to other people. Here is another one that says, "Designing things." Again, some people may find that very meaningful and others may take it or leave it. There are 52 cards in the deck. (*Hands the deck to the patient.*)

PATIENT: OK.

THERAPIST: Now, look through the deck and read all the cards. As you do this, I am going to ask you to form three piles in front of you with these cards. The first pile you will build with cards that are of utmost importance to you. These are things that you cannot imagine missing from your life. The second pile will be made of cards that have values on them that are of moderate importance to you. These are things that you know you value, but they are not the first priorities. The third pile is made up of things that are not important to you. These are things that are not at all essential for you to find your life meaningful. You would be totally fine with a life missing those things.

PATIENT: OK. Let's see . . . (*Immediately begins sorting through the pile and continues until he has made three piles—it takes about 5 minutes.*) Done!

THERAPIST: Terrific! You looked like you were really focused on that. What was it like to do that?

PATIENT: I was surprised. I have felt so blah for so long, I didn't think I would be too interested in any of these cards. I am glad I saw things here that matter to me.

THERAPIST: So how many cards are in your "utmost importance" pile?

PATIENT: (*Counts the cards.*) Twenty-seven.

THERAPIST: Wow! That gives you a lot to work with. OK, now the next step is sort of hard; at least that's what other people have told me when they've done this exercise. Take that pile of 27 cards and try to narrow it down to your most important 10. Go through it as many times as you need to and form a pile of your top 10 values.

PATIENT: Oh, boy! Hmm. OK. Let me try that. (*Goes through the cards more slowly, spending about 5 more minutes.*) This is it. That was hard. But I think these speak the best for my values.

The last step in this exercise involved a values rating scale. Based on a version designed by Whiting (2012), a worksheet was presented that had 10 sets of boxes that each looked like this:

Value:									
How important is this value?					How consistently are you acting in accordance with this value?				
Not at all				Very much	Not at all				Very much
0	1	2	3	4	0	1	2	3	4

For each of the 10 values Edwin picked from the deck as his most important ones, he was asked to transpose the phrase in the blank spot, then do two ratings. First he would rate the degree of importance the value holds, then rate the degree to which he is currently living in accordance with it. This list represents the data he entered on the sheet:

Having genuine and close friends	Importance: 4	Accordance: 3
Being loyal to friends, family, and/or my group	Importance: 4	Accordance: 2
Experiencing positive mood states	Importance: 3	Accordance: 0
Being competent and effective	Importance: 3	Accordance: 0
Being honest	Importance: 3	Accordance: 4
Having relationships involving love and affection	Importance: 4	Accordance: 2
Being self-sufficient	Importance: 4	Accordance: 0
Figuring things out, solving problems	Importance: 2	Accordance: 0
Gaining wisdom and a mature understanding of life	Importance: 3	Accordance: 1
Engaging in clearly defined work	Importance: 3	Accordance: 0

This sheet was used to inform the goals of treatment. It was explained to Edwin that congruence between the level of importance of one's values and level of action in service of those values is associated with mental health and a sense of well-being, one of the assumptions behind the ACT model. Two of his values were rated as being fairly congruent: having genuine and close friends and being honest. Seeing this was pleasing to him and he reported that he felt more hopeful because of it. The values that showed the greatest discrepancy between the importance score and accordance score became areas of focus while building the treatment plan. So, the goals that were set were informed by Edwin's desire to work toward experiencing positive mood states more often, becoming more competent and effective, becoming more self-sufficient, and engaging in clearly defined work.

This exercise can be done in a variety of ways and there are several other rating methods available in the sources provided throughout this section. My preference for the card-sort approach is because of the multimodal presentation of materials. Anecdotally speaking, the movement that is required to manipulate the cards seems to have an activating effect on patients, even those who are severely depressed. Edwin, for example, had a Beck Depression Inventory (BDI) score of 42 at the time that he performed this exercise, yet he was able to engage fully in this task.

In sum, values clarification is a useful way to help adults with ASD to access and express their deeply felt principles for living. The list that results from a values exercise becomes a useful tool to bolster other treatment components aimed at improving ER abilities. Because the values are coming from the patient, using them to guide the treatment enhances compliance. When the therapist asks the patient to do something that is difficult, or that involves acceptance and tolerance of painful situations, the patient is more likely to participate because his or her values are at the basis of the rationale.

Chapter Summary and Conclusions

This chapter provided a rationale for considering mindfulness and acceptance-based strategies for inclusion in the CBT treatment plan for some adults with ASD. ER impairments are associated with both the core symptoms of ASD as well as common comorbid mental health problems. Mindfulness-based CBT approaches that are efficacious for specific mental health problems in the general population were reviewed, along with their applicability for adults with ASD. Examples of methods to offer these strategies to adults with ASD were provided through case illustrations.

Due to the complex nature of the problems experienced by adults with ASD, the treatment strategies that were detailed in this and the last two intervention chapters are rarely implemented in isolation because the patient often has other treatment providers from other disciplines involved. The next chapter describes how adjunctive therapies can be integrated into the overall treatment plan.

CHAPTER 9

Adjunctive Therapies
and Interdisciplinary Collaboration

As previously described, patients with ASD often have multiple treatment needs, some of which cannot be addressed by an individual psychotherapist. After the initial assessment and identification of treatment needs, the patient should be referred for other indicated services in which he or she is not already involved. It is likely that these other therapies will enhance the patient's responsiveness to CBT. Therapists must be able to communicate effectively with members of diverse professional disciplines. This chapter provides general guidelines for *collaboration* and integration of treatment, followed by a list and descriptions of *adjunctive services*.

Guidelines for Referral
and Collaboration with Other Service Providers

When to Refer

Generally, an individual therapist refers a patient to another provider to obtain a specialized *evaluation* or to begin an *additional course of treatment* different from the individual psychotherapy already provided.

Evaluation

During the intake and assessment process, the therapist asks many questions to determine the various factors contributing to the problems for which the patient is seeking help. Many times, additional evaluations—such as those performed by other mental health, medical, or rehabilitation specialists—will be necessary to answer those questions. The specialties are described later in this chapter to help readers consider the different types of assistance that can be offered to these patients.

Initiate Additional Course of Treatment

The answers to the questions raised during the assessment often lead the therapist to treatment goals that can be met only by an outside professional. Sometimes patients are reluctant to accept a referral because they may already feel overwhelmed by the number of appointments they must make each week. Others may question why the service being recommended was never needed before (e.g., speech therapy). It is the therapist's job to describe in lay terms why these adjunctive services are necessary and how they may improve the patient's quality of life. The brief descriptions provided later in this chapter can be used as the basis of any discussion with an individual patient.

Collaboration

At the point of intake, many patients are already involved in other therapies. Sometimes it will be one of those other professionals who referred the patient for individual psychotherapy. Whether the patient is continuing with ongoing treatments or will be initiating new ones at the recommendation of the therapist, effective collaboration with other providers is crucial for the treatment plan to be effective. This collaboration involves a balancing act between the need to maintain confidentiality and the need to facilitate ongoing communication so that all involved parties can secure important information.

Maintaining Confidentiality

Every psychotherapist should be well versed in the ethical and legal requirements regarding confidentiality, set forth by the guidelines of his or her discipline and the state in which he or she is practicing. A discussion of those issues is outside the scope of this volume. However, special challenges arise when serving adults with ASD because they customarily have multiple providers and caregivers involved in their lives.

The therapist must be mindful of the need to get the patient's signed authorization for communication with every professional involved. Obtaining this authorization can be a matter of routine during the intake or after a referral is made, but it also may become cumbersome if the patient is involved in a program where there is a lot of staff turnover. For example, if a patient signs an authorization form for the therapist to speak to his or her case manager, and then that case manager is replaced by a new one who calls the therapist several months later, the therapist will not be able to speak to that person about the patient's care until a new authorization form has been signed by the patient.

In addition, in terms of the need to preserve confidentiality, caregivers and providers often do not understand how the role of the psychotherapist differs from that of other professionals with whom the patient is involved. The case manager mentioned in the example above may not understand why a spontaneous conversation cannot take place over the phone about the patient, as it can when he or she calls the patient's vocational counselor, for instance.

Most people accept the confidentiality constraints once they understand them. Therapists working with adults who have ASD should be prepared to explain confidentiality to patients and other providers more often than they might when working with typical adults.

Facilitating Regular Communication

Despite the confidentiality issues, most therapists should have ongoing communication with other providers once proper authorization has been obtained. It is crucial to set the tone of collaboration from the point of intake with patients by explaining to them the importance of having authorization to contact all involved providers. The frequency of contact with other providers will be determined by the nature of the services, but the main objectives of making regular calls are listed below:

- Discuss assessment findings and diagnosis.
- Inform other provider(s) of treatment goals.
- Become familiar with the treatment goals of the other provider(s).
- Ensure that the treatment goals are compatible with your own.
- Gain information about how the patient presents in other settings.
- Gain information about the patient's impact on others.
- Provide psychoeducation on ASD and mental health diagnoses.

All of the information obtained can be used to reevaluate and modify the psychotherapy goals. By participating in an integrated treatment approach, the effectiveness of the individual psychotherapy is enhanced. This type of information exchange also helps to avoid duplication or gaps in service.

Adjunctive Services and Their Roles

The following sections describe the other types of treatment in which the patient may be involved during the course of CBT. The benefits of each are described, along with precautionary notes where applicable.

Adjunctive Psychotherapy, Counseling, and Support

There are a number of reasons other types of psychotherapy or counseling may be indicated for a patient who is also receiving CBT.

Individual Therapy with Other Goals

In general, it is not advisable for a patient to work with two individual therapists concurrently. However, there are times when a patient may have a preexisting, ongoing relationship with a therapist at the time of the intake, and an agreement may be reached between both therapists for that service to continue even during CBT. For instance, a patient may have been receiving supportive counseling from a therapist for many years prior to the ASD diagnosis, but that therapist may not offer the skill-building strategies that are warranted. Because patients with ASD so often have a paucity of supportive relationships, terminating with the other therapist may put undue stress on the patient, and the benefits of continuing that relationship can outweigh any risks of duplicating services. Both therapists must communicate regularly to ensure that each is working on different treatment goals. In other cases, the patient may see a specialist with expertise in treating a specific psychological condition (e.g., eating disorders, substance use disorders), who lacks an understanding of ASD. Acting as an adjunctive therapist for the patient and consultant to the therapist, the therapist with expertise in ASD can provide, even on a temporary basis, psychoeducation about ASD and related skill-building strategies.

Family Therapy

Some patients have difficulty responding to CBT because they are living with family members who engage them in maladaptive interactions. Occasionally, it is helpful to invite family members into sessions to address minor issues of communication and support. Obviously, the patient must consent to this step. Because the involvement of family members is sporadic and its only purpose is to further the individual work with the patient, it is not true family therapy. When the family relationships appear to be severely dysfunctional, the therapist should refer the entire family, including the patient with ASD, to a trained family therapist. In extreme cases, wherever individual treatment would be completely futile, an agreement to provide individual treatment should be contingent upon the family entering outside treatment.

Marital Therapy

Some adults with ASD, especially those newly diagnosed, want to involve a spouse or partner in their treatment, as they gain a new understanding of their roles in their relationships. The partners are usually motivated to participate, as well, given that they have had to cope with many "quirks" for which they had no previous explanations. CBT practioners trained in marital therapy may opt to treat the couple rather than the individual as a means to address their social problems, with the accompanying depression and anxiety. In other cases, however, the person with ASD may want individual therapy to address problems not involving the relationship, but may want marital therapy with a different practitioner, in addition. Again, this arrangement is feasible, as long as the patient allows the two therapists to communicate with each other.

Sexuality Education or Therapy

Patients with ASD may present with a wide range of sexual problems, as mentioned earlier. Some can be addressed in CBT along with other goals related to social functioning or anxiety reduction. However, depending on the nature of the problem and the level of expertise of the CBT clinician, a referral can be made to a sexuality expert. The psychosexual assessment and treatment continuum model for adults with developmental disabilities (Matich-Maroney et al., 2005), discussed in Chapter 3, can be useful in determining the type of expert the patient needs to see. The model offers guidelines for deciding among providers of psychoeducation, interpersonal skills training, trauma treatment, sexuality disorders treatment, or forensic treatment.

Addictive Disorders Treatment

Patients who meet criteria for a comorbid substance use disorder or gambling disorder may benefit from specialized treatment for those problems either before or during the course of CBT that is focused on other ASD issues. At intake, the therapist will determine, as with any new patient, to what degree the addictive disorder symptoms will interfere with other treatment goals. If the therapist and patient agree to pursue CBT after an inpatient addictive disorders program, or simultaneous to a course of outpatient addiction treatment, coordination between treatment providers is essential.

It is not uncommon for a patient with ASD to be participating in a 12-step program to address an addictive disorder (e.g., Alcoholics Anonymous, Narcotics Anonymous, Gamblers Anonymous) while also engaging in CBT. Because the meetings are not treatment groups, and are anonymous peer-run support groups, there is no need or means to coordinate with the facilitators. In my practice, I have seen some patients with ASD benefit greatly from being in these groups, while others have struggled with managing various aspects of the program. Not unlike patients in the general population, individual therapists can be most helpful by building in time to discuss the patient's ongoing experience with the meetings. If the patient is generally motivated to attend a group, CBT therapists can support the effort by helping with ASD-related problems that may make the 12-step group more difficult. Examples include anxiety about speaking in front of a group, stress related to the confrontational style of some group members, and extremely literal interpretation of the 12-step principles and rules.

Collateral Therapy for Family Members

Some patients have parents or siblings who are highly involved in their day-to-day lives, providing varying levels of guidance and support. Others are in a caretaking role themselves as they raise their children or care for elderly parents. Relationships can be strained, either directly or indirectly, by the features of ASD, and there are times when family members may be referred for their own individual treatment. Common reasons for making such a recommendation are outlined below.

Unless there is psychopathology or severe family dysfunction present, supporting parents and siblings typically share the individual's desire for him or her to achieve more independence. Sometimes parents are near or at retirement age and are anxious to enjoy their later years without having to support or worry about an adult child who is not yet self-sufficient. The stress involved in trying to help their son or daughter can be difficult to cope with year after year, and some parents report a sense of being "burnedout" and tired of repeating strategies that do not seem to lead to improvement. These individuals can benefit from therapy that is geared toward coping, problem solving, and sometimes behavior management issues. Individual treatment of the patient with ASD is enhanced because the parents' therapy will reduce stress and tension, and the parents will learn strategies that better foster independence in their adult child.

Collateral therapy can also be offered to parents when their adult child with ASD does not want to enter therapy at all. Again, providing parents with coping, problem-solving, and behavior management strategies can indirectly help the ASD individual who is dependent on them.

Children of a parent on the spectrum may be referred for their own therapy if they appear to be having difficulty coping with any aspect of family life. Depending on the age, cognitive ability, and diagnostic status of the child (with or without ASD), psychoeducation about ASD may be considered. It is important to note, however, that there is no reason to assume that the features of ASD necessarily adversely affect the children they are raising. If there are psychosocial stressors challenging the family, such as financial problems or marital discord, then there are obvious pressures on children, as there would be for any patient population. These factors, along with relationship functioning, are examined during a thorough intake. However, if such issues are not present and the patient is not reporting relationship strain with his or her children, the therapist should not assume that the children of a parent on the spectrum are in need of extra support.

The individual therapist must be clear about his or her role with a given family. Once collateral therapy has begun with a family member, that person is the designated patient. If the individual with ASD decides to enter therapy at another point, he or she should be referred to a different therapist. If a therapist tries to shift roles between parents and an adult child with ASD, for example, the individual with ASD may see the therapist as an agent of the parent and will, with reason, have difficulty trusting the relationship. This point must be made clear to parents at the outset because some enter treatment hoping to encourage their son or daughter into coming for treatment later. It should be explained that if they choose to come for individual therapy themselves, their son or daughter would be referred to someone else. Some parents may choose not to start treatment, hoping to get the child into treatment with the therapist at a later point.

Group Therapy

Patients with ASD can benefit from being involved in group therapy concurrently with individual treatment. Some patients may already be in a group when individual therapy begins. As long as the patient likes the group and authorizes regular communication between therapists, ongoing participation should be encouraged. Adult social skills groups for people with ASD, though surprisingly scarce, can be very helpful, if run by a therapist well versed in autism spectrum issues, and can serve as a useful adjunct to individual CBT. As mentioned in Chapter 8, concomitant participation in a DBT skills training group or MBSR program can also enhance the effectiveness of individual therapy.

Support Groups

Chapter 5 discussed the growing number of support and advocacy networks for cognitively able people with ASD (a list of the well-established organizations can be found in the Appendix). The sense of belongingness that can be gained by attending such a group can be a powerful source of support and encouragement for patients with ASD. However, therapists must be sensitive to the fact that support groups are very different from therapy groups, and some patients may need to discuss adverse reactions to experiences there in their individual sessions. Support groups are open (anyone can come at any time) and, therefore, less predictable than a therapy group. Facilitators may have varying levels of experience and training, and meetings may not follow an agenda. Because, by definition, the attendees have difficulty with social skills, some patients may be offended or put off by the behavior of others in the group, even though they understand that everyone there has ASD. Other patients may not be ready to discuss their ASD diagnosis so openly or may dislike being associated with others who are known to have a disability. Overall, I have found support groups to be an invaluable adjunct to the treatment plan. Even negative experiences can become "grist for the mill" in session because they bring opportunities for further growth.

Medical and Rehabilitation Services

Many of the core problems of ASD have a neurobiological basis. CBT can be helpful in teaching patients new skills and to manage anxiety and depression, but many areas of impaired functioning must be addressed by medical and rehabilitation profession-als.

Psychiatry

In my practice, at the time of intake, approximately 75% of patients with ASD are tak-ing psychotropic medication. Usually the medications are prescribed by a psychiatrist, although on rare occasions, by the primary care physician. The pharmacological treat-ment of the symptoms of ASD and comorbid mental illness is a vast and ever-growing field that falls outside the scope of this volume. Readers are referred to Ghaziuddin (2005) and Westphal, Kober, Voos, and Volkmar (2014) for overviews of psychopharma-cology in the treatment of people on the autism spectrum.

The cognitive-behavioral therapist who is not a physician will need to establish a collaborative relationship with the professional who is prescribing psychotropic medi-cation to the patient. With complex cases, I have found the psychiatrists to be my most important contacts because they not only prescribe medication but also have their own therapy relationship with the patient. When the symptoms are severe and the progress is slow, it is helpful to have the support of another professional. In the most optimal situation, the psychiatrist and therapist benefit from an ongoing "peer supervision" relationship.

At times, a patient who is not on medication may be referred to a psychiatrist for an evaluation. This referral is warranted only if comorbid mental health symptoms are so severe that they interfere with the CBT process, cause significant distress in the patient's day-to-day life without improvement after CBT is well under way, or present a direct threat to the safety of the patient and/or others.

Primary Medical Care

The intake should include a brief assessment of the patient's medical status, such as the date of his or her last physical exam and any known physical problems. Sometimes the therapist may recommend a medical consultation to rule out biological causes for the patient's problems. For example, sleep irregularity is a common problem triggering a referral. Many patients have erratic sleep patterns and complain of a wide range of sleep problems, even in the absence of other mood symptoms. Patients should be strongly encouraged to meet with their primary care physician to discuss this issue so that a referral to a sleep disorders clinic can be considered, if indicated. The anxiety that is so prevalent in these patients can also have physical sequelae warranting medical atten-tion (e.g., gastrointestinal problems, exacerbation of allergies). For patients presenting with depressive symptoms, thyroid function must be evaluated because hypothyroid-ism is a frequent cause of depression.

Speech Therapy

Many cognitively able people with ASD tend to have verbal strengths and rarely show problems with speech or the mechanics of language. For this reason, many of them have never been referred for speech therapy before. Yet, speech–language pathologists have the expertise to help individuals who have auditory-processing difficulties as well as problems with social language and pragmatics. I have referred numerous patients for speech therapy because I suspected auditory-processing problems. Despite the fact that they were well spoken and had never been previously identified as having language difficulties, I noticed problems in our sessions. For example, they would struggle to answer when I asked for a "recap" of a point we had covered or to explain their understanding of a homework assignment. When probed, they acknowledged that they were having difficulty understanding what people were saying to them. This is particularly problematic when teachers or employers gave them multistep instructions, or when they try to interact socially in a group situation. While some patients may be skeptical about their need for this service, once the rationale is understood, an evaluation can be fruitful. Finding a speech–language pathologist who works with adults is a crucial resource for any psychotherapist working with adult ASD cases.

Occupational Therapy

People with ASD have sensory–motor functioning deficits that can interfere with self-care and self-management. Sensitivities to light, sound, movement, and touch, though less severe in adulthood, can continue to cause problems for the patient with ASD. Problems with motor planning, or *dyspraxia*, can interfere with the initiation or shifting of motor tasks, including grooming and housekeeping responsibilities. Organizational deficits can interfere with budgeting and time management. All of these issues can be improved by an occupational therapist, who can either remediate some of the problems or teach the individual to compensate. Again, finding an occupational therapist who works with adults on the spectrum is a worthwhile pursuit for the psychotherapist.

Adult Disability Services

ASD is considered a disability by many states and may qualify a patient to receive various types of support and services. In some states it is considered a developmental disability, in others a psychiatric disability, and in some states it is considered neither. The rules and regulations can be very confusing, but it is worthwhile for newly diagnosed patients to investigate the services for which they may be eligible by visiting the appropriate state government websites. The generic categories of support services from which patients may benefit are listed below, with a reminder that the terminology and eligibility criteria will vary from state to state.

Case Management

The case manager or "service coordinator" has the responsibility of ensuring that the individual gets all of services he or she needs. Usually there is a requirement to meet monthly, and the case manager will help the patient access financial and therapeutic supports. At the time of intake, the patient may already have a case manager, who will become an important contact for the therapist. Other times, a referral to case management may be made by the therapist. This referral is particularly helpful to parents who have been bearing the burden of doing much of the "legwork" involved in applying to programs and services and who may not know that case management services exist.

Vocational Training/Job Coaching

Most patients with ASD are either unemployed or underemployed, despite achieving high levels of education and talent. The development of employment programs tailored to the adult ASD population is in its infancy in the United States (see Gerhardt, Cicero, & Mayville, 2014, for a review). A referral to vocational counseling can be made, but this service will be helpful only if the counselor understands ASD or is willing to learn about it. Some states supply "job coaches" to adults with disabilities; these are workers assigned to accompany the adult on job interviews and/or on the job site, if necessary. Again, a job coach will be effective only if he or she truly understands the special needs and challenges of an individual with ASD. Unfortunately, job coaches are often trained to work with disabilities other than ASD (e.g., ID, substance abuse) and may not always have the level of experience necessary to adapt to the unique needs of an adult with ASD. Nevertheless, the referral should be made for a patient who is reporting repeated job losses or job dissatisfaction. Sometimes, through collaboration, the therapist can assist in designing appropriate vocational training and supports for the patient. Recommending the book *Developing Talents: Careers for Individuals with Asperger Syndrome and High-Functioning Autism* (Grandin & Duffy, 2004), *Social Thinking at Work: Why Should I Care?* (Winner & Crooke, 2011), and/or *An Employer's Guide to Managing Professionals on the Autism Spectrum* (Scheiner & Bogden, 2017) to a newly appointed vocational counselor can be a good way to start the relationship.

Assisted Living

Most states support supervised residential programs that allow adults with disabilities to live in the community as independently as possible. Again, the types of services and eligibility criteria will vary greatly from state to state. The generic service models are listed below, starting with the lowest level of staff supervision and ending with the highest.

- Housing programs that offer only subsidized rent.
- Counseling services that provide workers (e.g., "community habilitative specialists") who visit the individual in his or her own home or apartment for several hours a week to teach higher-level skills and to monitor the individual's status.
- Supportive apartment programs in which there are staff nearby at all times, but who may visit the individual only for brief daily meetings.
- Group homes that are located in the community and may be staffed 24 hours a day. The staff-to-resident ratio will vary according to the severity of disability in the residents.

The population of adults with ASD is very heterogeneous in terms of their need for residential support. Some need no support and may have lived on their own for years with spouses or partners, supporting children of their own. At the other end of the spectrum are those who, despite a high level of intelligence, have needed 24-hour super-vised group homes, usually because of chronic comorbid psychiatric problems. Most patients, however, are somewhere in between, needing a minimum to moderate level of support on a weekly basis.

Legal Services

The last type of outside service a patient with ASD may need from time to time is legal. There are two types of legal problems to which a person with ASD may be prone, and appropriate referrals to attorneys may be necessary in either case. They are *service eligibility appeals* and *criminal defense*.

Service Eligibility Appeals

Because ASD is an ever-shifting concept, many state agencies have inconsistent meth-ods for evaluating its eligibility for various supports and services. If patients are denied services to which they believe they are entitled, referrals to an attorney who has exper-tise in disability law and health care issues may be warranted.

Criminal Defense

Unfortunately, people with ASD can be vulnerable to negative encounters with law enforcement, as mentioned earlier in this book. Their unusual social behaviors, poor social judgment, and reactions to stress that can look bizarre may lead people in the community to either provoke them or report them as a threat. Also, their lack of under-standing of the importance of certain social norms may lead them to break the law outright. The books *Autism, Advocates, and Law Enforcement Professionals: Recognizing and Reducing Risk Situations for People with Autism Spectrum Disorders* (Debbaudt, 2002) and *The Autism Spectrum, Sexuality and the Law* (Attwood et al., 2014) are useful texts for patients and their families when high-risk behavior is present. Despite prevention efforts, some patients may find themselves facing various criminal charges and will need to be referred to a defense attorney who is well versed in disability and/or autism spectrum issues.

Chapter Summary and Conclusions

This chapter highlighted how the CBT therapist usually works collaboratively with other providers in treating the adult patient with ASD. Guidelines for preserving con-fidentiality while encouraging interdisciplinary communication were presented. The options for adjunctive services were identified and the rationale for including each one in the treatment plan was discussed. The next chapter presents strategies for handling obstacles to implementing the treatment plan.

CHAPTER 10

Obstacles to Treatment
and How to Address Them

S ome of the challenges the therapist faces when treating adults with ASD are unique to the population, whereas others may be found in any patient group where problems are complex. The obstacles and their solutions have been interwoven with the topics throughout this book. To clarify and highlight this topic, this chapter summarizes those issues and expands on points that were only briefly mentioned previously.

Due to the complicated nature of this patient population, people with ASD may have multiple problems in several areas of their lives. Some of these can interfere with treatment implementation or hinder progress. Throughout the course of treatment, therapists need to address these obstacles through adjustments within the therapy sessions and/or by making the appropriate phone calls and referrals to other practitioners. The problems addressed in this chapter include social interaction problems within session, problems completing homework, low motivation for treatment, family members not supporting treatment, substance abuse, social isolation, financial problems, untreated health problems, and polypharmacy.

Social-Interaction Difficulties as Challenges
in the Psychotherapy Session

As mentioned many times in this book, people with ASD have atypical ways of processing information, particularly during social interactions. Therapy sessions are, obviously, one type of social interaction. Special considerations therapists must make for patients who perceive interpersonal exchanges in such a unique way were discussed in Chapter 3. In some cases, these problems persist even after precautions have been taken; this section presents examples as well as strategies for minimizing their negative impact.

Behavioral Issues

Patients with ASD display behaviors that would be considered odd by most people, including hand gestures, postures, facial grimaces, atypical use of eye contact, or in some cases, poor hygiene. These are often manifestations of the sensory problems inherent in ASD (e.g., sensitivity to light, specific sounds, or movements), or ER problems (e.g., high arousal in the session). Some of these behaviors can interfere with therapy sessions if they are not addressed. The therapist should first make every effort to help the individual feel comfortable and relaxed in the room being used for the sessions.

One way to ensure comfort is to have a flexible office environment that can accommodate different sensory issues. If possible, include different seating choices, a variety of light fixtures (incandescent, fluorescent, and LED), and white noise machines that can be turned on or left off. Remembering that these individuals may not report that a sensory issue is at play, the therapist should pay extra attention to the noises or lighting in the office. Each patient is different in terms of sensitivities, so the therapist may spend more time than he or she would with typical adults asking questions such as "Does this light bother you?" or "Is that noise bothering you?"

The therapist must address any behavior that is interfering with the session and that does not seem to improve when accommodations are made. This intervention should be done in a direct, clear, but nonjudgmental fashion. For example, one patient who preferred to sit in a sprawled posture, almost lying down, put his muddy shoes onto the upholstery. I said to him in a pleasant tone, "You can sit however you want, but I am going to ask that you keep your feet off the upholstery." In another example, a patient's sensory problems led him to avoid taking showers. Although this problem had implications that had to be addressed in the overall treatment plan, I needed immediate relief from the odor in the sessions, so I said in a calm and nonjudgmental way, "I cannot sit in a room with you when you have not showered because the smell is aversive to me. I have to ask you to take a shower on the days you are coming to see me."

By combining strategies to ensure the patient's comfort with clear feedback about imposing behaviors, therapists can usually conduct successful sessions despite eccentric behavior.

Language and Communication Issues

The language and communication issues described earlier can obviously impede the therapy process. A therapist needs to be aware of these issues so that a lack of progress is not misattributed to other factors.

In the receptive communication domain, patients may have auditory-processing abilities that are discrepant with their expressive skills. For example, a person who appears to be very articulate, using a wide vocabulary and complex sentences, may not necessarily *understand* that level of language when the therapist is speaking. Many of these individuals interpret language in a very literal way and may miss the meaning of abstract concepts or idioms. The therapist should never assume a patient has comprehended ideas or instructions, even if the person is behaving as if he or she did. Therapists can avoid miscommunication by checking in more often than they might with other adult patients to see whether the information conveyed is being received and asking patients to reiterate or summarize what has been covered.

In the case of Andrew, as an example, I had been working with him for several months before I realized he had extensive auditory-processing problems. I had erroneously assumed he understood some simple homework instructions, and when he repeatedly failed to carry them out, I attributed his behavior to a lack of motivation. His academic history and comorbid mental health problems contributed to a sense of shame about his failure to understand others and a reluctance to ask people to repeat or to clarify, and he had "mastered the art" of pretending he was listening and understanding (he made good eye contact and nodded his head at key points). I referred him to a speech–language pathologist, who helped him improve his listening skills and increase his willingness to ask for clarification.

In the expressive communication domain, alexithymia, or lack of access to words describing mental states, can interfere with therapy. These patients may have difficulty reporting important emotional experiences to the therapist, and information about these is crucial to CBT. As suggested in Chapter 3, it is helpful to adopt a common language with the patient, which may include some of his or her unusual word choices. Also, using multimodal communication tools, such as the Talk Blocks (Innovative Interactions, 2000) described in Chapter 8, can overcome the obstacles that language problems can create.

Finally, in the interactive communication domain, patients may show problems with the social use of language (pragmatics) that can interfere with the therapy process. Patients' failure to demonstrate reciprocity in their interactions with the therapist is a common obstacle. Patients may appear to be having a one-sided conversation at times, describing an issue at length and in detail, but not responsive to the therapist's questions, interjections, or attempts to move on to another topic. They will also tend to miss any nonverbal cues the therapist may be using to communicate.

Sometimes this problem can be rectified by adjusting the pace, as mentioned above. The therapist may need to simply give the patient a bit of extra time to finish making a point and then that person may actually be responsive to the therapist's contribution to the conversation. However, if that does not work, therapists will need to interrupt more often than they might with typical patients. For some therapists, including me, this may be difficult at first, for fear of being "rude" to the patient. However, it is necessary for certain patients in order to accomplish the tasks of therapy. It is important to participate in "metacommunication" with patients who have this problem—that is, to communicate about the communication issues taking place in the session. For example, if a therapist finds that many interruptions are necessary, it might help to say something like the following:

"I noticed you have a difficult time stopping what you are saying about a topic. At times I want to say something to you about your point, but you tend to talk over me and I don't get to share with you what I am thinking. From now on, if I have an important question or comment for you, I am going to raise my hand and say, 'I am going to stop you for a moment.' I am not doing this to be rude, but only so we can get the most out of what you are saying. Is that acceptable to you?"

Another pragmatics problem is found when the patient fails to notice nonverbal cues and/or the invisible interpersonal boundaries of the therapist. The patient may not recognize the limits in the relationship with the therapist, such as the need to end a session at a particular time, for the therapist to protect the privacy of him- or herself, or to protect the privacy of other patients. This lack of recognition may be exhibited when the patient asks questions that most people would deem intrusive or personal. Examples include questions about the therapist's schedule for the rest of the day, other patients encountered in the waiting room, what kind of car the therapist drives, personal financial issues, or personal family matters. I have observed that these questions are usually asked because the person is trying to make "small talk" and does not recognize boundaries, not because he or she has an excessive interest in the therapist's personal life. I assume this behavior mirrors the way they behave with most people in their social environment, which makes it very important to address. Frank and non-judgmental feedback about the difference between "polite" and "personal" questions can help the patient shape more adaptive ways to "chat."

Cognitive Issues

The primary cognitive issue that can pose a challenge in therapy for patients with ASD is their difficulty with cognitive shifting. As mentioned several times, they have problems shifting attention, perspectives, and ideas, and these problems can interfere during basic CBT interventions. By definition, CBT is aimed at helping people modify their thoughts, so patients who are prone to rigid thinking may not respond as quickly as typical patients to the interventions. In my experience, however, people with ASD have shown that they *can* shift, they just need more time to do it. The guideline about pacing and setting realistic time frames for change applies to this problem.

EF Problems Interfering with Homework Completion

Patients who have EF problems have difficulty with planning and organization. Those who have mild-to-moderate problems with task organization may actually appreciate the structure provided by homework worksheets and are very compliant for those reasons. However, some patients are so overwhelmed by the simplest tasks of daily living that they cannot focus on standard CBT homework between sessions. The therapist can use several strategies to help these patients. One is to break the homework into smaller units than what may be assigned in CBT for a typical adult. In Bob's case, for example, the thought record was introduced to him gradually, in subcomponents, across several weeks. Another strategy is providing the individual with visual cues. For example, Andrew, who tended to let things "pile up" in his apartment, lost his homework sheets several times. Giving him a bright red folder in which to keep his worksheets increased compliance because the folder stood out among his other papers and cued him to remember to do his homework. If modifications do not increase compliance, it may be necessary to do all of the written work in session and assign homework that involves simple observations that the patient can report from memory. As a reminder, if a patient's EF deficits are severe and pervasive, referring him or her to an occupational therapist can be helpful.

Low Motivation to Be in Treatment or Rejection of the Cognitive Model

As with any adult population, sometimes patients enter treatment for reasons other than genuine motivation to work toward improvement. The most common reason seen in this population is that they are being urged to come by a third party—either a family member or another professional. Chapter 3 presented the importance of doing a thorough telephone screening to ensure that patients are not being pressured by someone else, and that they have their own reasons for entering treatment. Despite that prevention strategy, patients may show low motivation in therapy for other reasons.

One reason can be found when a patient has unrealistic expectations for the therapy and/or does not understand roles the therapist and patient will play in working toward goals. For example, some patients may think that they can play a passive role in the treatment and that the therapist can make their problems disappear just by talking to them. Others may think that progress can happen faster than it does and will get frustrated if significant change is not seen early in treatment. If the therapist does a thorough orientation to therapy, these problems can be caught and addressed. After roles and expectations are clarified, the patient may or may not choose to continue.

Another obstacle to motivation can be seen when a patient has so many stressors in his or her life that the process of making and keeping appointments is not manageable for him or her. Sometimes incorporating stress management strategies into the treatment early on can help the patient with this area, whereas other times a referral to additional support services may be necessary to help him or her manage the demands of daily living. Therapy may be able to continue with those supports in place or may be suspended until practical constraints are addressed.

Finally, in rare cases, the patient does not accept the cognitive model, once it is introduced and understood. Sometimes this stance leads to termination or a referral to a therapist with a different orientation, but not necessarily. For example, one patient with whom I worked rejected the model because he believed that by accepting that thoughts and beliefs influence mood, he would be accepting blame for his lifelong problems with depression. Despite numerous clarification discussions, he persistently reiterated that idea. I made the decision to continue meeting with him because he was very willing to engage in an ongoing dialogue about this topic. Over the course of several months, he was able to challenge his belief that he was at fault for his depression, leading him to be more accepting of the cognitive model. In another case, the individual rejected the cognitive model but had recently suffered a loss (his mother died) and was in need of supportive counseling. While offering support, I gradually began using the cognitive model to help him understand his thoughts and feelings about losing his mother. He was later more willing to apply the model to address other life problems.

Family Issues That Interfere with Treatment

Family members are often involved in the lives of adults with ASD, especially if they are having difficulties with unemployment and daily living tasks. Many of them live with one or both parents. Those who have achieved independence may have spouses and/ or children of their own. In the majority of cases, families are supportive of the therapy process and many want to be involved, as mentioned earlier. However, several family issues can interfere with the therapy.

One challenge is when very dysfunctional interactions between the patient and his or her family members are damaging to CBT, either directly or indirectly. Some family members have difficulty understanding and accepting the ASD diagnosis as an explanation for the struggles faced by the patient and take an invalidating or blaming stance, or continue to exert pressure on the patient to "act normal" and "fit in." Another unfortunate scenario can be seen in the families of some young adults, when parents have negative reactions to patients' progress toward independence. Most parents who have raised a child with a disability feel apprehensive about "launching" him or her into the world, and concerns about vulnerability are typical even in the most healthy families. However, in families where one or both parents have some form of psychopathology, an adult son's or daughter's dependence on the family is resulting in secondary gain for the parent(s). In those cases, the parent may discourage or sabotage the young adult's steps toward self-reliance.

Some patients can be taught skills to cope with unhealthy family relationships or conflict, but there are often too many factors over which the patient has no control. The therapist who faces this problem may urge the patient to bring one or more family members in to discuss the treatment. In a treatment planning session, the patient and therapist can explain to the family member(s) the rationale and goals of treatment and address any interfering behaviors. If this intervention does not lead to improvement, a referral to family therapy must be made.

Another family issue can arise when the patient is a parent. Child care responsibilities can interfere with sessions. A patient's problems with time management and task organization may be responsible, and sometimes therapy can address these issues. Other times the family obligations may lead to premature termination. This happened in the case of Lorraine, the young woman introduced in Chapter 1, who became pregnant soon after starting treatment. She stopped coming to therapy after her baby was born because she was overwhelmed by her new responsibilities and could not manage to coordinate her schedule to keep our therapy appointments. Several problem-solving strategies were attempted, but she finally ended treatment. She was referred to a case manager with a plan to continue sessions once she had more supports in place.

Trauma History or "Complex" PTSD

Chapter 3 discussed how many adults with ASD have a history of being mistreated repeatedly throughout their lives. At best, this involves frequent episodes of verbal teasing in childhood, and at worst, could be severe physical violence. While the risk of comorbid PTSD and the need for therapists to assess for it was covered earlier in this book, the issue is raised here to bring attention to scenarios in which the PTSD symptoms can interfere with therapy sessions. For patients whose trauma histories involved ongoing abuse or domestic violence within their family homes, the symptoms of PTSD can be particularly severe and pervasive. PTSD that results from repeated, ongoing traumatic experiences that have occurred in the context of relationships with caregivers is sometimes called "complex" PTSD (Ford & Courtois, 2013; Herman, 1992), and people with ASD are at least as prone if not more so than the general population (King, 2010).

Patients with this problem may have reexperiencing symptoms (flashbacks, intrusive thoughts) in session, for example, that can interfere with the CBT work, especially if the therapist is not aware of it. The collaborative process that is inherent in CBT can be a perceived threat to a patient who has been mistreated by caregivers in the past. ER impairments can further complicate this, as an adult with ASD may be more prone to arousal and less equipped to report it to the therapist than a typical person. Therapists can minimize these barriers by screening for trauma history at intake and doing more comprehensive PTSD assessment when warranted.

Substance Use

As with the general population, a patient with ASD who is actively abusing or dependent on a substance will not benefit very well from CBT. If the patient is forthright about substance use in the intake, the therapist can encourage the individual to either stop or reduce that behavior, explaining how it may interfere with progress. If the patient agrees, it can become a goal of therapy. If the patient does not agree, it can be a barrier to treatment progress.

I have observed, anecdotally, that alcohol and marijuana seem to have a particularly disorganizing effect on people with ASD. For this reason, it is even more important for the therapist to know whether the patient is using because the disorganized behavior may be misattributed to other psychiatric issues. As an example, I had a new patient where ASD was suspected, but his behavior was particularly bizarre and chaotic, causing a diagnostic dilemma. Thinking he might be experiencing a comorbid psychotic episode, I referred him to a trusted colleague who is a psychiatrist. It was only through this process and collaboration with the psychiatrist that it was revealed that the patient was smoking marijuana daily—a fact he had withheld during my initial intake. When he temporarily stopped, the most extreme bizarre behaviors dissipated, and his symptoms fit a more classic ASD profile.

Isolation and Lack of Supports

Although all patients with ASD report some sense of isolation, some have fewer supports in their lives than others. A weak social support system can contribute to practical constraints. Transportation to sessions could be affected, for example, if a patient has no driver's license and must find someone to bring him or her. Child care responsibilities could interfere with attendance if a patient has children but no friends or family to babysit.

Extreme isolation is not only a risk factor for depression, but it can also interfere with some aspects of CBT. As a person learns social skills in session, for example, he or she needs real-life situations and relationships within which to practice those new skills. If a patient has almost no contact with others in between sessions, the progress will be slower. A referral to either a therapy group or a support group may be warranted. In addition, case management services may also be considered so that the patient will have further help in connecting to other support services such as appropriate recreational activities.

Financial Problems

It has been mentioned numerous times that adults with ASD are often unemployed or underemployed. This status has obvious financial implications, such as low income and lack of adequate health insurance coverage, which can be obstacles to psychotherapy. Therapists who serve this population must be prepared to address the same issues they would for any patient group with low income and/or long-term disability.

Ideally a patient's financial status and ability to pay for psychotherapy is known at intake, and a therapist can make a suitable arrangement or, if necessary, a referral to another provider at that point. Many variables affect the sorts of fee agreements that can be made, including the type of setting in which the therapist is practicing (e.g., hospital, outpatient clinic, private group practice, private sole proprietorship), whether or not the therapist is a provider for the patient's third-party reimbursement source (e.g., Medicaid, Medicare, private health insurance), whether or not the third-party source will reimburse for out-of-network services, and whether or not the therapist can apply a sliding scale when setting the fee. These are general practice management issues, and a description of each possible arrangement falls beyond the scope of this book. However, common obstacles that arise for patients with ASD, which can sometimes interrupt psychotherapy services even after a viable fee agreement was established at intake, should be mentioned. Some example scenarios are outlined below.

Employment Status Changes

Any time a patient loses a job or changes jobs it can have significant implications for access to health insurance coverage and ability to pay for therapy. Some patients with ASD are not only underemployed but *erratically* employed. In some ways, frequent changes in status can be more problematic than stable *unemployment* when it comes to accessing third-party reimbursement for psychotherapy services.

Take Janine's case as an example. At the time of her psychotherapy intake she was unemployed, receiving long-term disability benefits, and accessing medical coverage through Medicaid. This coverage had enabled her to get psychotherapy services at an outpatient clinic that exclusively served people who had disabilities and Medicaid. Several months into treatment, she found a full-time job, which meant she was no longer eligible for Medicaid and therefore unable to continue with her therapist at the clinic. She was referred to a private therapist who would accept the health insurance she would be getting at her new job. Typical for many adults with ASD, interpersonal difficulties led to her being fired after 5 months, leaving her with no income, no health insurance, and no Medicaid. She was worse off than she had been before she got the job, facing the all-too-common dilemma of "Should I try to get another job (and risk another termination) or reapply for government assistance?" Fortunately, to avoid a second interruption in her therapy, her private therapist was able to apply a sliding scale to reduce her fee, while referring her to a case manager to deal with her larger financial and employment service needs.

Janine's case is typical and points to the need for therapists to incorporate problem-solving strategies into sessions whenever patients face employment or financial decisions. The services outlined in Chapter 9, including case management and employment counseling, are also important to consider when patients face these issues.

Life Circumstance Changes

Some unemployed patients rely on "natural supports" (e.g., material and financial assistance from family members) instead of government assistance to get their daily living needs met. Many rely on parents or siblings for housing, food, and health care costs. Psychotherapy fees for these individuals may be paid by family members, either through direct pay or by the parents' health insurance company (if coverage is provided to disabled dependents). Although these adults with ASD are more fortunate than peers who do not have such resources, their financial security can be lost abruptly when there are major life transitions in the family. They can be significantly affected, for example, if a primary supporter becomes seriously ill, retires, moves residences, or dies.

Henry's case is one illustration. At the time of his intake, his financial status was stable, and he had no difficulty paying for psychotherapy. He was 56 years old, lived with both parents, and had a full-time job with a health insurance plan that reimbursed him for half of his psychotherapy fees. His salary was relatively low, and he was over-qualified for his job (he held a master's degree in English literature and was working as a shipping clerk). However, the support of his parents, who allowed him to live in their large suburban home for a nominal rent, enabled him to live very comfortably and to save a small amount of money. Within the first 6 months of his treatment, his father passed away. His mother became medically frail soon after and was forced to sell the house and move into an assisted-living facility. Henry used his savings to put a down payment on a condominium, but then had mortgage and maintenance payments that he could barely manage. Suddenly, the half of his therapy fee that he was responsible for was impossible for him to pay. In order to ensure continuation of the therapy that he needed now more than ever, the therapist agreed to accept the assigned amount specified by his insurance company and to waive his co-payment.

Henry represents the segment of the adult ASD population that has the most independence potential. In that regard, he was fortunate to be able to purchase his own home despite his struggles. Nevertheless, his therapy would have been interrupted without some modifications to his fee agreement. Therapists working with this population must be prepared to encounter these types of changes in financial status and to have various options available to offer patients in order to avoid disruption of treatment.

Limits Set by Private Insurance

The restrictions that are placed on mental health services by private insurance companies and HMOs create a large problem that does not just affect patients with ASD. Because it is such a broad topic, this discussion focuses only on two specific issues that patients with ASD may encounter when seeking reimbursement from a carrier.

One problem can arise when a private insurance company defines ASD as a condition not warranting "talk therapy." For example, one patient was denied reimbursement because her company stated that "any form of autism is a medical condition warranting treatment from a physician, only." Psychotherapy from a psychologist was deemed inappropriate by the representative reviewing her case. Although I had included a diagnosis of GAD in her treatment plan, it had not been listed as primary. This case illustrates the need for therapists to be aware of how a particular insurance company defines ASD: as a *medical, neurobiological,* or *mental health* problem. Unfortunately, these terms have not been standardized to date, and they vary from state to state and even from insurance company to insurance company. The decision by a therapist to list ASD as primary or secondary to a comorbid psychiatric disorder should be based on familiarity with these differences.

A second common problem can arise when an insurance company rejects the notion of "skill building" if it appears in a treatment plan. The strengths-based *habilitation* model that this book has emphasized, especially in Chapter 6, is not necessarily embraced by health insurance companies. In one example, a patient's sessions were cut off by his HMO because I had emphasized the notion of *skill building* more strongly than *symptom reduction* in the treatment plan, as the patient's goals were focused on increasing social skills. This problem can be avoided if a therapist, when writing a treatment plan for an insurance company, remains mindful of the illness model to which many companies adhere.

Finally, many insurance companies put limits on the number of sessions allowed per year for psychotherapy sessions. For patients whose needs are ongoing, these restrictions can be prohibitive to effective treatment. Knowing the limits at the beginning of treatment can be helpful, even if the therapist is not a participating provider on the insurance panel. Sometimes making a plan to meet every other week, for example, can ensure ongoing treatment throughout the year.

Untreated Health Problems

As a standard practice for any patient, with ASD or not, it is essential to rule out medical causes for presenting problems. Even when special attention is paid to this area during assessment, there are still times when a patient is struggling with a medical problem that has not been properly treated, or for which the individual has been noncompliant with care. The case of Bob and his diabetes is one example. As mentioned before, medical symptoms can simulate mood or anxiety problems and can slow down progress in CBT. Encouraging physician visits is obviously important. If the patient has behavioral and emotional obstacles to complying with physician visits, then goals can be incorporated into the treatment plan to address them.

Polypharmacy: Multiple Psychiatric Medications without a Rationale

Some adults with ASD have long histories of mental health treatment that has been carried out by multiple providers. Because ASD may not have come to light for them until recently, they may be carrying a collection of different diagnoses that may or may not be accurate. Along with those diagnoses, unfortunately, may come a collection of psychotropic medications that may not be appropriate for the patient. If the therapist is not a physician, then he or she obviously cannot evaluate this area. However, coordinating treatment with the prescribing physician is an important part of the planning process. It is crucial during conversations with the physician to clarify the rationale for each medication for both the therapist and the patient. If the patient has not had a recent psychiatric evaluation because, for instance, the primary care physician is refilling prescriptions, the therapist may want to recommend a referral to a psychiatrist and to discuss this idea with the patient and the primary care physician.

Lack of Cooperation from Other Providers

Without regular communication between providers about the patient's problems and treatment goals, progress in therapy can be hindered. Duplication of services can be one result, where two providers are working on the same goal. For example, it would be unnecessary for a psychotherapist to teach assertive communication while a speech–language pathologist is already addressing that need. Without any coordination between these clinicians, it would be a waste of resources and could also send confusing messages to the patient if the two providers use different approaches to achieve the goal. The opposite problem is a gap in service, when each of two providers neglects to attend to an issue, assuming that the other is already addressing it. For example, one patient who lived in a supervised apartment had been gradually gaining weight over several months. The residential staff believed he was overeating as a response to increased stress, and instructed the patient to bring it up to the psychotherapist. The psychotherapist, who had asked the patient about his increased weight, had been told by the patient that he was on a diet and was being assisted by the residential staff. When the gap was discovered during a phone conversation between the staff and the therapist, it was agreed by all, including the patient, that more frequent phone contact was warranted in this case.

Unfortunately, there are instances when another provider is unresponsive to the therapist's attempts to collaborate, or worse, expresses disagreement to the patient about therapy goals without a willingness to discuss it with the therapist. This type of behavior can hinder or even sabotage the CBT process. In rare cases, it is necessary to explain to the patient that the treatment cannot be provided when two clinicians are expressing competing views. The patient can be asked to encourage the other provider to participate in coordination of care efforts. If that strategy does not bring about cooperation, the therapist may elect to ask the patient to choose between the two clinicians.

Chapter Summary and Conclusions

This chapter outlined the most common obstacles to progress in CBT for adults with ASD. Suggestions for strategies to address each were also made. Some of these issues are not specific to this population, and others have been discussed elsewhere in this book. Nevertheless, the best advice to the therapist is to anticipate and prevent as many obstacles as possible because doing so usually involves less work than reacting to a problem that is well under way.

CHAPTER 11

Ending Treatment and Looking Ahead

This chapter provides guidelines for the various ways a treatment plan can come to a close. Some of the points covered in Chapter 9, about interdisciplinary collaboration, and in Chapter 10, about obstacles, will be mentioned again here because both relate to different aspects of terminating therapy. Beyond those special considerations, ending treatment is done in much the same way as it is with a patient from any population with complex problems. Numerous scenarios can lead to the end of a treatment plan, and this chapter divides these scenarios into two categories: situations in which *the goals have been met* and situations where *the goals have not been met* at the time of termination.

When the Goals of Treatment Are Met

Naturally, the most gratifying scenario for both patient and therapist is when there has been progress and all of the objectives set forth in the treatment plan have been met. At this point, the relationship can terminate, may continue with new goals, or may continue with an ongoing supportive function.

Therapy Ends

When the goals have been met and the patient reports that the initial presenting problems have dissipated, sessions can stop. The termination process should take place across several sessions and should focus on ensuring that the patient can identify risk factors for recurrence of anxiety or depression symptoms, and can articulate a set of strategies he or she can use to prevent escalation. Some patients may benefit from a gradual reduction in the frequency of appointments so that they can "try out" new skills without the therapist's help and report back on what it was like. Of course, such a plan would be individualized, but an example of a fading procedure would involve meeting every other week for several months, then once a month for several months, and then terminate completely.

269

A termination that is "nice and neat," as described here, is seen only when a patient has fewer risk factors for mental illness that were mentioned throughout this book. For example, a patient who has mild symptoms of ASD, a good social support system, a generally optimistic attitude about life, and only a single acute episode of a comorbid anxiety or mood disorder is going to be the best candidate for a "clean" termination. Although I have had such cases, they are not the majority.

Therapy Continues with New Goals

The most common scenario that occurs when goals are met is that new ones are established. Adults with ASD often have multiple problems, and the initial treatment plan usually focuses on the highest priorities. As improvement occurs in those areas, the patient often identifies other areas in which he or she would like to see improvement. This process continues until the patient and therapist agree that the presenting problems have been adequately addressed. Sometimes symptom remission in one domain uncovers chronic problems that were previously undetected because they were overshadowed by an acute crisis. Setting these new goals can be a positive experience because such patients are usually quite motivated by their own success with the initial goals.

One example of this is Bob, the case that was discussed more than any other in this book. At the time of this writing, I have been working with him for more than 16 years. The goals have changed several times since the initial plan was made. Each time he achieves a goal, there is a dual benefit. There is obviously the improvement in the issue named in the goal (e.g., increased frequency of exercise), *and* the experience serves a schema-changing function. The reader may recall that Bob's core beliefs about himself are "I am helpless," "I cannot take care of myself," "I am powerless," and "I am defective." Each time he achieves a therapy goal, it provides evidence that contradicts his self-schema because he is the one who is bringing about the changes in his life.

Sessions Continue for Maintenance of Gains and Ongoing Monitoring

Another common scenario occurs when the goals of therapy are met, but the patient has so many risk factors for chronic anxiety or depression that the regular contact with the therapist is a crucial relapse prevention tool. Usually in such cases, the therapist alternates between periods of active treatment (working on goals) and periods in which sessions focus on support and reinforcement of adaptive skills. The latter would occur when the patient is not in a significant amount of distress, but the therapist has judged that he or she will not be able to identify and respond to triggers in an adaptive way on his or her own. The sessions therefore allow the therapist to be a source of social reinforcement for strengthening skills that have been learned, while also "keeping an eye" on potential triggers for relapse. If a symptom-activating event does occur, the therapist can quickly initiate active treatment and hopefully minimize the severity of the impact.

The case of Seth falls in this category. At the time of this writing, I have been working with him for 22 years and he is now 67 years old. His case does not represent the majority of adult ASD cases any more than the "clean terminations" mentioned earlier. However, his symptoms of ASD are significant, he has very little family support, and he has a severe and chronic anxiety disorder. He has made vast improvements in his social life, as he now has a network of several friends and he has recreational plans almost every weekend. Like several of my clients in his age range, he has taken on care-taking responsibilities for an elderly parent. This has represented an increase in daily stressors, while at the same time bolstered his confidence in his own judgment and competence. By meeting regularly with the therapist, even during periods of relative calm, Seth is able to prevent stressful events from becoming catastrophic. Despite the progress he has made over the years, he is not likely to be able to maintain his current level of functioning without this ongoing support.

When Treatment Is Interrupted before Goals Are Met

Unfortunately, a fair number of cases face unexpected interruptions or endings. The situations described below can arise in any adult psychotherapy practice, but some may be more prevalent in the ASD adult population, again because of the complex nature of their problems. Complications may lead to an unplanned suspension from treatment, transfer to another therapist, or premature termination.

Temporary Suspension of Treatment

There may be both practical and therapeutic reasons to temporarily suspend treatment, with the intention of both patient and therapist to resume at some point.

Practical Reasons to Suspend Sessions

Practical or logistical factors may unexpectedly change, leading to a gap in appointments while the situation is resolved. Examples include:

- A long illness or injury of either the patient or the therapist.
- Transportation problems.
- Temporary third-party payment problems (e.g., patients who rely on Medicaid may face periodic gaps in coverage, during which they may opt not to come until coverage is reinstated).
- Scheduling conflicts (e.g., change in the patient's job schedule).

Therapeutic Reasons to Suspend Sessions

Therapeutic reasons to put psychotherapy on hold are usually related to the patient's participation in some other intensive program or intervention that is going to support the overall treatment plan but which interferes with attendance. Examples are:

- Time-limited job training program.
- Psychiatric day treatment program.
- Inpatient psychiatric or addiction treatment program.
- Summer recreational program (similar to camp).
- Extended travel.

Any of these programs may have a schedule or location that does not allow the patient to come to regular therapy appointments. Even if the schedule would permit continuing sessions, some patients ask to suspend the treatment simply because having too many places to go each week increases anxiety. It is important to keep in mind that these adults do not adapt well to change and are easily overwhelmed by multiple demands. If a patient is joining a new activity that the therapist believes is going to help him or her move toward their agreed-upon mental health goals, then taking a break from therapy will likely facilitate, rather than hinder, the patient's progress.

The decision to keep a case open during an absence is a judgment call that a therapist will make on a case-by-case basis, considering many factors. Some of these factors are summarized in the questions listed below:

- Has the patient shown motivation in treatment up to this point?
- Is the absence due to an obstacle that is unavoidable?
- Does the patient seem genuinely motivated to return after the absence?
- Does the absence have a clear time frame defined?
- Is the absence for an activity that will enhance quality of life or support the goals of the therapy treatment plan?

Even after a decision is made to suspend treatment, there are times when a case ultimately has to be closed. Some of those issues are discussed next.

Transfer to Another Therapist

Chapter 9 described the reasons a therapist may refer a patient with ASD to adjunctive psychotherapy services. There are other times when a therapist and patient agree that a complete transfer should be made. Listed below are some of the factors that could lead up to that decision:

- The patient does not feel comfortable with the therapist. This discomfort could be due to the therapist's style, philosophy of therapy, or gender. As in any population, some patients feel more comfortable working with one gender over the other. Of course, the therapist will be able to make the best referral if the patient is able to be specific about his or her reasons for wanting to change, and such a discussion should be encouraged.

- The patient has a comorbid condition with the ASD that is outside the therapist's scope of practice. In some cases, adjunctive therapy for the comorbid condition is not practical (e.g., eating disorder, addictive disorder), and a transfer to an expert is warranted.

- The patient experiences a change in his or her personal or work schedule that is not temporary, and the therapist cannot accommodate the new schedule.

- The patient cannot afford the therapy or is reliant on using a health insurance plan in which the therapist does not participate.

- There is a change in obligations to family. In the example of Lorraine, mentioned earlier, she ended treatment after having a baby.

- The patient moves and can no longer commute comfortably to the therapist.

Some of these issues arise early in treatment, whereas others can crop up at any time. As with any patient population, obtaining the patient's authorization to speak to the new therapist can be a helpful step in easing the transition.

Premature Termination of Treatment

Unfortunately, there are cases for which a temporary suspension or transfer is not feasible, but treatment ends nonetheless. Sometimes the termination is driven by the patient, and other times the therapist may decide to end the relationship. Naturally, these are all least desirable scenarios for therapists. Listed below are the typical ways in which premature termination occurs:

- The patient drops out without explaining why and is unresponsive to the therapist's attempts to reach out by phone, e-mail, or text messages.

- The patient suspends treatment for one of the reasons listed above, but does not return despite the original plan.

- The patient is agitated or offended in response to some part of the treatment and terminates abruptly. There are times when a patient cannot tolerate the aspects of CBT that involve self-evaluation and will withdraw from the process, even when the therapist is flexible and tries to minimize pressure.

- The therapist initiates the termination because the patient continually engages in behavior that interferes with therapy and is not amenable to intervention. These problems include, but are not limited to, repeated no-shows, persistent extreme hostility expressed toward the therapist, or active substance abuse (e.g., the patient mentioned in the previous chapter who was smoking marijuana was never able to completely stop, and the disorganizing effect it had on him grossly limited his ability to focus in sessions).

- The therapist initiates the termination because the patient is not engaging in a collaborative process (e.g., is noncompliant with treatment goals and unwilling to participate in a dialogue to revise the plan). Some patients do not accept or understand the cognitive model, which in and of itself is not a reason to discharge. However, if the patient is not willing to engage in an honest dialogue about it by expressing his or her beliefs and opinions, then no progress can be made.

- The therapist initiates the termination because the patient is noncompliant with recommendations to initiate crucial adjunctive treatment. At times, the therapist refers a patient to another professional to address a serious threat to the patient's health and well-being. If a patient is unwilling to follow up on one of those problems and the consequence interferes with the treatment plan, it may be necessary for the therapist to at least suspend treatment until the matter is addressed. For example, one patient with whom I worked complained about severe headaches that were interfering with daily functioning. Despite repeated urging by me, she would not go to her physician. I explored the reasons for her reluctance in session (e.g., ruled out fear of doctors, financial constraints), but she would only say that she did not think the problem was medically based. She was otherwise motivated to work on therapy goals. I suspended appointments with the condition that sessions could resume after she was medically evaluated. She ultimately went to a physician, and our sessions resumed. In another case, significant family dysfunction was interfering with a patient's progress in individual CBT. After several meetings with the family, I decided that CBT would not be effective in addressing the patient's presenting problems without co-occurring family therapy. The patient and family were unwilling to take that step, so I terminated the treatment and referred the patient to a colleague with a different orientation.

Whenever the therapist initiates the termination, it is good practice to discuss the decision with colleagues, a supervisor, and/or a mental health risk management professional (e.g., a lawyer with expertise in the legal and ethical aspects of mental health practice). It is always a very difficult decision to end a therapy relationship before the goals have been met. However, a therapist is doing a disservice to the patient if he or she continually applies a therapy approach that he or she knows is not going to be effective.

So far, this chapter has outlined the various ways in which therapy comes to an end. Ideally, all therapists hope to end after goals have been achieved, and that was discussed at the beginning of the chapter. More often, however, therapy will continue even after the initial goals have been met because of the complex nature of this population, or will end prematurely, as the examples illustrated. I bring this book to an end by describing my hopes for the future in the science and treatment of ASD.

Looking Ahead for Adults with ASD

I hope your interest in this book reflects a desire to begin or continue accepting adults with ASD into your practice. These individuals are among the people who seek help in a variety of mental health treatment settings, whether for issues that are directly related to their ASD or for comorbid mental health problems (Maddox & Gaus, 2018). This book was meant to serve as a framework for conceptualizing adult cases using evidence-based practices, despite the paucity of clinical research to guide us. If we, as members of a mental health community, are to serve our patients appropriately, we will need to see a growth in both basic and applied research on many subjects. When the first edition of this book was published in 2007, I listed the areas of research that I hoped would develop more to benefit CBT therapists working with adult ASD. In the 11 years that have passed since then, there has been some growth in these areas, but not nearly enough. My wish list for future research directions has remained largely the same, with the addition of the subject of aging. The topics are outlined below, with comments about progress as well as further needs.

Cognitive Dysfunction in ASD

In my conceptual model of adult ASD, I cite the evidence base for core cognitive dysfunction and hypothesize the causal role these information-processing impairments play in the clinical problems seen in psychotherapy cases. Generating these hypotheses has clinical utility while trying to understand an individual case, but the causal connections have not been established through controlled investigations. Key empirical questions that have yet to be answered are:

- Which *cognitive* deficits cause the maladaptive *behavior* that differentiates people with ASD from typical people? For example, what social-cognition impairments are causing the "social skill deficits" observed in people with ASD? Are EF deficits truly causing self-direction problems in practical, everyday life?
- Are *emotion regulation* impairments the cause, the consequence, or bidirectionally related to ASD symptoms? Similarly, how are ER impairments related to the comorbid anxiety and depression so often seen in these adults?
- Which behaviors are most associated with which types of peer rejection? What specific behavioral changes are most closely related to improvements in perceived social support and satisfaction in relationships?
- Are people with ASD subject to particular types of schemas or core beliefs, as per Beck's (1976) cognitive model?

Comorbidity

Clinical descriptions of adult ASD cases, in this book and elsewhere, refer to the high risk and incidence of comorbid psychiatric disorders. Some epidemiological studies have corroborated these observations, as described in Chapter 1. Nevertheless, more up-to-date incidence and prevalence data are needed, especially since the publication of DSM-5 (American Psychiatric Association, 2013), which not only redefined ASD but also changed the definitions of other conditions that commonly co-occur in adult patients.

Stress

The importance of stress factors in the scientific and clinical understanding of ASD has received little attention in the autism spectrum literature, with the exception of the decades of pioneering work by the Groden Center group. Their edited book (Baron et al., 2006) called for more research in this critical area, but the number of studies since then that have appeared in the literature is surprisingly small. As a practitioner, I find it impossible not to consider stress factors when assessing a patient's presenting problems, so I look forward to seeing more efforts toward a clear definition of stress as well as the development of a larger evidence base on the role of stress in ASD.

Cognitive-Behavioral Therapy

This book presented an evidence-based rationale—from an integration of research from multiple sources—for providing CBT to adults with ASD. While there is a growing evidence base for the use of CBT with children, adolescents, and emerging adults, I would like to see more intervention studies using adults with ASD of all ages, including protocols for specific clinical issues. These include:

- Protocols designed to improve the core cognitive deficits of ASD (e.g., those targeting social cognition or EF) in adults.
- Protocols designed to improve the ER difficulties that are closely associated with both ASD symptoms, as well as comorbid anxiety and depressive disorders in adults.

- Protocols for specific comorbid disorders as they occur in adults with ASD, such as social anxiety disorder, obsessive–compulsive disorder, generalized anxiety disorder, agoraphobia, PTSD, and major depressive disorder.
- Mechanisms of change in CBT and treatment components most associated with positive outcomes in adults with ASD.
- CBT in different modalities, such as couple therapy when one or both members has ASD, or group applications of CBT, which have shown promise for youth with ASD and could be a cost-effective alternative for adults who have limited finances.

Gender

Because the prevalence of ASD is higher in males than in females, most research on these disorders has been done using male subjects, leaving us with very little information about affected females. Recent attention has been paid to gender differences in symptom manifestation (e.g., Kreiser & White, 2014)—these issues were presented in Chapter 1. Clinicians serving adults with ASD need accurate information about the similarities and differences between the needs of men and women seeking treatment, for both assessment and intervention purposes.

Aging

ASD is a condition that affects people across the lifespan. As Wright and Wadsworth (2016) point out, focusing on adulthood should not stop with the "aging-out" population of emerging adults in their late teens and early 20s. Older people with autism have been living among us for as long as the diagnostic entity has existed, yet they have rarely been the focus of research or clinical work. Thankfully, in an edited book by Wright (2016), researchers and scholars from multiple disciplines have summarized the most relevant research about ASD and aging. With that, they defined a direction for the autism community in terms of meeting the needs of adults with ASD who are in mid-to-late life right *now*. It is not enough to discuss the population of young adults who will *eventually* be old and to talk about meeting the needs of aging people with ASD as if it is a problem the field *will* face one day. For a very large number of people, the challenges of aging in daily life are very current. Nothing could illustrate this better than the recent best-selling book *In a Different Key* (Donvan & Zucker, 2016), which details the history of autism in America through the eyes of two journalists. As part of their investigation, the authors tracked down the very first person who was ever diagnosed with autism in the United States: Leo Kanner's "Case #1." The child, who was described along with several other boys in Kanner's (1943) seminal article that coined the term *autism*, was found to be alive and well, living as an elderly man in the town where he spent his whole life. Now 83 years old, Donald Triplett not only reminds us that people with ASD can thrive and lead a meaningful life but that people with ASD have already been growing old for a very long time.

Support Service Models

Adults with ASD are grossly underserved by disability service agencies. Many of these adults need specialized training in *vocational* and *independent living* skills, but there is a paucity of employment and adult residential services that are appropriate to serve those adults who need them. ASD is not viewed as a "legitimate" disability in some states. Even in states where the syndrome does qualify for funding, the individual will be hard-pressed to find an employment training or residential program that is designed to meet his or her unique needs. Existing vocational training centers, for example, are designed to serve distinct populations, such as those with chronic mental illness, substance abuse, or ID. A person with ASD typically has needs that are very different from each of those groups and would therefore be ill served in those settings. Gerhardt, Cicero, and Mayville (2014) have made specific recommendations for the kinds of changes that are needed to improve this problem; these changes would involve people in government, educational systems, and adult disability services agencies, as well as potential employers of these individuals. Adults with ASD would have fewer mental health needs if they could work in satisfying careers and live independently.

Concluding Comments

Whether you already have patients with ASD on your caseload or are looking to begin treating these adults, I hope you will consider using an individualized case conceptualization approach like the one presented here. If you do, it should lead you to the vast literature on evidence-based CBT interventions that are readily available for typical adults, and which can easily be applied to people with ASD. I have been continually fascinated with the peculiar workings of the ASD mind ever since I met Joe in 1995, and I wish for you to equally enjoy working with these unusual and delightful patients.

Therapy Resources

Professional Overviews

Attwood, T. (2015). *The complete guide to Asperger's syndrome.* London: Jessica Kingsley.
McPartland, J. C., Klin, A., & Volkmar, F. R. (Eds.). (2014). *Asperger syndrome: Assessing and treating high-functioning autism spectrum disorders* (2nd ed.). New York: Guilford Press.
Stoddardt, K. P., Burke, L., & King, R. (2012). *Asperger syndrome in adulthood.* New York: Norton.

Therapy Tools and Workbooks

This list includes tools and sources of worksheets that are useful in an adult psychotherapy setting.

Attwood, T. (2004). *Exploring feelings: Cognitive behaviour therapy to manage anger.* Arlington, TX: Future Horizons.
Attwood, T., & Garnett, M. (2016). *Exploring depression, and beating the blues: A CBT self-help guide to understanding and coping with depression in Asperger's syndrome (ASD-Level 1).* London: Jessica Kingsley.
Attwood, T., Hénault, I., & Dubin, N. (2014). *The autism spectrum, sexuality, and the law: What every parent and professional needs to know.* London: Jessica Kingsley.
Buron, K. D., & Curtis, M. (2012). *The Incredible 5-Point Scale: Assisting students in understanding social interactions and controlling their emotional responses.* Shawnee Mission, KS: Autism Asperger.
Cambridge University. (2007). *Mind reading: The interactive guide to emotions* [DVD]. London: Jessica Kingsley.
Faherty, C. (2000). *Asperger's: What does it mean to me?* Arlington, TX: Future Horizons.
Gaus, V. L. (2011). *Living well on the spectrum: How to use your strengths to meet the challenges of Asperger syndrome/high-functioning autism.* New York: Guilford Press.
Gray, C. (1994). *Comic strip conversations.* Arlington, TX: Future Horizons.
Gray, C. (2015). *The new social story book, revised and expanded 15th anniversary edition: Over 150 social stories that teach everyday social skills to children and adults with autism and their peers* (3rd ed.). Arlington, TX: Future Horizons.
Groden, J., Weidenman, L., & Diller, A. (2016). *Relaxation: A comprehensive manual for children and adults with autism and other developmental disabilities.* Champaign, IL: Research Press.

Hamilton, I. S. (2004). *An Asperger dictionary of everyday expressions.* London: Jessica Kingsley.

Hénault, I. (2005). *Asperger's syndrome and sexuality: From adolescence through adulthood.* London: Jessica Kingsley.

Innovative Interactions. (2000). *Talk Blocks for work.* Seattle, WA: Author. (Available only from third-party sellers)

Myles, B. S., Trautman, M. L., & Schelvan, R. L. (2004). *The hidden curriculum: Practical solutions for understanding unstated rules in social situations.* Shawnee Mission, KS: Autism Asperger.

Scheiner, M., & Bogden, J. (2017). *An employer's guide to managing professionals on the autism spectrum.* London: Jessica Kingsley.

Winner, M. G. (2000). *Inside out: What makes a person with social cognitive deficits tick?* San Jose, CA: Author.

Winner, M. G. (2002). *Thinking about you thinking about me.* San Jose, CA: Author.

Winner, M. G., & Crooke, P. J. (2011). *Social thinking at work: Why should I care?* Great Barrington, MA: North River Press.

Autobiographical and Self-Help Books by Authors on the Autism Spectrum

Several hundred books have been written by individuals or family members of individuals on the autism spectrum. This short list comprises my preferences for patients who are newly diagnosed or reading about ASD for the first time.

Finch, D. (2910). *The journal of best practices: A memoir of marriage, Asperger syndrome, and one man's quest to be a better husband.* New York: Scribner.

Grandin, T. (2006). *Thinking in pictures and other reports from my life with autism: Expanded edition.* New York: Vintage.

Grandin, T. (2008). *Developing talents: Careers for individuals with Asperger syndrome and high functioning autism.* Shawnee Mission, KS: Autism Asperger.

Newport, J. (2001). *Your life is not a label: A guide to living fully with autism and Asperger syndrome.* Arlington, TX: Future Horizons.

Paridiz, V. (2002). *Elijah's cup: A family's journey into the community and culture of high-functioning autism and Asperger syndrome.* London: Jessica Kingsley.

Prince-Hughes, D. (2004). *Songs of the gorilla nation: My journey through autism.* New York: Harmony Books.

Robison, J. E. (2007). *Look me in the eye: My life with Asperger's.* New York: Random House.

Robinson, J. E. (2011). *Be different: My adventures with Asperger's and my advice for fellow Aspergians, misfits, families and teachers.* New York: Crown.

Shore, S. M. (2001). *Beyond the wall: Personal experiences with autism and Asperger syndrome.* Shawnee Mission, KS: Autism Asperger.

Shore, S. (Ed.). (2004). *Ask and tell: Self-advocacy and disclosure for people on the autism spectrum.* Shawnee Mission, KS: Autism Asperger.

Wiley, L. H. (2001). *Asperger syndrome in the family: Redefining normal.* London: Jessica Kingsley.

Wiley, L. H. (2015). *Pretending to be normal: Living with Asperger's syndrome (autism spectrum disorder).* London: Jessica Kingsley.

Zaks, Z. (2006). *Life and love: Positive strategies for autistic adults.* Shawnee Mission, KS: Autism Asperger.

Websites of Education, Advocacy, and Support Organizations for AS and ASD

These organizations deal specifically with ASD or cover the whole autism spectrum but *include* information about ASD in more cognitively able individuals.

Asperger/Autism Network (AANE)
www.aane.org

Asperger Autism Spectrum Education Network (ASPEN)
www.aspennj.org

Asperger Syndrome and High Functioning Autism Association (AHA)
www.ahany.org

Autism Society of America
www.autism-society.org

Autism Speaks
www.autismspeaks.org

Autism Spectrum Coalition
www.aspergersyndrome.org

Global and Regional Asperger Syndrome Partnership (GRASP)
www.grasp.org

Integrate Autism Employment Advisors
www.integrateadvisors.org

National Association for the Dually Diagnosed (NADD)
www.thenadd.org

The National Autistic Society (NAS; United Kingdom)
www.autism.org.uk

Organization for Autism Research (OAR)
www.researchautism.org

References

Alvarez-Fernandez, S., Brown, H. R., Zhao, Y., Raithel, J. A., Bishop, S. L., Kern, S. B., et al. (2017). Perceived social support in adults with autism spectrum disorder and attention-deficit/hyperactivity disorder. *Autism Research, 10*(5), 866–877.

Ambery, F. Z., Russell, A. J., Perry, K., Morris, R., & Murphy, D. G. (2006). Neuropsychological functioning in adults with Asperger syndrome. *Autism, 10*(6), 551–564.

American Psychiatric Association. (1987). *Diagnostic and statistical manual of mental disorders* (3rd ed., rev.). Washington, DC: Author.

American Psychiatric Association. (1994). *Diagnostic and statistical manual of mental disorders* (4th ed.). Washington, DC: Author.

American Psychiatric Association. (2000). *Diagnostic and statistical manual of mental disorders* (4th ed., text rev.). Washington, DC: Author.

American Psychiatric Association. (2013). *Diagnostic and statistical manual of mental disorders* (5th ed.). Arlington, VA: Author.

Anholt, G. E., Cath, D. C., Van Oppen, P., Eikelenboom, M., Smit, J. H., Van Megen, H., et al. (2010). Autism and ADHD symptoms in patients with OCD: Are they associated with specific OC symptoms dimensions or OC symptom severity? *Journal of Autism and Developmental Disorders, 45*(12), 3949–3960.

Asperger, H. (1944). Die "autischen Psychopathen" im Kindeshalter. *Archiv für Psychiatrie und Nervenkrankenheiten, 117,* 76–136.

Attwood, T. (1998). *Asperger's syndrome: A guide for parents and professionals.* London: Jessica Kingsley.

Attwood, T. (2004a). Cognitive behaviour therapy for children and adults with Asperger's syndrome. *Behaviour Change, 21*(3), 147–162.

Attwood, T. (2004b). *Exploring feelings: Cognitive behavior therapy to manage anger.* Arlington, TX: Future Horizons.

Attwood, T. (2004c). *Exploring feelings: Cognitive behavior therapy to manage anxiety.* Arlington, TX: Future Horizons.

Attwood, T. (2006). Asperger's syndrome and problems related to stress. In M. G. Baron, J. Groden, G. Groden, & L. P. Lipsitt (Eds.), *Stress and coping in autism* (pp. 351–370). New York: Oxford University Press.

Attwood, T. (2007). *The complete guide to Asperger's syndrome.* London: Jessica Kingsley.

Attwood, T. (2015). *The complete guide to Asperger's syndrome* (rev. ed.). London: Jessica Kingsley.

Attwood, T., & Garnett, M. (2016). *Exploring depression, and beating the blues: A CBT self-help guide to understanding and coping with depression in Asperger's syndrome (ASD-Level 1)*. London: Jessica Kingsley.

Attwood, T., Hénault, I., & Dubin, N. (2014). *The autism spectrum, sexuality, and the law: What every parent and professional needs to know.* London: Jessica Kingsley.

Baker, E. K., & Richdale, A. L. (2017). Examining the behavioural sleep–wake rhythm in adults with autism spectrum disorder and no comorbid intellectual disability. *Journal of Autism and Developmental Disorders, 47*(4), 1207–1222.

Baldwin, S., Costley, D., & Warren, A. J. (2014). Employment activities and experiences of adults with high-functioning autism and Asperger's disorder. *Journal of Autism and Developmental Disorder, 44*(10), 2440–2449.

Baranek, G. T., Parham, L. D., & Bodfish, J. W. (2005). Sensory and motor features in autism: Assessment and intervention. In F. R. Volkmar, R. Paul, A. Klin, & D. Cohen (Eds.), *Handbook of autism and pervasive developmental disorders: Vol. 2. Assessment, interventions and policy* (3rd ed., pp. 831–857). Hoboken, NJ: Wiley.

Barlow, D. H. (2001). *Anxiety and its disorders: The nature and treatment of anxiety and panic* (2nd ed.). New York: Guilford Press.

Baron, M. G., Groden, J., Groden, G., & Lipsitt, L. P. (Eds.). (2006). *Stress and coping in autism.* New York: Oxford University Press.

Baron-Cohen, S. (1995). *Mindblindness: An essay on autism and theory of mind.* Boston: MIT Press.

Baron-Cohen, S., Jolliffe, T., Mortimore, C., & Robertson, M. (1997). Another advanced test of theory of mind: Evidence from very high functioning adults with autism or Asperger syndrome. *Journal of Child Psychology and Psychiatry, 38*, 813–822.

Baron-Cohen, S., Leslie, A. M., & Frith, U. (1985). Does the autistic child have a "theory of mind"? *Cognition, 21*, 37–46.

Baron-Cohen, S., & Wheelwright, S. (2004). The empathy quotient: An investigation of adults with Asperger syndrome or high functioning autism, and normal sex differences. *Journal of Autism and Developmental Disorders, 34*, 163–175.

Baron-Cohen, S., Wheelwright, S., Skinner, R., Martin, J., & Clubley, E. (2001). The autism spectrum quotient (AQ): Evidence from Asperger syndrome/high functioning autism, males and females, scientists and mathematicians. *Journal of Autism and Developmental Disorders, 31*, 5–17.

Beck, A. T. (1963). Thinking and depression. *Archives of General Psychiatry, 9*, 324–333.

Beck, A. T. (1976). *Cognitive therapy and the emotional disorders.* New York: International Universities Press.

Beck, A. T. (1990). *Beck Anxiety Inventory.* San Antonio, TX: Psychological Corp.

Beck, A. T. (1996). *Beck Depression Inventory* (2nd ed.). San Antonio, TX: Psychological Corp.

Beck, A. T., Epstein, N., Brown, G., & Steer, R. A. (1988). An inventory for measuring clinical anxiety: Psychometric properties. *Journal of Consulting and Clinical Psychology, 56*, 893–897.

Beck, A. T., Freeman, A., Davis, D. D., & Associates. (2004). *Cognitive therapy of personality disorders* (2nd ed.). New York: Guilford Press.

Beck, A. T., Rush, J. A., Shaw, B. F., & Emery, G. (1979). *Cognitive therapy for depression.* New York: Guilford Press.

Beck, J. S. (1995). *Cognitive therapy: Basics and beyond.* New York: Guilford Press.

Begeer, S., Bouk, S. E., Boussaid, W., Terwogt, M. M., & Koot, H. M. (2009). Underdiagnosis and referral bias of autism in ethnic minorities. *Journal of Autism and Developmental Disorders, 39*, 142–148.

Bejerot, S., Eriksson, J. M., & Mörtberg, E. (2014). Social anxiety in adult autism spectrum disorder. *Psychiatry Research, 220*(1–2), 705–707.

Bejerat, S., Nylander, L., & Lindstrom, E. (2001). Autistic traits in obsessive–compulsive disorders. *Nordic Journal of Psychiatry, 55,* 169–176.

Bennetto, L., Pennington, B. F., & Rogers, S. J. (1996). Intact and impaired memory functions in autism. *Child Development, 67,* 1816–1835.

Bernstein, D. A., & Borkovec, T. D. (1973). *Progressive relaxation training: A manual for the helping professions.* Champaign, IL: Research Press.

Berthoz, S., & Hill, E. L. (2005). The validity of using self-reports to assess emotion regulation abilities in adults with autism spectrum disorder. *European Psychiatry, 20*(3), 291–298.

Bird, G., Press, C., & Richardson, D. C. (2011). The role of alexithymia in reduced eye-fixation in autism spectrum conditions. *Journal of Autism and Developmental Disorders, 41*(11), 1556–1564.

Bishop-Fitzpatrick, L., Mazefsky, C. A., Minshew, N. J., & Eack, S. M. (2015). The relationship between stress and social functioning in adults with autism spectrum disorder and without intellectual disability. *Autism Research, 8*(2), 164–173.

Bishop-Fitzpatrick, L., Mineshew, N. J., Mazefsky, C. A., & Eack, S. M. (2017). Perception of life as stressful, not biological response to stress, is associated with greater social disability in adults with autism spectrum disorder. *Journal of Autism and Developmental Disorders, 47*(1), 1–16.

Bishop-Fitzpatrick, L., Smith DaWalt, L., Greenberg, J. S., & Mailick, M. R. (2017). Participation in recreational activities buffers the impact of perceived stress on quality of life in adults with autism spectrum disorder. *Autism Research, 10*(5), 973–982.

Brown, J. (2016). *The Emotion Regulation Skills System for cognitively challenged clients: A DBT-informed approach.* New York: Guilford Press.

Brownell, K. D. (2000). *The LEARN program for weight management.* Dallas, TX: American Health.

Brugha, T. S., McManus, S., Bankart, J., Scott, F., Purdon, S., Smith, J., et al. (2011). Epidemiology of autism spectrum disorders in adults in the community in England. *Archives of General Psychiatry, 68*(5), 459–465.

Brukner-Wetman, Y., Laor, N., & Golan, O. (2016). Social (pragmatic) communication disorder and its relation to the autism spectrum: Dilemmas arising from the DSM-5 classification. *Journal of Autism and Developmental Disorders, 46*(8), 2821–2829.

Bryan, C. J., & Rudd, M. D. (2016). The importance of temporal dynamics in the transition from suicidal thought to behavior. *Clinical Psychology: Science and Practice, 23*(1), 21–25.

Buck, T. R., Viskochil, J., Farley, M., Coon, H., McMahon, W. H., Morgan, J., et al. (2014). Psychiatric comorbidity and medication use in adults with autism spectrum disorder. *Journal of Autism and Developmental Disorders, 44*(12), 3063–3071.

Buhler, E., Bachmann, C., Goyert, H., Heinzel-Gutenbrunner, M., & Kamp-Becker, I. (2011). Differential diagnosis of autism spectrum disorder and attention deficit hyperactivity disorder by means of inhibitory control and "theory of mind." *Journal of Autism and Developmental Disorders, 41*(12), 1718–1726.

Burns, D. D. (1980). *Feeling good: The new mood therapy.* New York: Avon Books.

Burns, D. D. (1999). *Feeling good: The new mood therapy* (rev.). New York: Avon Books.

Burns, D. D. (2009). *Feeling good: The new mood therapy* (Vol. 1). New York: Avon Books.

Buron, K. D., & Curtis, M. (2012). *The Incredible 5-Point Scale: Assisting students in understanding social interactions and controlling their emotional responses.* Shawnee Mission, KS: Autism Asperger.

Butler, A. C., Chapman, J. E., Forman, E. M., & Beck, A. T. (2006). The empirical status of cognitive-behavior therapy: A review of meta-analyses. *Psychology Review, 26*(1), 17–31.

Butwicka, A., Långström, N., Larsson, H., Lundström, S., Serlachius, E., Almqvist, C., et al. (2017). Increased risk for substance use-related problems in autism spectrum disorders:

A population-based cohort study. *Journal of Autism and Developmental Disorders, 47*(1), 80–89.

Byers, E. S., & Nichols, S. (2014). Sexual satisfaction of high-functioning adults with autism spectrum disorder. *Sexuality and Disability, 32*(3), 365–382.

Byers, E. S., Nichols, S., & Voyer, S. D. (2013). Challenging stereotypes: Sexual functioning of single adults with high functioning autism spectrum disorder. *Journal of Autism and Developmental Disorders, 43*(11), 2617–2627.

Byers, E. S., Nichols, S., Voyer, S. D., & Reilly, G. (2013). Sexual well-being of a community sample of high-functioning adults on the autism spectrum who have been in a romantic relationship. *Autism, 17*(4), 418–433.

Cambridge University. (2004). *Mind reading: The interactive guide to emotions* [DVD]. London: Jessica Kingsley.

Campbell, J. M., James, C. L., & Vess, S. F. (2014). Evidence-based assessment of Asperger syndrome: A selective review of screening and diagnostic instruments. In J. C. McPartland, A. Klin, & F. R. Volkmar (Eds.), *Asperger syndrome: Assessing and treating high-functioning autism spectrum disorders* (2nd ed., pp. 43–70). New York: Guilford Press.

Cardaciotto, L., & Herbert, J. D. (2004). Cognitive behavior therapy for social anxiety disorder in the context of Asperger's syndrome: A single subject report. *Cognitive and Behavioral Practice, 11*, 75–81.

Cassidy, S., Bradley, P., Robinson, J., Allison, C., McHugh, M., & Baron-Cohen, S. (2014). Suicidal ideation and suicide plans or attempts in adults with Asperger's syndrome attending a specialist diagnostic clinic: A clinical cohort study. *Lancet, 1*(2), 142–147.

Cautela, J. R., & Groden, J. (1978). *Relaxation: A comprehensive manual for adults, children, and children with special needs.* Champaign, IL: Research Press.

Chambless, D. L., Baker-Ericzen, M., Baucom, D., Beutler, L. E., Calhoun, K. S., Crits-Christoph, P., et al. (1998). Update on empirically validated therapies: II. *The Clinical Psychologist, 51*, 3–16.

Channon, S., Charman, T., Heap, J., Crawford, S., & Rios, P. (2001). Real-life-type problem solving in Asperger's syndrome. *Journal of Autism and Developmental Disorders, 31*(5), 461–469.

Chiesa, A., & Serretti, A. (2009). Mindfulness-based stress reduction for stress management in healthy people: A review and meta-analysis. *Journal of Alternative and Complementary Medicine, 15*(5), 593–600.

Christensen, D. L., Baio, J., Van Naarden Braun, K., Bilder, D., Charles, J., Constantino, J. N., et al. (2016). Prevalence and characteristics of autism spectrum disorder among children aged 8 years—Autism and Developmental Disabilities Monitoring Network, 11 sites, United States, 2012. *Morbidity and Mortality Weekly Report Surveillance Summaries, 65*(SS-3), 1–23.

Ciarrochi, J., & Bailey, A. (2008). *A CBT-practitioner's guide to ACT: How to bridge the gap between cognitive behavioral therapy and acceptance and commitment therapy.* Oakland, CA: New Harbinger.

Clarke, T., Tickle, A., & Gillott, A. (2016). Substance use disorder in Asperger syndrome: An investigation into the development and maintenance of substance use disorder by individuals with a diagnosis of Asperger syndrome. *International Journal of Drug Policy, 27*, 154–163.

Cohen, M. C. (2011). *Social literacy: A social skills seminar for young adults with ASDs, NLDs, and social anxiety.* Baltimore: Brookes.

Cohen, S., & Wills, T. A. (1985). Stress, social support, and the buffering hypothesis. *Psychological Bulletin, 98*(2), 310–357.

Conner, C. M., & White, S. W. (2018). Brief report: Feasibility and preliminary efficacy of individual mindfulness therapy for adults with autism spectrum disorder. *Journal of Autism and Developmental Disorders, 48*(1), 290–300.

Constantino, J. N., & Gruber, C. P. (2012). *Social Responsiveness Scale* (2nd ed.). Los Angeles: Western Psychological Services.

Cook, R., Brewer, R., Shah, P., & Bird, G. (2013). Alexithymia, not autism, predicts poor recognition of emotional facial expressions. *Psychological Science, 24*(5), 723–732.

Cooper, K., Loades, M. E., & Russell, A. (2018). Adapting psychological therapies for autism. *Research in Autism Spectrum Disorders, 45*(1), 43–50.

Cottle, K. J., McMahon, W. M., & Farley, M. (2016). Adults with autism spectrum disorders: Past, present, and future. In S. D. Wright (Ed.), *Autism spectrum disorder in mid and later life* (pp. 30–51). London: Jessica Kingsley.

Courchesne, E., Akshoomoff, N. A., & Ciesielski, K. (1990). Shifting attention abnormalities in autism: ERP and performance evidence. *Journal of Clinical and Experimental Neuropsychology, 12,* 77.

Craig, F., Lamanna, A. L., Margari, F., Matera, E., Simone, M., & Margari, L. (2015). Overlap between autism spectrum disorders and attention deficit hyperactivity disorder: Searching for distinctive/common clinical features. *Autism Research, 8*(3), 328–337.

Crane, R. S., Brewer, J., Feldman, C., Kabat-Zinn, J., Santorelli, S., Williams, J. M. G., et al. (2016). What defines mindfulness-based programs?: The warm and the weft. *Psychological Medicine, 47*(6), 990–999.

Crespi, B., & Badcock, C. (2008). Psychosis and autism and diametrical disorders of the social brain. *Behavioral and Brain Sciences, 31*(3), 241–261.

Crooke, P. J., Winner, M. G., & Oswang, L. B. (2016). Thinking socially: Teaching social knowledge to foster social behavioral change. *Topics in Language Disorders, 36*(3), 284–298.

Davis, M. H. (1980). A multidimensional approach to individual differences in empathy. *JSAS Catalog of Selected Documents in Psychology, 10,* 85.

Dawson, P., & Guare, R. (2016). *The smart but scattered guide to success: How to use your brain's executive skills to keep up, stay calm, and get organized at work and at home.* New York: Guilford Press.

Debbaudt, D. (2002). *Autism, advocates, and law enforcement professionals: Recognizing and reducing risk situations for people with autism spectrum disorders.* London: Jessica Kingsley.

Debbaudt, D. (2009). Patients with autism and other high risks: A growing challenge for healthcare security. *Journal of Healthcare Protection Management, 25*(1), 14–26.

DeLong, R., & Nohria, C. (1994). Psychiatric family history and neurological disease in autism spectrum disorders. *Developmental Medicine and Child Neurology, 36,* 441–448.

Dobson, K. S., & Dozois, D. J. A. (2010). Historical and philosophical bases of the cognitive-behavioral therapies. In K. S. Dobson (Ed.), *Handbook of cognitive-behavioral therapies* (3rd ed., pp. 3–38). New York: Guilford Press.

Donvan, J., & Zucker, C. (2016). *In a different key: The story of autism.* New York: Crown.

Duijkers, J. C. L. M., Vissers, C. T. W. M., Verbeeck, W., Arntz, A., & Egger, J. I. M. (2014). Social cognition in the differential diagnosis of autism spectrum disorders and personality disorders. *Clinical Neuropsychiatry, 11*(5), 118–129.

Duncan, J. (1986). Disorganisation of behaviour after frontal lobe damage. *Cognitive Neuropsychology, 3,* 271–290.

Durkin, M. S., Maenner, M. J., Baio, J., Christensen, D., Daniels, J., Fitzgerald, R., et al. (2017). Autism spectrum disorder among US children (2002–2010): Socioeconomic, racial, and ethnic disparities. *American Journal of Public Health, 107,* 1818–1826.

Dziobek, I., Fleck, S., Kalbe, E., Rogers, K., Hassenstab, J., Brand, M., et al. (2006). Introducing MASC: A movie for the assessment of social cognition. *Journal of Autism and Developmental Disorders, 36,* 623–636.

Dziobek, I., Rogers, K., Fleck, S., Bahnemann, M., Heekeran, H. R., Wolf, O. T., et al. (2008). Dissociation of cognitive and emotional empathy in adults with Asperger syndrome using the Multifaceted Empathy Test (MET). *Journal of Autism and Developmental Disorders, 38*(3), 464–473.

D'Zurilla, T. J. (1986). *Problem-solving therapy: A social competence approach to clinical intervention.* New York: Springer.

D'Zurilla, T. J. (1988). Problem-solving therapies. In K. S. Dobson (Ed.), *Handbook of cognitive-behavioral therapies* (pp. 85–135). New York: Guilford Press.

D'Zurilla, T. J., & Goldfried, M. R. (1971). Problem solving and behavior modification. *Journal of Abnormal Psychology, 78,* 107–126.

Ehrenreich-May, J., Storch, E. A., Queen, A. H., Rodriguez, J. H., Ghilain, C. S., Alessandri, M., et al. (2014). An open trial of cognitive-behavioral therapy for anxiety disorders in adolescents with autism spectrum disorders. *Focus on Autism and Other Developmental Disabilities, 29*(3), 145–155.

Ellis, A. (1962). *Reason and emotion in psychotherapy.* New York: Stuart.

Eriksson, J. M., Anderson, L. M. J., & Bejerot, S. (2013). RAADS–14 Screen: Validity of a screening tool for autism spectrum disorder in an adult psychiatric population. *Molecular Autism, 4*(49), 1–11.

Evans, S., Ferrando, S., Findler, M., Stowell, C., Smart, C., & Haglin, D. (2008). Mindfulness-based cognitive therapy for generalized anxiety disorder. *Journal of Anxiety Disorders, 22*(4), 716–721.

Fiske, S. T., & Taylor, S. E. (1984). *Social cognition.* New York: Random House.

Fitzgerald, M., & Bellgrove, M. A. (2006). The overlap between alexithymia and Asperger's syndrome. *Journal of Autism and Developmental Disorders, 36*(4), 573–576.

Fletcher, R. J., & Dosen, A. (Eds.). (1993). *Mental health aspects of mental retardation.* New York: Lexington Books.

Ford, J. D., & Courtois, C. A. (Eds.). (2013). *Treating complex traumatic stress disorders in children and adolescents: Scientific foundations and therapeutic models.* New York: Guilford Press.

Frank, E. (2005). *Treating bipolar disorder: A clinician's guide to interpersonal and social rhythm therapy.* New York: Guilford Press.

Frank, R. I., & Davidson, J. (2014). *The transdiagnostic road map to case formulation and treatment planning: Practical guidance for clinical decision making.* Oakland, CA: New Harbinger.

Frith, U. (1989). *Autism: Explaining the enigma.* Oxford, UK: Blackwell.

Gardner, W. I., & Sovner, R. (1994). *Self-injurious behaviors: A functional approach.* Willow Street, PA: Vida Press.

Garfinkel, S. N., Tiley, C., O'Keeffe, S., Harrison, N. A., Seth, A. K., & Critchley, H. D. (2016). Discrepancies between dimensions of interoception in autism: Implications for emotion and anxiety. *Biological Psychology, 114*(1), 117–126.

Gaus, V. L. (2007). *Cognitive-behavioral therapy for adult Asperger syndrome.* New York: Guilford Press

Gaus, V. L. (2011). *Living well on the spectrum: How to use your strengths to meet the challenges of Asperger syndrome/high-functioning autism.* New York: Guilford Press.

Gaus, V. L. (2016). Psychotherapy with older adults on the spectrum. In S. D. Wright (Ed.), *Autism spectrum disorder in mid and later life* (pp. 193–206). London: Jessica Kingsley.

Gaus, V. L., & Tanaka-Matsumi, J. (1987). *Cross-situational assessment of the behavioral repertoire of an autistic child.* Paper presented at the annual meeting of the American Psychological Association, New York.

Gelfand, D. M., & Hartmann, D. P. (1984). *Child behavior analysis and therapy.* New York: Pergamon Press.

Geller, L. (2003). *Autism spectrum disorders and organizational management issues: How to facilitate executive function skills for independent living.* Paper presented at the annual conference of Advocates for Individuals with High Functioning Autism, Asperger's Syndrome and Other Pervasive Developmental Disorders, Woodbury, NY.

Geller, L. (2005, Summer). Emotion regulation and autism spectrum disorders. *Autism Spectrum Quarterly*, pp. 8–11.

Gerhardt, P. F., Cicero, F., & Mayville, E. (2014). Employment and related services for adults with autism spectrum disorders. In F. R. Volkmar, B. Reichow, & J. C. McPartland (Eds.), *Adolescents and adults with autism spectrum disorders* (pp. 105–119). New York: Springer.

Ghaziuddin, M. (2005). *Mental health aspects of autism and Asperger's syndrome.* London: Jessica Kingsley.

Ghaziuddin, M., Weidmer-Mikhail, E., & Ghaziuddin, N. (1998). Comorbidity of Asperger syndrome: A preliminary report. *Journal of Intellectual Disability Research, 42*(4), 279–283.

Ghaziuddin, M., & Zafar, S. (2008) Psychiatric comorbidity of adults with autism spectrum disorders. *Clinical Neuropsychiatry, 5*(1), 9–12.

Gillberg, I. C., & Gillberg, C. (1989). Asperger syndrome—some epidemiological considerations: A research note. *Journal of Child Psychology and Psychiatry, 30*(4), 631–638.

Gillberg, I. C., Helles, A., Billstedt, E., & Gillberg, C. (2016). Boys with Asperger syndrome grow up: Psychiatric and neurodevelopmental disorders 20 years after initial diagnosis. *Journal of Autism and Developmental Disorders, 46*(1), 74–82.

Global and Regional Asperger Syndrome Partnership. (2003). *GRASP informational brochure.* New York: Author.

Goel, V., & Grafman, J. (1995). Are the frontal lobes implicated in planning functions?: Interpreting data from the Tower of Hanoi. *Neuropsychologia, 33*, 623–642.

Goldfried, M. (1971). Systematic desensitization as training in self-control. *Journal of Consulting and Clinical Psychology, 37*, 228–234.

Goldfried, M. (1977). The use of relaxation and cognitive relabeling as coping skills. In R. B. Stuart (Ed.), *Behavioral self-management: Strategies, techniques and outcomes* (pp. 82–116). New York: Brunner/Mazel.

Gotlib, I. H., & Hammen, C. L. (Eds.). (2014). *Handbook of depression* (3rd ed.). New York: Guilford Press.

Grandin, T. (1995). *Thinking in pictures and other reports from my life with autism.* New York: Doubleday.

Grandin, T. (2003, March). *My experiences with autism, visual thinking, learning language and getting a job.* Lecture presented at the meeting of Advocates for Individuals with High Functioning Autism, Asperger's Syndrome and Other Pervasive Developmental Disorders, Brookville, NY.

Grandin, T., & Duffy, K. (2004). *Developing talents: Careers for individuals with Asperger syndrome and high-functioning autism.* Shawnee Mission, KS: Autism Asperger.

Gray, C. (1994). *Comic strip conversations.* Arlington, TX: Future Horizons.

Gray, C. (1995). *The original social story book.* Arlington, TX: Future Horizons.

Gray, C. (1998). Social stories and comic strip conversations with students with Asperger syndrome and high-functioning autism. In E. Schopler, G. B. Mesibov, & L. J. Kunce (Eds.), *Asperger syndrome or high functioning autism?* (pp. 167–198). New York: Plenum Press.

Gray, C. (2015). *The new social story book, revised and expanded 15th anniversary edition: Over 150 social stories that teach everyday social skills to children and adults with autism and their peers* (3rd ed.). Arlington, TX: Future Horizons.

Green, J., Gilchrist, A., Burton, D., & Cox, A. (2000). Social and psychiatric functioning in adolescents with Asperger syndrome compared with conduct disorder. *Journal of Autism and Developmental Disorders, 30*, 279–293.

Grice, H. (1975). Logic and conversation. In D. Davidson & G. Harmon (Eds.), *The logic of grammar* (pp. 64–74). Encino, CA: Dickenson.

Grodberg, D., & Mount Sinai School of Medicine. (2011). *The Autism Mental Status Examination.* New York: Authors.

Grodberg, D., Weinger, P. M., Halpern, D., Parides, M., Kolvzon, A., & Buxbaum, J. D. (2014). The Autism Mental Status Exam: Sensitivity and specificity using DSM-5 criteria for autism spectrum disorder in verbally fluent adults. *Journal of Autism and Developmental Disorders, 44*(3), 609–614.

Grodberg, D., Weinger, P. M., Kolevzon, A., Soorya, L., & Buxbaum, J. D. (2012). The Autism Mental Status Examination: Development of a brief autism-focused exam. *Journal of Autism and Developmental Disorders, 42*(3), 455–459.

Groden, J., Baron, M. G., & Groden, G. (2006). Assessment and coping strategies. In M. G. Baron, J. Groden, G. Groden, & L. P. Lipsitt (Eds.), *Stress and coping in autism* (pp. 15–41). New York: Oxford University Press.

Groden, J., Cautela, J. R., Prince, S., & Berryman, J. (1994). The impact of stress and anxiety on individuals with autism and developmental disabilities. In E. Schopler & G. B. Mesibov (Eds.), *Behavioral issues in autism* (pp. 177–194). New York: Plenum Press.

Groden, J., Weidenman, L., & Diller, A. (2016). *Relaxation: A comprehensive manual for children and adults with autism and other developmental disabilities.* Champaign, IL: Research Press.

Gross, J. J., & John, O. P. (2003). Individual differences in two emotional regulation processes: Implications for affect, relationships, and well-being. *Journal of Personality and Social Psychology, 85*(2), 348–362.

Gross, J. J., & Thompson, R. A. (2007). Emotion regulation: Conceptual foundations. In J. J. Gross (Ed.), *Handbook of emotion regulation* (pp. 3–24). New York: Guilford Press.

Grossman, P., Niemann, L., Schmidt, S., & Walach, H. (2004). Mindfulness-based stress reduction and health benefits: A meta-analysis. *Journal of Psychosomatic Research, 57*(1), 35–43.

Gutstein, S. E., & Sheely, R. K. (2002). *Relationship development intervention with children, adolescents and adults.* London: Jessica Kingsley.

Happé, F. G. (1994). An advanced test of theory of mind: Understanding of story characters' thoughts and feelings by able autistic, mentally handicapped, and normal children and adults. *Journal of Autism and Developmental Disorders, 24,* 129–154.

Happé, F. G. (2005). The weak central coherence account of autism. In F. R. Volkmar, R. Paul, A. Klin, & D. Cohen (Eds.), *Handbook of autism and pervasive developmental disorders: Vol. 1. Diagnosis, development, neurobiology, and behavior* (3rd ed., pp. 640–649). Hoboken, NJ: Wiley.

Happé, F. G., & Booth, R. D. (2008). The power of the positive: Revisiting weak coherence in autism spectrum disorders. *Quarterly Journal of Experimental Psychology, 61*(1), 50–63.

Happé, F. G., & Frith, U. (2006). The weak coherence account: Detail-focused cognitive style in autism spectrum disorders. *Journal of Autism and Developmental Disorders, 36*(1), 5–25.

Hare, D. J., & Paine, C. (1997). Developing cognitive behavioural treatments for people with Asperger's syndrome. *Clinical Psychology Forum, 110,* 5–8.

Harris, R. (2008). *The happiness trap: How to stop struggling and start living.* Boston: Trumpeter Books.

Harris, R., & Aisbett, B. (2013). *The illustrated happiness trap: How to stop struggling and start living.* Boston: Shambhala.

Harrison, A. J., Long, K. A., Tommet, D. C., & Jones, R. N. (2017). Examining the role of race, ethnicity, and gender on social and behavioral ratings within the Autism Diagnostic Observation Schedule. *Journal of Autism and Developmental Disorders, 47,* 2770–2782.

Hartmann, K., Urbano, M., Manser, K., & Okwara, L. (2012). Modified dialectical behavior therapy to improve emotion regulation in autism spectrum disorders. In C. E. Richardson & R. A. Wood (Eds.), *Autism spectrum disorders* (pp. 41–72). Hauppauge, NY: Nova Science.

Hatchard, T., Mioduszweski, O., Zambrana, A., O'Farrell, E., Caluyong, M., Poulin, P. A., et al. (2017). Neural changes associated with mindfulness-based stress reduction (MBSR): Current knowledge, limitations, and future directions. *Psychology and Neuroscience, 10*(1), 41–56.

Hayes, S. C., & Smith, S. (2005). *Get out of your mind and into your life: The new acceptance and commitment theory.* Oakland, CA: New Harbinger.

Hayes, S. C., Strosahl, K. D., & Wilson, K. G. (1999). *Acceptance and commitment therapy: An experiential approach to behavior change.* New York: Guilford Press.

Hayes, S. C., & Wilson, K. G. (1994). Acceptance and commitment therapy: Altering the verbal support for experiential avoidance. *The Behavior Analyst, 17*(2), 289–303.

Haynes, S. N., Kaholokula, J. K., & Nelson, K. (1999). The idiographic application of nomothetic, empirically based treatments. *Clinical Psychology: Science and Practice, 6,* 456–461.

Hefter, R. L., Manoach, D. S., & Barton, J. J. S. (2005). Perception of facial expression and facial identity in subjects with social developmental disorders. *Neurology, 65,* 1620–1625.

Hénault, I. (2005). *Asperger's syndrome and sexuality: From adolescence through adulthood.* London: Jessica Kingsley.

Herman, J. L. (1992). Complex PTSD: A syndrome in survivors of prolonged and repeated trauma. *Journal of Traumatic Stress, 5*(3), 377–391.

Hill, E. L., & Bird, C. M. (2006). Executive processes in Asperger syndrome: Patterns of performance in a multiple case series. *Neuropsychologia, 44*(14), 2822–2835.

Hingsburger, D., Griffiths, D., & Quinsey, V. (1991). Detecting counterfeit deviance: Differentiating sexual deviance from sexual inappropriateness. *Habilitative Mental Healthcare Newsletter, 10,* 51–54.

Hirvikoski, T., & Blomqvist, M. (2015). High self-perceived stress and poor coping in intellectually able adults with autism spectrum disorder. *Autism, 19*(6), 752–757.

Hobson, P. (2005). Autism and emotion. In F. R. Volkmar, R. Paul, A. Klin, & D. Cohen (Eds.), *Handbook of autism and pervasive developmental disorders: Vol. 1. Diagnosis, development, neurobiology, and behavior* (3rd ed., pp. 406–422). Hoboken, NJ: Wiley.

Hoffman, W. L., & Prior, M. R. (1982). Neuropsychological dimensions of autism in children: A test of the hemispheric dysfunction hypothesis. *Journal of Clinical Neuropsychology, 4,* 27–41.

Hofmann, S. G., Asnaani, A., Vonk, I. J. J., Sawyer, A. T., & Fang, A. (2012). The efficacy of cognitive behavioral therapy: A review of meta-analyses. *Cognitive Therapy and Research, 36*(5), 427–440.

Hofmann, S. G., Sawyer, A. T., & Fang, A. (2010). The empirical status of the "new wave" of cognitive behavioral therapy. *Psychiatric Clinics of North America, 33*(3), 701–710.

Hofvander, B., Delorme, R., Chase, P., Nyden, A., Wentz, E., Stahlberg, O., et al. (2009). Psychiatric and psychosocial problems in adults with normal-intelligence autism spectrum disorders. *BMC Psychiatry, 9*(35).

Holwerda, A., van der Klink, J. J., Groothoff, J. W., & Brouwer, S. (2012). Predictors for work participation in individuals with an autism spectrum disorder: A systematic review. *Journal of Occupational Rehabilitation, 22,* 333–352.

Hughes, C., Russell, J., & Robbins, T. W. (1994). Evidence for executive dysfunction in autism. *Neuropsychologia, 32,* 477–492.

Ingram, R. E., Miranda, J., & Segal, Z. V. (1999). *Cognitive vulnerability to depression.* New York: Guilford Press.

Innovative Interactions. (2000). *Talk Blocks for work.* Seattle, WA: Author.

Jacobsen, P. (2003). *Asperger syndrome and psychotherapy.* London: Jessica Kingsley.

Jeste, S. S., & Nelson, C. A. (2009). Event related potentials in the understanding of autism spectrum disorders: An analytical review. *Journal of Autism and Developmental Disorders, 39*(3), 495–510.

Joliffe, T., & Baron-Cohen, S. (1997). Are people with autism and Asperger syndrome faster than normal on the Embedded Figures Test? *Journal of Child Psychology and Psychiatry, 38,* 527–534.

Joliffe, T., & Baron-Cohen, S. (2001). A test of central coherence theory: Can adults with high-functioning autism or Asperger's syndrome integrate fragments of an object? *Cognitive Neuropsychiatry, 6,* 193–216.

Joshi, G., Biederman, J., Petty, C., Goldin, R. L., Furtak, S. L., & Wozniak, J. (2013). Examining the comorbidity of bipolar disorder and autism spectrum disorders: A large controlled analysis of phenotypic and familial correlates in a referred population of youth with bipolar I disorder with and without autism spectrum disorders. *Journal of Clinical Psychiatry, 74*(6), 578–586.

Joshi, G., Wozniak, J., Petty, C., Martelon, M. K., Fried, R., Bolfek, A., et al. (2012). Psychiatric comorbidity and functioning in a clinically referred population of adults with autism spectrum disorders: A comparative study. *Journal of Autism and Developmental Disorders, 43*(6), 1314–1325.

Kabat-Zinn, J. (1982). An outpatient program in behavioral medicine for chronic pain patients based on the practice of mindfulness mediation: Theoretical considerations and preliminary results. *General Hospital Psychiatry, 41*(1), 33–47.

Kabat-Zinn, J. (1990). *Full catastrophe living: Using the wisdom of your body and mind to face stress, pain, and illness.* New York: Bantam Books.

Kanner, L. (1943). Autistic disturbances of affective contact. *Nervous Child, 2,* 217–253.

Kaur, S., Mikramanayake, M., Kolli, S., Shahper, S., Jefferies-Sewell, J., Reid, J., et al. (2016). Autistic spectrum disorder in adults with obsessive compulsive disorder: Results from a UK survey. *European Neuropsychopharmacology, 26*(5), 886–887.

Kerns, C. M., Roux, A. M., Connell, J. E., & Shattuck, P. T. (2016). Adapting cognitive behavioral techniques to address anxiety and depression in cognitively able emerging adults on the autism spectrum. *Cognitive Behavior Practice, 23*(3), 329–340.

Khoury, B., Lecomte, T., Fortin, G., Masse, M., Therien, P., Bouchard, V., et al. (2013). Mindfulness-based therapy: A comprehensive meta-analysis. *Clinical Psychology Review, 33*(6), 763–771.

Kiep, M., Spek, A. A., & Hoeben, L. (2015). Mindfulness-based therapy in adults with an autism spectrum disorder: Do treatment effects last? *Mindfulness, 6*(3), 637–644.

King, R. (2010). Complex post-traumatic stress disorder: Implications for individuals with autism-spectrum disorders—Part I. *Journal on Developmental Disabilities, 16*(3), 198–206.

Kingdon, D. G., & Turkington, D. (2005). *Cognitive therapy of schizophrenia.* New York: Guilford Press.

Kleinhans, N., Akshoomoff, N., & Delis, D. C. (2005). Executive functions in autism and Asperger's disorder: Flexibility, fluency, and inhibition. *Developmental Neuropsychology, 27*(3), 379–401.

Kliemann, D., Dziobek, I., Hatri, A., Steimke, R., & Heekeren, H. R. (2010). Atypical reflexive gaze patterns on emotional faces in autism spectrum disorders. *Journal of Neuroscience, 30*(37), 12281–12287.

Klin, A., Jones, W., Schultz, R., & Volkmar, F. (2005). The enactive mind—from actions to cognition: Lessons from autism. In F. R. Volkmar, R. Paul, A. Klin, & D. Cohen (Eds.), *Handbook of autism and pervasive developmental disorders: Vol. 1. Diagnosis, development, neurobiology, and behavior* (3rd ed., pp. 682–703). Hoboken, NJ: Wiley.

Klin, A., Jones, W., Schultz, R., Volkmar, F., & Cohen, D. (2002a). Defining and quantifying the social phenotype in autism. *American Journal of Psychiatry, 159*(6), 895–908.

Klin, A., Jones, W., Schultz, R., Volkmar, F., & Cohen, D. (2002b). Visual fixation patterns during viewing of naturalistic social situations as predictors of social competence in individuals with autism. *Archives of General Psychiatry, 59*(9), 809–816.

Klin, A., Volkmar, F. R., & Sparrow, S. S. (Eds.). (2000). *Asperger syndrome*. New York: Guilford Press.

Koenig, K., & Levine, M. (2011). Psychotherapy for individuals with autism spectrum disorders. *Journal of Contemporary Psychotherapy, 41*(1), 29–36.

Koenig, K., & Tsatsanis, D. (2005). Pervasive developmental disorders in girls. In D. G. Bell & S. L. Foster (Eds.), *Handbook of behavioral and emotional problems in girls* (pp. 211–237). New York: Kluwer Academic/Plenum Press.

Koller, R. (2000). Sexuality and adolescents with autism. *Sexuality and Disability, 18,* 125–135.

Koszycki, D., Benger, M., Shlik, J., & Bradwejn, J. (2007). Randomized trial of a meditation-based stress reduction program and cognitive behavior therapy in generalized social anxiety disorder. *Behaviour Research and Therapy, 45*(1), 2518–2526.

Kreiser, N. L., & White, S. W. (2014). ASD in females: Are we overstating the gender difference in diagnosis? *Clinical Child Family Psychology Review, 17*(1), 67–84.

Kring, A. M., & Sloan, D. M. (2010). Introduction and overview. In A. M. Kring & D. M. Sloan (Eds.), *Emotion regulation and psychopathology: A transdiagnostic approach to etiology and treatment* (pp. 1–9). New York: Guilford Press.

Kroese, B. S., Dagnan, D., & Loumidis, K. (Eds.). (1997). *Cognitive-behaviour therapy for people with learning disabilities*. London: Routledge.

Lai, M., Baron-Cohen, S., & Buxbaum, J. D. (2015). Understanding autism in the light of sex/gender. *Molecular Autism, 6*(24), 1–5.

Landa, R. (2000). Social language use in Asperger syndrome and high-functioning autism. In A. Klin, F. R. Volkmar, & S. S. Sparrow (Eds.), *Asperger syndrome* (pp. 125–155). New York: Guilford Press.

Laugeson, E. A. (2017). *PEERS for young adults: Social skills training for adults with autism spectrum disorder and other social challenges*. New York: Taylor & Francis.

Laugeson, E. A., & Park, M. N. (2014). Using a CBT approach to teach social skills to adolescents with autism spectrum disorder and other social challenges: The PEERS method. *Journal of Rational-Emotive and Cognitive-Behavior Therapy, 32*(1), 85–95.

Leoni, M., Corti, S., & Cavagnola, R. (2015). Third generation behavioural therapy for neurodevelopmental disorders: Review and trajectories. *Advances in Mental Health and Intellectual Disabilities, 9*(5), 265–274.

Lerner, M. D., Haque, O. S., Northrup, E. C., Lawer, L., & Bursztajn, H. J. (2012). Emerging perspectives on adolescents and young adults with high-functioning autism spectrum disorders, violence, and criminal law. Correction. *Journal of the American Academy of Psychiatry and the Law, 40*(3), 445.

Lerner, M. D., McPartland, J. C., & Morris, J. P. (2013). Multimodal emotion processing in autism spectrum disorders: An event-related potential study. *Developmental Cognitive Neuroscience, 3,* 11–21.

Levant, R. F., Halter, M. J., Hayden, E. W., & Williams, C. M. (2009). The efficacy of alexithymia reduction treatment: A pilot study. *Journal of Men's Studies, 17*(1), 75–84.

Lever, A. G., & Geurts, H. M. (2016). Psychiatric co-occurring symptoms and disorders in young, middle-aged, and older adults with autism spectrum disorder. *Journal of Autism and Developmental Disorders, 46*(6), 1916–1930.

Limoges, É., Bolduc, C., Berthiaume, C., Mottron, L., & Godbout, R. (2013). Relationship between poor sleep and daytime cognitive performance in young adults with autism. *Research in Developmental Disabilities, 34*(4), 1322–1335.

Limoges, É., Mottron, L., Bolduc, C., Berthiaume, C., & Godbout, R. (2005). Atypical sleep architecture and the autism phenotype. *Brain, 128*(5), 1049–1061.

Linehan, M. M. (1993a). *Cognitive-behavioral treatment of borderline personality disorder*. New York: Guilford Press.

Linehan, M. M. (1993b). *Skills training manual for treating borderline personality disorder.* New York: Guilford Press.

Linehan, M. M. (2015). *DBT skills training manual* (2nd ed.). New York: Guilford Press.

Linehan, M. M., Armstrong, H. E., Suarez, A., Allmon, D., & Heard, H. L. (1991). Cognitive-behavioral treatment of chronically parasuicidal borderline patients. *Archives of General Psychiatry, 48*(12), 1060–1064.

Linkenauger, S. A., Lerner, M. D., Ramenzoni, V. C., & Proffitt, D. R. (2012). A perceptual motor deficit predicts social and communicative impairments in individuals with autism spectrum disorders. *Autism Research, 5*(5), 352–362.

Lord, C., & Corsello, C. (2005). Diagnostic instruments in autistic spectrum disorders. In F. R. Volkmar, R. Paul, A. Klin, & D. Cohen (Eds.), *Handbook of autism and pervasive developmental disorders: Vol. 2. Assessment, interventions, and policy* (3rd ed., pp. 730–771). Hoboken, NJ: Wiley.

Lord, C., Rutter, M., DiLavore, P. C., Risi, S., Gotham, K., & Bishop, S. (2012). *Autism Diagnostic Observation Schedule, Second edition.* Torrance, CA: Western Psychological Services.

Lugnegård, T., Hällerback, M. U., & Gillberg, C. (2011). Personality disorders and autism spectrum disorders: What are the connections? *Comprehensive Psychiatry, 53*(4), 333–340.

Maddox, B. B., & Gaus, V. L. (2018). Community mental health services for autistic adults: Good news and bad news. *Autism in Adulthood, 1*(1). [Epub ahead of print]

Maddox, B. B., Miyazaki, Y., & White, S. W. (2016). Long-term effects of CBT on social impairment in adolescents with ASD. *Journal of Autism and Developmental Disorders, 47,* 1–11.

Maddox, B. B., & White, S. W. (2015). Comorbid social anxiety disorder in adults with autism spectrum disorder. *Journal of Autism and Developmental Disorders, 45*(12), 3949–3960.

Maisel, M. E., Stephenson, K. G., South, M., Rodgers, J., Freeston, M. H., & Gaigg, S. B. (2016). Modeling the cognitive mechanisms linking autism symptoms and anxiety in adults. *Journal of Abnormal Psychology, 125*(5), 692–703.

Marans, W. D., Rubin, E., & Laurent, A. (2005). Addressing social communication skills in individuals with high-functioning autism and Asperger syndrome: Critical priorities in educational programming. In F. R. Volkmar, R. Paul, A. Klin, & D. Cohen (Eds.), *Handbook of autism and pervasive developmental disorders: Vol. 2. Assessment, interventions, and policy* (3rd ed., pp. 977–1002). Hoboken, NJ: Wiley.

Matich-Maroney, J., Boyle, P., & Crocker, M. M. (2005). The psychosexual assessment and treatment continuum: A tool for conceptualizing the range of sexuality-related issues and support needs of individuals with developmental disabilities. *Mental Health Aspects of Developmental Disabilities, 8,* 77–90.

Matson, J. L., Ancona, M. N., & Wilkins, J. (2008). Sleep disturbances in adults with autism spectrum disorders and severe intellectual impairments. *Journal of Mental Health Research in Intellectual Disabilities, 1*(3), 129–139.

Matson, J. L., & Barrett, R. P. (Eds.). (1993). *Psychopathology in the mentally retarded.* Boston: Allyn & Bacon.

Matson, J. L., & Williams, L. W. (2014). Depression and mood disorders among persons with autism spectrum disorders. *Research in Developmental Disabilities, 35*(9), 2003–2007.

Matsuo, J., Kamio, Y., Takahashi, H., Ota, M., Teraishi, T., Hori, H., et al. (2015). Autistic-like traits in adult patients with mood disorders and schizophrenia. *PLOS ONE, 10*(4), e0122711.

Mattila, M., Kielinen, M., Jussila, K., Linna, S., Bloigu, R., Ebeling, H., et al. (2007). An epidemiological and diagnostic study of Asperger syndrome according to four sets of diagnostic criteria. *Journal of the American Academy of Child and Adolescent Psychiatry, 46*(5), 636–646.

Mazefsky, C. A., Herrington, J., Siegel, M., Scarpa, A., Maddox, B. B., Scahill, L., et al. (2013).

The role of emotion regulation in autism spectrum disorder. *Journal of the American Academy of Child and Adolescent Psychiatry, 52*(7), 679–688.

McDougle, C., Kresch, L., Goodman, W. K., Naylor, S. T., Volkmar, F. R., Cohen, D. J., et al. (1995). A case-controlled study of repetitive thoughts and behavior in adults with autistic disorder and obsessive–compulsive disorder. *American Journal of Psychiatry, 152*(3), 772–777.

McPartland, J. C., Klin, A., & Volkmar, F. R. (Eds.). (2014). *Asperger syndrome: Assessing and treating high-functioning autism spectrum disorders* (2nd ed.). New York: Guilford Press.

Meichenbaum, D. (1985). *Stress inoculation training.* New York: Pergamon Press.

Miller, A. L., & Rathus, J. H. (2000). DBT for adolescents: Dialectical dilemmas and secondary treatment targets. *Cognitive and Behavioral Practice, 7*(4), 425–434.

Miller, A. L., Rathus, J. H., & Linehan, M. M. (2007). *Dialectical therapy with suicidal adolescents.* New York: Guilford Press.

Miller, A. L., Rathus, J. H., Linehan, M. M., Wetzler, S., & Leigh, E. (1997). Dialectical behavior therapy adapted for suicidal adolescents. *Journal of Psychiatric Practice, 3*(2), 78.

Murphy, N. A., & Elias, E. R. (2006). Sexuality of children and adolescents with developmental disabilities. *Pediatrics, 118,* 398–403.

Myles, B. S., Hagen, K., Holverstott, J., Hubbard, A., Adreon, D., & Trautman, M. (2005). *Life journey through autism: An educator's guide to Asperger syndrome.* Arlington, VA: Organization for Autism Research.

Myles, B. S., Trautman, M., & Schelvan, R. L. (2004). *The hidden curriculum: Practical solutions for understanding unstated rules in social situations.* Shawnee Mission, KS: Autism Asperger.

Nezu, C. M., & Nezu, A. M. (1994). Outpatient psychotherapy for adults with mental retardation and concomitant psychopathology: Research and clinical imperatives. *Journal of Consulting and Clinical Psychology, 62,* 34–42.

Nezu, C. M., Nezu, A. M., & Gill-Weiss, M. J. (1992). *Psychopathology with mental retardation: Clinical guidelines for assessment and treatment.* Champaign, IL: Research Press.

Nichols, S., & Blakeley-Smith, A. (2010). "I'm not sure we're ready for this . . .": Working with families toward facilitating healthy sexuality for individuals with autism spectrum disorders. *Social Work in Mental Health, 1,* 72–91.

Nichols, S., & Byers, E. S. (2016). Sexual well-being and relationships in adults with autism spectrum disorder. In S. D. Wright (Ed.), *Autism spectrum disorder in mid and later life* (pp. 248–262). London: Jessica Kingsley.

Nichols, S., Sheehan, A. H., & Zito, D. (2017, April). *Learning to live a personally meaningful life: Acceptance and commitment therapy (ACT) for individuals on the spectrum.* Paper presented at the annual conference of the Asperger Syndrome and High Functioning Autism Association, Garden City, NY.

Norbury, C. F. (2014). Practitioner review: Social (pragmatic) communication disorder conceptualization, evidence, and clinical implications. *Journal of Child Psychology and Psychiatry, 55*(3), 204–216.

Nord, D. K., Stancliffe, R. J., Nye-Lengerman, K., & Hewitt, A. S. (2016). Employment in the community for people with and without autism: A comparative analysis. *Research in Autism Spectrum Disorders, 24,* 11–16.

Nummenmaa, L., Glerean, E., Hari, R., & Hietanen, J. K. (2014). Bodily maps of emotions. *Proceedings of the National Academy of Sciences of the USA, 111*(2), 646–651.

Öst, L. G. (2014). The efficacy of acceptance and commitment therapy: An updated systematic review and meta-analysis. *Behaviour Research and Therapy, 61,* 105–121.

Ozonoff, S. (2012). Editorial: DSM-5 and autism spectrum disorders—two decades of perspectives from the JCPP. *Journal of Child Psychology and Psychiatry, 53*(9), e4–e6.

Ozonoff, S., & Griffith, E. M. (2000). Neuropsychological function and the external validity of Asperger syndrome. In A. Klin, F. R. Volkmar, & S. S. Sparrow (Eds.), *Asperger syndrome* (pp. 72–96). New York: Guilford Press.

Ozonoff, S., & McEvoy, R. E. (1994). A longitudinal study of executive function and theory of mind development in autism. *Development and Psychopathology, 6,* 415–431.

Ozonoff, S., Rogers, S. J., & Pennington, B. F. (1991). Asperger's syndrome: Evidence of an empirical distinction from high-functioning autism. *Journal of Child Psychology and Psychiatry, and Allied Disciplines, 32,* 1107–1122.

Ozonoff, S., South, M., & Provencal, S. (2005). Executive functions. In F. R. Volkmar, R. Paul, A. Klin, & D. Cohen (Eds.), *Handbook of autism and pervasive developmental disorders: Vol. 1. Diagnosis, development, neurobiology, and behavior* (3rd ed., pp. 606–627). Hoboken, NJ: Wiley.

Ozonoff, S., & Strayer, D. L. (1997). Inhibitory function in nonretarded children with autism. *Journal of Autism and Developmental Disorders, 27,* 59–77.

Ozonoff, S., & Strayer, D. L. (2001). Further of intact working memory in autism. *Journal of Autism and Developmental Disorders, 31,* 257–263.

Padesky, C. A. (1994). Schema change processes in cognitive therapy. *Clinical Psychology and Psychotherapy, 1,* 267–278.

Pahnke, J., Lundgren, T., Hursti, T., & Hirvikoski, T. (2014). Outcomes of an acceptance and commitment therapy-based skills training group for students with high-functioning autism spectrum disorder: A quasi-experimental pilot study. *Autism, 18*(8), 953–964.

Palmer, R. F., Walker, T., Mandell, D., Bayles, B., & Miller, C. S. (2010). Explaining low rates of autism among Hispanic schoolchildren in Texas. *American Journal of Public Health, 100*(2), 270–272.

Paul, R., Landa, R., & Simmons, E. (2014). Communication in Asperger syndrome. In J. C. McPartland, A. Klin, & F. R. Volkmar (Eds.), *Asperger syndrome: Assessing and treating high-functioning autism spectrum disorders* (2nd ed., pp. 103–143). New York: Guilford Press.

Pennington, B. F., & Ozonoff, S. (1996). Executive functions and developmental psychopathologies. *Journal of Child Psychology and Psychiatry, 37,* 51–87.

Persons, J. B. (2008). *The case formulation approach to cognitive-behavior therapy.* New York: Guilford Press.

Persons, J. B., Davidson, J., & Tompkins, M. A. (2000). *Essential components of cognitive-behavior therapy for depression.* Washington, DC: American Psychological Association.

Philip, R., Whalley, H., Stanfield, A., Sprengelmeyer, R., Santos, I., Young, A. W., et al. (2010). Deficits in facial, body movement and vocal emotional processing in autism spectrum disorders. *Psychological Medicine, 40*(11), 1919–1929.

Pocnet, C., Antonietti, J. P., Strippoli, M. F., Glaus, J., Preisig, M., & Rossier, J. (2016). Individuals' quality of life linked to major life events, perceived social support, and personality traits. *Quality of Life Research, 25*(11), 2897–2908.

Powers, M. D., & Loomis, J. W. (2014). Asperger syndrome in adolescence and adulthood. In J. C. McPartland, A. Klin, & F. R. Volkmar (Eds.), *Asperger syndrome: Assessing and treating high-functioning autism spectrum disorders* (2nd ed., pp. 311–367). New York: Guilford Press.

Rathus, J. H., & Miller, A. L. (2015). *DBT skills training manual for adolescents.* New York: Guilford Press.

Ratto, A. B., Anthony, B. D., Kenworthy, L., Armour, A. C., Dudley, K., & Anthony, L. G. (2016). Are non-intellectually disabled black youth with ASD less impaired on parent report than their white peers? *Journal of Autism and Developmental Disorders, 46*(3), 773–781.

Ratto, A. B., Reznick, J. S., & Turner-Brown, L. (2016). Cultural effects on the diagnosis of autism spectrum disorder among Latinos. *Focus on Autism and Other Developmental Disabilities, 31*(4), 275–283.

Reid, G. M., Holt, M. K., Bowman, C. E., Espelage, D. L., & Green, J. G. (2016). Perceived social support and mental health among first-year college students with histories of bullying victimization. *Journal of Child and Family Studies, 25*(11), 3331–3341.

Reisinger, L. M., Cornish, K. M., & Fombonne, E. (2011). Diagnostic differentiation of autism spectrum disorders and pragmatic language impairment. *Journal of Autism and Developmental Disorders, 41*(12), 1694–1704.

Reiss, S., & Szyszko, J. (1983). Diagnostic overshadowing and professional experience with mentally retarded persons. *American Journal of Mental Deficiency, 87,* 396–402.

Reynolds, W. M. (1999). *Multidimensional Anxiety Questionnaire.* Odessa, FL: Psychological Assessment Resources.

Richdale, A. L., & Prior, M. R. (1995). The sleep/wake rhythm in children with autism. *European Child and Adolescent Psychiatry, 4,* 175–186.

Richdale, A. L., & Schreck, K. A. (2009). Sleep problems in autism spectrum disorders: Prevalence, nature, and possible biopsychological etiologies. *Sleep Medicine Reviews, 13*(6), 403–411.

Ritvo, R. A., Ritvo, E. R., Guthrie, D., Ritvo, M. J., Hufnagel, D. H., McMahon, W., et al. (2011). The Ritvo Autism Asperger Diagnostic Scale—Revised (RAADS-R): A scale to assist the diagnosis of autism spectrum disorder in adults: An international validation study. *Journal of Autism and Developmental Disorders, 41*(8), 1076–1089.

Rogers, K., Dziobek, I., Hassenstab, J., Wolf, O. T., & Convit, A. (2007). Who cares?: Revisiting empathy in Asperger syndrome. *Journal of Autism and Developmental Disorders, 37*(4), 709–715.

Ross, A. O. (1981). *Child behavior therapy: Principles, procedures, and empirical basis.* New York: Wiley.

Roux, A. M., Shattuck, P. T., Cooper, B. P., Anderson, K. A., Wagner, M., & Narendorf, S. C. (2013). Postsecondary employment experiences among young adults with an autism spectrum disorder. *Journal of the American Academy of Child and Adolescent Psychiatry 52*(9), 931–939.

Rudd, M. D. (2006). Fluid vulnerability theory: A cognitive approach to understanding the process of acute and chronic suicide risk. In T. E. Ellis (Ed.), *Cognition and suicide: Theory, research, and therapy* (pp. 355–368). Washington, DC: American Psychological Association.

Rumsey, J. M. (1985). Conceptual problem-solving in highly verbal, nonretarded autistic men. *Journal of Autism and Developmental Disorders, 15,* 23–36.

Rumsey, J. M., & Hamburger, S. D. (1988). Neuropsychological findings in high-functioning men with infantile autism, residual state. *Journal of Clinical and Experimental Neuropsychology, 10,* 210–221.

Rumsey, J. M., & Hamburger, S. D. (1990). Neuropsychological divergence of high-level autism and severe dyslexia. *Journal of Autism and Developmental Disorders, 20,* 155–168.

Russell, A. J., Jassi, A., Fullana, M. A., Mack, H., Johnston, K., Heyman, I., et al. (2013). Cognitive behavior therapy for comorbid obsessive–compulsive disorder in high functioning autism spectrum disorders: A randomized controlled trial. *Depression and Anxiety, 30*(8), 697–708.

Russell, A. J., Mataix-Cols, D., Anson, M., & Murphy, D. G. (2005). Obsessions and compulsions in Asperger syndrome and high-functioning autism. *British Journal of Psychiatry, 186,* 525–528.

Russell, A. J., Mataix-Cols, D., Anson, M. A. W., & Murphy, D. G. M. (2009). Psychological treatment for obsessive–compulsive disorder in people with autism spectrum disorders: A pilot study. *Psychotherapy and Psychosomatics, 78*(1), 59–61.

Rutherford, M. D., Baron-Cohen, S., & Wheelwright, S. (2002). Reading the mind in the voice:

A study with normal adults and adults with Asperger syndrome and high-functioning autism. *Journal of Autism and Developmental Disorders, 32,* 189–194.

Rutter, M., LeCouteur, A., & Lord, C. (2003). *Autism Diagnostic Interview—Revised.* Los Angeles: Western Psychological Services.

Rydén, E., & Bejerot, S. (2008). Autism spectrum disorders in an adult psychiatric population: A naturalistic cross-sectional controlled study. *Clinical Neuropsychiatry, 5*(1), 13–21.

Samson, A. C., Huber, O., & Gross, J. J. (2012). Emotion regulation in Asperger's syndrome and high-functioning autism. *Emotion, 12*(4), 659–665.

Santomauro, D., Sheffield, J., & Sofronoff, K. (2016). Depression in adolescents with ASD: A pilot RCT of group intervention. *Journal of Autism and Developmental Disorders, 46,* 572–588.

Sarason, I. G., & Sarason, B. R. (Eds.). (1985). *Social support: Theory, research and applications.* Dordrecht, The Netherlands: Martinus Nijhof.

Scheiner, M., & Bogden, J. (2017). *An employer's guide to managing professionals on the autism spectrum.* London: Jessica Kingsley.

Schmidt, L., Kirchner, J., Strunz, S., Brozus, J., Ritter, K., Roepke, S., et al. (2015). Psychosocial functioning and life satisfaction in adults with autism spectrum disorder without intellectual impairment. *Journal of Clinical Psychology, 71*(12), 1259–1268.

Segal, Z. V., Williams, J. M. G., & Teasdale, J. D. (2001). *Mindfulness-based cognitive therapy for depression: A new approach to preventing relapse.* New York: Guilford Press.

Segers, M., & Rawana, J. S. (2014). What do we know about suicidality in autism spectrum disorders?: A systematic review. *Autism Research, 7*(4), 507–521.

Seligman, M. E., & Csikzentmihalyi, M. (2000). Positive psychology: An introduction. *American Psychologist, 55*(1), 5–14.

Seligman, M. E., & Peterson, C. (2003). Character strengths before and after September 11. *Psychological Science, 14*(4), 381–384.

Shah, A., & Frith, U. (1983). An islet of ability in autistic children: A research note. *Child Psychology and Psychiatry, 24,* 613–620.

Shah, P., Hall, R., Catmur, C., & Bird, G. (2016). Alexithymia, not autism, is associated with impaired interoception. *Cortex, 81,* 215–220.

Shattuck, P. T., Narendorf, S. C., Cooper, B., Sterzing, P. R., Wagner, M., & Taylor, J. L. (2012). Postsecondary education and employment among youth with an autism spectrum disorder. *Pediatrics, 129*(6), 1042–1049.

Shore, S. (Ed.). (2004). *Ask and tell: Self-advocacy and disclosure for people on the autism spectrum.* Shawnee Mission, KS: Autism Asperger.

Silverman, W. K., & Hinshaw, S. P. (2008). The second special issue on evidence-based psychosocial treatments for children and adolescents: A 10-year up-date. *Journal of Clinical Child and Adolescent Psychology, 37,* 1–7.

Simms, M. D., & Jin, X. M. (2015). Autism, language disorder, and social (pragmatic) communication disorder: DSM-V and differential diagnoses. *Pediatric Review, 36*(8), 355–362.

Simonoff, E., Pickles, A., Charman, T., Chandler, S., Loucas, T., & Baird, G. (2008). Psychiatric disorders in children with autism spectrum disorders: Prevalence, comorbidity, and associated factors in a population-derived sample. *Journal of the American Academy of Child and Adolescent Psychiatry, 47*(8), 921–929.

Sizoo, B. B., & Kuiper, E. (2017). Cognitive behavioral therapy and mindfulness based stress reduction may be equally effective in reducing anxiety and depression in adults with autism spectrum disorders. *Research in Developmental Disabilities, 64,* 47–55.

Sizoo, B., van den Brink, W., Gorissen van Eenige, M., & van der Gaag, R. J. (2009). Personality characteristics of adults with autism spectrum disorders or attention deficit hyperactivity disorder with and without substance use disorders. *Journal of Nervous and Mental Diseases, 197*(6), 450–454.

Skokauskas, N., & Frodl, T. (2015). Overlap between autism spectrum disorder and bipolar affective disorder. *Psychopathology, 48*(4), 209–216.

Snowling, M., & Frith, U. (1986). Comprehension in "hyperlexic" readers. *Journal of Experimental Child Psychology, 42*, 392–415.

Solomon, M., Olsen, E., Niendam, T., Ragland, J. D., Yoon, J., Minzenberg, M., et al. (2011). From lumping to splitting and back again: Atypical social and language development in individuals with clinical-high-risk for psychosis, first episode of schizophrenia, and autism spectrum disorders. *Schizophrenia Research, 131*(1–3), 146–151.

South, M., Carr, A. W., Stephenson, K. G., Maisel, M. E., & Cox, J. C. (2017). Symptom overlap on the SRS-2 Adult Self-Report between adults with ASD and adults with high anxiety. *Autism Research, 10*(7), 1215–1220.

South, M., & Rodgers, J. (2017). Sensory, emotional and cognitive contributions to anxiety in autism spectrum disorders. *Frontiers in Human Neuroscience, 11*, 20.

Spain, D., Sin, J., Chalder, T., Murphy, D., & Happé, F. G. (2015). Cognitive behaviour therapy for adults with autism spectrum disorders and psychiatric co-morbidity: A review. *Research in Autism Spectrum Disorders, 9*, 151–162.

Spek, A. A., van Ham, N. C., & Nyklíček, I. (2013). Mindfulness-based therapy in adults with an autism spectrum disorder: A randomized controlled trial. *Research in Developmental Disabilities, 34*(1), 246–253.

Spielberger, C. D., Gorsuch, R. L., Lushene, R., Vagg, P. R., & Jacobs, G. A. (1983). *Manual for the State–Trait Anxiety Inventory.* Palo Alto, CA: Consulting Psychologists Press.

Strohmer, D. C., & Prout, H. T. (Eds.). (1994). *Counseling and psychotherapy with persons with mental retardation and borderline intelligence.* Brandon, VT: Clinical Psychology.

Sturm, A., Kuhfeld, M., Kasari, C., & McCracken, J. T. (2017). Development and validation of an item response theory-based Social Responsiveness Scale—Short Form. *Journal of Child Psychology and Psychiatry, 58*(9), 1053–1061.

Swain, D., Scarpa, A., White, S., & Laugeson, E. (2015). Emotion dysregulation and anxiety in adults with ASD: Does social motivation play a role? *Journal of Autism and Developmental Disorders, 45*(12), 3971–3977.

Tager-Flusberg, H. (1991). Semantic processing in the free recall of autistic children: Further evidence for a cognitive deficit. *British Journal of Developmental Psychology, 9*, 417–430.

Talari, S., Balaji, K., & Stansfield, A. J. (2017). What is the association between ADI-R scores and final diagnosis of autism in an all IQ adult autism diagnostic service? *Advances in Autism, 3*(4), 250–262.

Tani, P., Lindberg, N., Nieminen-von Wendt, T., von Wendt, L., Virkkala, J., Appelberg, G., et al. (2004). Sleep in young adults with Asperger syndrome. *Neuropsychobiology, 50*(2), 147–152.

Taurines, R., Schwenck, C., Westerwald, E., Sachse, M., Siniatchkin, M., & Freitag, C. (2012). ADHD and autism: Differential diagnosis or overlapping traits?: A selective review. *Attention Deficit and Hyperactivity Disorders, 4*(3), 115–139.

Teasdale, J. D., Segal, Z. V., & Williams, J. M. G. (1995). How does cognitive therapy prevent depressive relapse and why should attentional control (mindfulness) training help? *Behaviour Research and Therapy, 33*, 25–39.

Teasdale, J. D., Segal, Z. V., Williams, J. M. G., Ridgeway, V. A., Soulsby, J. M., & Lau, M. A. (2000). Prevention of relapse/recurrence in major depression by mindfulness-based cognitive therapy. *Journal of Consulting and Clinical Psychology, 68*(4), 615–623.

Tronick, E. Z. (1989). Emotions and emotional communication in infancy. *American Psychologist, 44*, 112–149.

Tsai, L. (2006). Diagnosis and treatment of anxiety disorders in individuals with autism spectrum disorder. In M. G. Baron, J. Groden, G. Groden, & L. P. Lipsitt (Eds.), *Stress and coping in autism* (pp. 388–440). New York: Oxford University Press.

Tsatsanis, K. D. (2005). Neuropsychological characteristics in autism and related conditions. In F. R. Volkmar, R. Paul, A. Klin, & D. Cohen (Eds.), *Handbook of autism and pervasive developmental disorders: Vol. 1. Diagnosis, development, neurobiology, and behavior* (3rd ed., pp. 365–381). Hoboken, NJ: Wiley.

Tsatsanis, K. D., & Powell, K. (2014). Neuropsychological characteristics of autism spectrum disorders. In F. R. Volkmar, S. J. Rogers, R. Paul, & K. A. Pelphrey (Eds.), *Handbook of autism and pervasive developmental disorders: Vol. 1. Diagnosis, development, and mechanisms* (4th ed., pp. 617–694). Hoboken, NJ: Wiley.

Twachtman-Cullen, D. (1998). Language and communication in high-functioning autism and Asperger syndrome. In E. Schopler, G. B. Mesibov, & L. J. Kunce (Eds.), *Asperger syndrome or high functioning autism?* (pp. 199–225). New York: Plenum Press.

Ung, D., Selles, R., Small, B. J., & Storch, E. A. (2015). A systematic review and meta-analysis of cognitive-behavioral therapy for anxiety in youth with high-functioning autism spectrum disorders. *Child Psychiatry and Human Development, 46*(4), 533–547.

Ünver, B., Öner, Ö., & Yurtbaşi, P. (2015.) Differential diagnosis between schizotypal personality disorder and autism spectrum disorders: A case report. *Turkish Journal of Psychiatry, 26*(1), 65–70.

Van Dijk, S., Jeffrey, J., & Katz, M. R. (2013). A randomized, controlled, pilot study of dialectical behavior therapy skills in a psychoeducational group for individuals with bipolar disorder. *Journal of Affective Disorders, 145*(3), 386–393.

Van Schalkwyk, G. I., Peluso, F., Qayyum, Z., McPartland, J. C., & Volkmar, F. R. (2015). Varieties of misdiagnosis in ASD: An illustrative case series. *Journal of Autism and Developmental Disorders, 45*(4), 911–918.

Van Wijngaarden-Cremers, P. J. M. (2016). Autism and substance use comorbidity: Screening, identification, and treatment. *European Psychiatry, 33*(Suppl.), S21–S22.

Volkmar, F. R., Klin, A., & McPartland, J. C. (2014). Asperger syndrome: An overview. In J. C. McPartland, A. Klin, & F. R. Volkmar (Eds.), *Asperger syndrome: Assessing and treating high-functioning autism spectrum disorders* (2nd ed., pp. 1–42). New York: Guilford Press.

Wainwright-Sharp, J. A., & Bryson, S. E. (1993). Visual orienting deficits in high-functioning people with autism. *Journal of Autism and Developmental Disorders, 23*, 1–13.

Walsh-Bender, D., & Kappenberg, C. F. (2016). *DBT-A+: An adapted DBT therapy approach for individuals with high functioning autism spectrum disorder (ASD) and related neurological conditions.* Paper presented at the meeting of the International Society for the Improvement and Teaching of Dialectical Behavior Therapy, New York.

Weiss, J. A., & Lunsky, Y. (2010). Group cognitive behaviour therapy for adults with Asperger syndrome and anxiety or mood disorder: A case series. *Clinical Psychology and Psychotherapy, 17*(5), 438–446.

Weston, L., Hodgekins, J., & Langdon, P. E. (2016). Effectiveness of cognitive behavioural therapy with people who have autistic spectrum disorders: A systematic review and meta-analysis. *Clinical Psychology Review, 4*, 41–54.

Westphal, A., Kober, D., Voos, A., & Volkmar, F. R. (2014). Psychopharmacological treatment of Asperger syndrome. In J. C. McPartland, A. Klin, & F. R. Volkmar (Eds.), *Asperger syndrome: Assessing and treating high-functioning autism spectrum disorders* (2nd ed., pp. 280–310). New York: Guilford Press.

White, S. W., Bray, B. C., & Ollendick, T. H. (2012). Examining shared and unique aspects of social anxiety disorder and autism spectrum disorder using factor analysis. *Journal of Autism and Developmental Disorders, 42*(5), 874–884.

White, S. W., Mazefsky, C. A., Dichter, G. S., Chiu, P. H., Richey, J. A., & Ollendick, T. H. (2014). Social-cognitive, physiological, and neural mechanisms underlying emotion regulation impairments: Understanding anxiety in autism spectrum disorder. *International Journal of Developmental Neuroscience, 39*, 22–36.

White, S. W., Ollendick, T., Albano, A. M., Oswald, D., Johnson, C., Southam-Gerow, M. A., et al. (2013). Randomized controlled trial: Multimodal anxiety and social skill intervention for adolescents with autism spectrum disorder. *Journal of Autism and Developmental Disorders, 43*(2), 382–394.

Whiting, D. (2012). Values Card Sort. Retrieved April 11, 2016, from *https://contextualscience.org/the_survey_of_guiding_principles_questionnaire_and*.

Wilson, C. E., Gillan, N., Spain, D., Robertson, D., Roberts, G., Murphy, C. M., et al. (2013). Comparison of ICD-10R, DSM-IV-TR and DSM-5 in an adult autism spectrum disorder diagnostic clinic. *Journal of Autism and Developmental Disorders, 43*(11), 2515–2525.

Wilson, C. E., Murphy, C. M., McAlonan, G., Robertson, D. M., Spain, D., Hayward, H., et al. (2016). Does sex influence the diagnostic evaluation of autism spectrum disorder in adults? *Autism, 20*(7), 808–819.

Wing, L. (1981). Asperger's syndrome: A clinical account. *Psychological Medicine, 11*, 115–130.

Wing, L. (2000). Past and future of research on Asperger syndrome. In A. Klin, F. R. Volkmar, & S. S. Sparrow (Eds.), *Asperger syndrome* (pp. 418–432). New York: Guilford Press.

Winner, M. G. (2000). *Inside out: What makes a person with social cognitive deficits tick?* San Jose, CA: Author.

Winner, M. G. (2002). *Thinking about you thinking about me.* San Jose, CA: Author.

Winner, M. G., & Crooke, P. J. (2011). *Social thinking at work: Why should I care?* Great Barrington, MA: North River Press.

Wolff, S. (1998). Schizoid personality in childhood: The links with Asperger syndrome, schizophrenia spectrum disorders, and elective mutism. In E. Schopler, G. B. Mesibov, & L. J. Kunce (Eds.), *Asperger syndrome or high-functioning autism?* (pp. 123–142). New York: Plenum Press.

Wolff, S. (2000). Schizoid personality in childhood and Asperger syndrome. In A. Klin, F. R. Volkmar, & S. S. Sparrow (Eds.), *Asperger syndrome* (pp. 278–305). New York: Guilford Press.

Wood, J. J., Ehrenreich-May, J., Alessandri, M., Fujii, C., Renno, P., Laugeson, E., et al. (2015). Cognitive behavioral therapy for early adolescents with autism spectrum disorders and clinical anxiety: A randomized control trial. *Behavior Therapy, 46*(1), 7–19.

World Health Organization. (1992). *International classification of diseases* (10th ed.). Geneva, Switzerland: Author.

World Health Organization. (1993). *The ICD-10 classification of mental and behavioural disorders: Diagnostic criteria for research.* Geneva, Switzerland: Author.

Wright, S. D. (Ed.). (2016). *Autism spectrum disorder in mid and later life.* London: Jessica Kingsley.

Wright, S. D., & Wadsworth, A. M. (2016). Introduction. In S. D. Wright (Ed.), *Autism spectrum disorder in mid and later life* (pp. 15–27). London: Jessica Kingsley.

Young, J. (1999). *Cognitive therapy for personality disorders: A schema-focused approach.* Sarasota, FL: Professional Resource Exchange.

Index

Note. *f* or *t* following a page number indicate a figure or a table.

Ability, 175
Academic documents. *See* Record review
Academic functioning, 4–5
Acceptance, 10, 153
Acceptance and commitment therapy (ACT), 152, 217–220
Acceptance-based strategies
    case examples illustrating, 237–238
    clarifying values and, 243–247, 245f
    improving emotion regulation skills and, 236–238, 242–243
    overview, 214, 217, 247
    Values Card Sort and, 244–247, 245f
    See also Interventions
Action based on values, 218
Activities of daily living, 48f, 50. *See also* Daily living consequences
Activity schedule, 199–201, 202f, 203f
Adaptation, 174–175, 215
Addiction, 251–252. *See also* Substance use disorders (SUD)
Adjunctive therapies
    collaboration and, 249–250
    before goals of treatment are met, 272–273
    as an obstacle to treatment, 268
    overview, 250–257
    referrals to other providers and, 248–250
    See also Treatment
Adult disability services, 255–257, 276–277
Advocacy, 12, 21, 281
Affordance perception, 68
Age issues, 20–22
Aging, 276

Agoraphobia, 74, 99
Alcohol use. *See* Substance abuse
Alexithymia
    alexithymia reduction treatment (ART) manual and, 230
    as an obstacle to treatment, 260
    overview, 63–64, 215
    See also Emotion regulation
All-or-nothing thinking, 191t. *See also* Cognitive distortions
Anger control problems, 80–82, 230–231
Antisocial personality disorder, 104–105
Anxiety
    acceptance and commitment therapy (ACT) and, 218
    case examples illustrating, 32–33
    cognitive-behavioral therapy (CBT) and, 74
    core problems in ASD and, 48f
    differential diagnosis and, 36–39
    emotion regulation and, 64–65, 215–216
    identifying and responding to dysfunctional automatic thoughts and, 190–198, 194f, 195f, 196f
    intake and, 88
    interventions and, 184, 230–231
    mental health needs of adults with ASD and, 11
    nomothetic formulation and, 154–155
    overview, 5–6
    schemas and, 76f
    See also Anxiety and related disorders
Anxiety and related disorders
    assessment and, 98–100
    cognitive-behavioral therapy (CBT) and, 74
    differential diagnosis and, 34, 36–39
    See also Anxiety

Arousal, emotional, 174–175, 182
Asperger syndrome (AS)
    classification systems and, 16t, 17t
    overview, 1, 10–11, 13–18, 16t, 17t
    psychoeducation regarding, 140–141
    terminology and, 3–4
Asperger's disorder, 14–18. *See also* Asperger
    syndrome
Asperger's Syndrome and Sexuality (Hénault), 169
Assertive communication skills, 174, 175
Assessment
    case formulation worksheet, 113f–114f
    comorbid mental health problems and, 97–108
    creating a problem list and setting preliminary
        goals for treatment, 111–112
    diagnosis and, 91–108, 92t, 93t, 95t
    instruments for, 94–97, 95t
    intake issues, 79–91
    interviewing strategies, 84–91
    nomothetic formulation and, 154–155
    overview, 79, 112
    referrals to other providers and, 248–249
    of strengths and resiliency factors, 108–111
    See also Intake
Assisted living, 256–257
Association for Contextual Behavioral Science
    (ACBS) website, 243
Attention deficit/hyperactivity disorder (ADHD)
    differential diagnosis and, 34, 35–36
    motor problems and, 68
    processing of information in nonsocial domains
        and, 69
Attentional control, 224
Attention-shifting ability, 70
Attitudes, 35. *See also* Intermediate beliefs
Auditory system, 67t
Autism Diagnostic Interview—Revised (ADI-R),
    94, 95t
Autism Diagnostic Observation Schedule, Second
    Edition (ADOS-2), 94, 95t
Autism Mental Status Exam (AMSE), 95t, 96
Autism spectrum disorder (ASD)
    acceptance and commitment therapy (ACT) and,
        219–220
    classification systems and, 14–18, 16t, 17t
    cognitive distortions in, 192
    diagnosis and, 91–108, 92t, 93t, 95t
    dialectical behavior therapy (DBT) and,
        222–223
    mindfulness-based programs (MBPs) and, 225
    myths about, 41–43, 41t
    overview, 1, 13, 45
    presentation of in adulthood, 18–33
    psychoeducation regarding, 140–142
    strengths and assets, 43–45, 44f
    symptom picture in adults and, 33–43, 40t, 41t
    terminology and, 3–4
Autism-Spectrum Quotient (AQ), 65, 95t, 96

Automatic thoughts
    acceptance and commitment therapy (ACT) and,
        218
    case examples illustrating, 193–198, 194f, 195f, 196f
    identifying and responding to, 190–198, 191t, 194f,
        195f, 196f
    overview, 184
    thought records to define, 185–190, 188f, 189f, 190f
    See also Cognitions; Cognitive distortions;
        Thoughts
Avoidance, 66
Avoidant personality disorder, 105

Beck Depression Inventory (BDI), 63, 103
Behavior
    case examples illustrating, 126–127, 137–138
    case formulation worksheet, 126–127
    cognitive model and, 74–75, 75f, 77f
    as an obstacle to treatment, 259
    thought records and, 187–190, 188f, 189f
    treatment plan and, 137–138
    See also Behavioral differences
Behavior Chain, 195–196. *See also* Downward arrow
    technique
Behavior management strategies, 252–253
Behavioral differences
    core problems in ASD and, 48f
    overview, 155
    schemas and, 76f
    skills training and, 156
    See also Behavior
Behavioral experiments, 199–201, 202f, 203f
Beliefs, core. *See* Core beliefs
Beliefs, intermediate. *See* Intermediate beliefs
Bermond and Vorst Alexithymia Questionnaire—
    Form B (BVAQ-B), 63
Biases in research, 19, 27–30
Biogenetic factors, 19–20
Biosocial theory, 220
Bipolar disorders, 39, 103
Bodily Map of Emotions, 232–234
Body language, 55, 93t, 260–261
Borderline personality disorder
    acceptance and commitment therapy (ACT) and,
        219
    assessment and, 104–105
    dialectical behavior therapy (DBT) and, 221
    differential diagnosis and, 40
Boundaries, 87–88, 260–261

Cancellation policies, 146
Case formulation
    case examples illustrating, 116–128, 117f–122f
    case formulation worksheet, 113f–114f, 115–128,
        117f–122f
    nomothetic formulation and, 154–155
    overview, 115–128, 117f–122f, 139
    See also Treatment plan

Case management, 255–256
Catastrophizing, 191*t. See also* Cognitive distortions
Causal factors, 124–127
Central coherence, 71
Change
    coping skills training and, 174–175
    philosophy of, 11–12
    treatment plan and, 128–131
Chronic pain, 152, 218, 223
Chronic stress, 73, 76*f*, 155. *See also* Stress
Classification systems, 14–18, 16*t*, 17*t*
Coaching, 221
Cognitions, 74–75, 75*f*, 77*f*, 189*f*
Cognitive distortions
    case examples illustrating, 193–198, 194*f*, 195*f*, 196*f*
    cognitive model and, 74–75, 75*f*
    identifying and responding to, 190–198, 191*t*, 194*f*, 195*f*, 196*f*
    See also Automatic thoughts
Cognitive dysfunction
    as an obstacle to treatment, 261
    overview, 5–6, 46, 50, 78, 274–275
    processing of information about self, 61–68, 67*t*
    processing of information in nonsocial domains, 69–71
    risk for mental health problems and, 71–77, 75*f*, 76*f*, 77*f*
    social cognition, 50–61
    See also Treatment
Cognitive model
    explaining to patients, 153, 184–190, 188*f*, 189*f*, 190*f*
    overview, 74–75, 75*f*
    rejection of as an obstacle to treatment, 262
    See also Cognitive-behavioral therapy (CBT)
Cognitive shifting, 87–88
Cognitive-behavioral therapy (CBT)
    for adults with ASD, 77–78
    comorbid mental health problems and, 183–184
    conceptualizing problems of ASD and, 74–77, 75*f*, 76*f*, 77*f*
    describing to patients, 152–153
    integration and, 5–6
    mindfulness-based interventions in, 216–225
    orientation to treatment and, 146–151
    overview, 1–2, 11–12, 46–47, 213, 275–276
    psychoeducation and, 143–145, 144*f*
    rationale for, 151–153
    See also Cognitive model; Interventions
Cognitive-emotional activity, 56–57
"Cognitively able" term, 4
Cohort issues, 20–22
Collaboration, 249–250, 257. *See also* Adjunctive therapies
Collateral therapy for family members, 252–253
Comic Strip Conversations (Gray), 168–169
Common sense, 4–5

Communication disorder. *See* Social (pragmatic) communication disorder (SCD)
Communication skills, 59, 84–85, 174, 259–261
Communicative intentions, 59–60
Comorbidity
    assessment and, 97–108
    cognitive-behavioral therapy (CBT) and, 74
    coping skills training and, 174–175
    dialectical behavior therapy (DBT) and, 221
    ending treatment before goals are met and, 272–273
    interventions and, 183–184, 213
    overview, 275
    thought records and, 185–190, 188*f*, 189*f*, 190*f*
Compensatory strategies, 11, 175–176
Complex PTSD, 263–264. *See also* Posttraumatic stress disorder (PTSD)
Compulsions, 38–39, 82
Confidentiality, 146, 249
Constructive feedback, 150–151
Context, 59–60. *See also* Social contexts
Continuum techniques, 206, 207–209
Coping skills training
    collateral therapy for family members and, 252–253
    compensatory strategies and, 175–176
    organizational skills, 176–177
    overview, 156, 174–182, 179*f*, 180*f*, 181*f*, 182
    problem-solving skills training, 178–182, 179*f*, 180*f*, 181*f*
    relaxation skills, 182
    See also Coping strategies; Skills training
Coping strategies
    intake and, 88
    rule development as, 198
    sensory problems and, 66
    strengths and resiliency factors and, 109
    See also Coping skills training
Core belief worksheet, 209–213, 212*f*
Core beliefs
    case examples illustrating, 207–209, 210–213, 212*f*
    cognitive model and, 74–75, 75*f*
    modifying, 206–213, 207*t*, 212*f*
    overview, 184
    See also Schemas
Core problems of ASD. *See* Behavioral differences; Chronic stress; Daily living consequences; Processing information about others; Processing information about the self; Processing of nonsocial information; Self-management problems; Social consequences; Social support; Symptoms
Corrective feedback, 88, 150–151
Counseling, 250–254
Counterfeit deviance, 106
Creativity, 43
Criminal defense, 257

Criminal justice system, 106–107
Crisis, 221
Cues, 52, 53–54, 56–57

Daily living consequences
  core problems in ASD and, 48f
  overview, 155
  risk for mental health problems and, 72
  schemas and, 76f
  skills training and, 156
Daily tasks, 109, 174–182, 179f, 180f, 181f, 276–277
Deficits, 175
Defusion technique, 239
Dementia, 69
Dependent personality disorder, 105
Depression
  acceptance and commitment therapy (ACT) and, 218
  adjunctive therapies and, 254
  case examples illustrating, 32–33
  cognitive-behavioral therapy (CBT) and, 74
  core problems in ASD and, 48f
  dialectical behavior therapy (DBT) and, 221
  differential diagnosis and, 39–40
  emotion regulation skills and, 215–216
  identifying and responding to dysfunctional
    automatic thoughts and, 190–198, 194f, 195f, 196f
  intake and, 80, 82
  interventions and, 183–184
  mental health needs of adults with ASD and, 11
  mindfulness-based programs (MBPs) and, 224–225
  nomothetic formulation and, 154–155
  overview, 5–6
  schemas and, 76f
  suicidality and, 108
Depressive disorders, 102–103. See also Depression
Developmental disorders (DD), 7–9, 20–21, 155
Diagnosis
  case examples illustrating, 123–124
  case formulation worksheet, 123–124
  classification systems and, 14–18, 16t, 17t
  comorbid mental health problems and, 97–108
  differential diagnosis, 34–41, 40t
  initial assessment and, 91–108, 92t, 93t, 95t
  overview, 112
  psychoeducation regarding, 140–142
  reactions to, 141–142
Diagnostic and Statistical Manual of Mental Disorders
    (DSM-IV), 13–14, 41
Diagnostic and Statistical Manual of Mental Disorders
    (DSM-IV-TR), 3–4, 17, 18
Diagnostic and Statistical Manual of Mental Disorders
    (DSM-5)
  differential diagnosis and, 34–41
  myths about ASD and, 41
  overview, 1–2, 14–18, 16t

psychoeducation regarding the diagnosis and, 140–142
  terminology and, 3–4
Dialectical behavior therapy (DBT)
  for adults with ASD, 77
  clarifying values and, 243–247, 245f
  explaining to patients, 152
  overview, 217, 220–223
  skills training manual used in, 226, 241
Differential diagnosis, 34–41, 40t. See also Diagnosis
Disability, 175
Disability services, 255–257, 276–277
Disclosure, 143–145, 144f
Discourse management, 59, 61
Distorted thoughts. See Automatic thoughts;
    Cognitive distortions
Distressing situations, 86–87, 128
Document review. See Record review
Downward arrow technique, 192–198, 194f, 195f, 196f
Drug use. See Substance abuse
Dysfunctional beliefs worksheet, 204–206, 205f
Dysfunctional thought record (DTR). See Thought
    records
Dysthymia. See Persistent depressive disorder
    (dysthymia)

Eating disorders, 221
Educational documents. See Record review
Ego dystonic obsessions and compulsions and, 38–39
Elaborate internal life, 35
Electroencephalogram (EEG), 55–56
Embedded Figures Test, 71
Emergency contact information, 146
Emotion, 74–75, 75f
Emotion perception, 62–65. See also Perception of
    information
Emotion recognition, 54–58, 55–56
Emotion regulation
  case examples illustrating, 229–230, 237–240, 241–243
  clarifying values, 243–247, 245f
  cognitive model and, 77f
  dialectical behavior therapy (DBT) and, 222–223
  differential diagnosis and, 39
  flexibility and, 240–243
  improving identification of one's own emotions
    and, 226–236, 227t, 228f, 229f, 232f, 233f, 235f
  interventions and, 236–243, 247
  mindfulness-based programs (MBPs) and, 225
  overview, 5–6, 62–65, 214–216, 275
Emotion Regulation Questionnaire (ERQ), 64
Emotion Regulation Skills System for Cognitively
    Challenged Clients, 231–232
Emotion vocabulary, 226
Emotional arousal, 174–175, 182
Emotional reasoning, 191t. See also Cognitive
    distortions
Emotional response, 57

Emotions
    acceptance and commitment therapy (ACT) and,
        218
    improving identification of, 226–236, 227t, 228f,
        229f, 232f, 233f, 234t, 235f
    psychoeducation regarding, 226, 227–230, 227t,
        228f, 229f
    thought records and, 187–190, 188f, 189f
Empathy, 42–43, 56–58, 64
Empathy Quotient (EQ), 57, 95t, 96
Employment issues. See Occupational functioning
Ending treatment, 269–274. See also Treatment
Environmental cues, 52, 59–60. See also Cues
Environmental modifications, 176, 221
Environmental stressors, 71–72
Ethical factors, 249
Ethnicity, 20
Evaluation, 248–249
Event-related potential (ERP), 55–56
Events, 77f, 189f
Evidence-based formulation-driven model, 46–47
Excoriation disorder, 101
Executive functions (EF)
    compensatory strategies and, 175
    core problems in ASD and, 49
    daily tasks and responsibilities and, 174–175
    differential diagnosis and, 35
    as an obstacle to treatment, 261
    orientation to treatment and, 149
    processing of information in nonsocial domains
        and, 69
Expectations
    increasing the fund of social knowledge, 161–168
    orientation to treatment and, 146–149
    social narrative and, 165
Exploring Depression, and Beating the Blues (Attwood
    & Garnett), 190
Exploring Feelings manuals, 230–231
Explosive outbursts, 39
Extrinsic skills, 62–63
Eye contact
    case examples illustrating, 158–161
    myths about ASD and, 42
    social inference and, 53–54
Eye-gaze patterns, 53–54

Face identification, 55
Facial expression, 52, 55, 59–60
Family factors, 262–263
Family participation in the therapy process
    collateral therapy for family members and,
        252–253
    intake and, 81–83, 88–91, 92, 93t
Family therapy, as an adjunctive therapy, 251
Fear of Negative Evaluation Scale (FNE), 65
Fee policies, 146
Feedback, 88, 150–151
Feedback cycle, 74–75, 75f
Feeling Good (Burns), 190

Financial factors, 25, 265–267. See also
    Socioeconomic status
Fine motor problems, 68
Five Facet Mindfulness Questionnaire (FFMQ), 65
Flat affect, 35, 39
Flexibility
    case examples illustrating, 241–243
    emotion regulation skills and, 240–243
    intake and, 85, 88
    processing of information in nonsocial domains
        and, 69–70
Full Scale IQ, 73
Fund of social knowledge, 161–168

Gender
    case examples illustrating, 27–30
    myths about ASD and, 42
    overview, 276
    presentation of ASD in adulthood, 18–20
Gender dysphoria, 106
"General population" term, 4
Generalized anxiety disorder (GAD), 74, 100
Gestures, 59–60
Global and Regional Asperger Syndrome
        Partnership (GRASP), 12, 128
Goal-directed behavior, 69
Goal-oriented approach, 111–112
Goals
    adjunctive therapies and, 250–251
    coping skills training and, 176
    creating, 111–112
    problem-solving skills training, 178–182, 179f,
        180f, 181f
    treatment plan and, 131, 136, 139
Grandin, Dr. Temple, 198
Group support/therapy, 142, 253
Gustatory system, 67t

Habilitation, 155–157, 182. See also Interventions;
        Skills training
Health problems. See Medical problems
Helpless core beliefs, 207t. See also Core beliefs
The Hidden Curriculum (Myles et al.), 162–163
"High functioning" term, 4
Histrionic personality disorder, 104–105
Hoarding disorder, 100–101
Hobbies, 110
Homework completion, 261
Honesty, 44
Humor, sense of, 44–45, 44f, 110
Hygiene, 83
Hypersensitivity problems, 66, 67t
Hypomania, 39
Hyposensitivity problems, 66, 67t

"If–then" statements, 194
The Illustrated Happiness Trap (Harris & Aisbett),
        237–238
Inappropriate affect, 35

Incredible 5-Point Scale, 231, 232f, 233f
Independence, desires for, 25
Independent living skills training, 276–277. *See also*
    Daily living consequences
Individual therapy, 250–251. *See also* Psychotherapy
Inference, social. *See* Social inference
Information processing
    core problems in ASD and, 47–49, 48f, 49f
    mental health needs of adults with ASD and, 11
    overview, 5–6, 78
    processing of information about self, 61–68, 67t
    processing of information in nonsocial domains,
        69–71
    schemas and, 76f
    social cognition, 50–61
    See also Processing information about others;
        Processing information about the self;
        Processing of nonsocial information
Inside Out (Winner), 169
Instrumental skills, 157, 158–161. *See also*
    Relationships; Social cognition
Insurance, as an obstacle to treatment, 265, 266–267
Intake
    case formulation worksheet, 113f–114f
    comorbid mental health problems and, 97–108
    creating a problem list and setting preliminary
        goals for treatment, 111–112
    diagnosis and, 91–108, 92t, 93t, 95t
    initial phone call and, 89–91
    interviewing strategies, 84–91
    overview, 112
    reasons for seeking treatment, 79–84
    record review and, 93
    referrals to other providers and, 248–249
    of strengths and resiliency factors, 108–111
    See also Assessment
Integration, 5–6
Intellectual disability (ID)
    Asperger syndrome (AS) and, 13
    dialectical behavior therapy (DBT) and, 222
    overview, 9
    presentation of ASD in adulthood, 18
Intelligence, 4, 43
Interests, 110
Intermediate beliefs, 184, 198–206, 202f, 203f, 205f
International Classification of Diseases (ICD-10)
    differential diagnosis and, 34–41
    overview, 13, 14–18, 17t
    presentation of ASD in adulthood, 18
International Society for the Improvement and Teaching
    of Dialectical Behavior Therapy (ISITDBT), 222
Interoception, 61–62
Interpersonal functioning, 4–5, 80–81
Interpersonal Reactivity Index (IRI), 57, 63–64
Interpreting information gathered, 54
Interventions
    case examples illustrating, 131, 132f–135f, 136–138,
        241–243
    case formulation worksheet, 131, 136–138

comorbid mental health problems and, 183–184
downward arrow technique, 192–198, 194f, 195f,
    196f
habilitation for core problems, 155–157
identifying and responding to dysfunctional
    automatic thoughts and, 190–198, 194f, 195f,
    196f
improving emotion regulation skills, 236–243
improving identification of one's own emotions
    and, 226–236, 227t, 228f, 229f, 232f, 233f, 235f
mental health needs of adults with ASD and, 5
modifying schemas, 206–213, 207t, 212f
nomothetic formulation and, 154–155
overview, 154, 213
recognizing and modifying intermediate beliefs,
    198–206, 202f, 203f, 205f
social language and, 58–59
social skills and, 157–174, 172f, 173f
social-interaction difficulties as challenges to,
    258–261
thought records and, 185–190, 188f, 189f, 190f
See also Cognitive-behavioral therapy (CBT);
    Mindfulness-based strategies; Skills training;
    Treatment; Treatment plan
Interviewing strategies, 84–91, 92, 92t, 93t
Intonation, 59–60
Intrinsic skills, 62–63
IQ, 73
Irritability, 39
Isolation, 264

Job coaching, 256. *See also* Occupational functioning
Judgment, 4–5, 51–52

Labeling, 191t, 198–199. *See also* Cognitive
    distortions
Labels, 15, 140
Lability, 39
Language
    intake and, 85–87
    as an obstacle to treatment, 259–261
    orientation to treatment and, 149–150
    social language and, 59
Language functioning, 4, 34, 49
Language pragmatics, 59
Learning styles
    identifying and responding to dysfunctional
        automatic thoughts and, 190–191
    psychoeducation regarding the diagnosis and,
        141
    skills training and, 156
Learning theory, 220
Legal factors, 83, 249, 257
Life circumstances, 81, 109, 266, 276–277. *See also*
    Daily living consequences
Likability, 129–131
Limitations, 175
Living Well on the Spectrum (Gaus), 175–176, 227–229,
    228f, 229f

Loneliness, 80
"Low functioning" term, 4

Maintenance factors, 124–127
Maintenance of gains, 270–271, 274–277
Major depressive disorder (MDD), 103
Mania, 39
Mannerisms, 49
Marital therapy, 251
Medical problems
    case examples illustrating, 124–125, 136
    case formulation worksheet, 124–125
    motor problems and, 68
    as an obstacle to treatment, 267
    treatment plan and, 136
Medical services, 254–255
Medication
    as an adjunctive therapy, 254
    as an obstacle to treatment, 267–268
Medication-induced movement disorders, 68
Mental filter/disqualifying the positive, 191t. See
    also Cognitive distortions
Mental health needs, 4–5, 8–9, 11
Mental health problems
    acceptance and commitment therapy (ACT) and,
        218–220
    assessment and, 97–108
    cognitive dysfunction and, 71–77, 75f, 76f, 77f
    core problems and, 47–50, 48f, 49f
Metaphors, 188–190
Mind reading, 54–58, 191t. See also Cognitive
    distortions
Mind Reading Software (Cambridge University), 169
Mindblindness, 54
Mindfulness-based cognitive therapy (MBCT),
    223–225
Mindfulness-based programs (MBPs), 224–225
Mindfulness-based strategies
    acceptance and commitment therapy (ACT) and,
        217–220
    for adults with ASD, 78
    clarifying values and, 243–247, 245f
    dialectical behavior therapy (DBT) and, 220–223
    explaining to patients, 153
    flexibility and, 241–243
    mindfulness-based stress reduction (MBSR), 152,
        217, 223–225
    overview, 214, 216–225, 247
    See also Interventions
Mindfulness-based stress reduction (MBSR), 152,
    217, 223–225
Mood, 74–75, 75f, 77f, 189f
Mood disorders
    assessment and, 102–103
    case examples illustrating, 32–33
    differential diagnosis and, 34, 39–40
    identifying and responding to dysfunctional
        automatic thoughts and, 190–198, 194f, 195f, 196f
    overview, 5–6

Motivation, lack of
    intake and, 82
    as an obstacle to treatment, 262
Motor problems, 68
Movie for the Assessment of Social Cognition
    (MASC), 56
Multifaceted Empathy Test (MET), 58
Multimodal teaching strategies, 168
Mutual regulation skills, 62–65

Narcissistic personality disorder, 104–105
Narrow interests, 82. See also Obsessional focus
National Association for the Dually Diagnosed
    (NADD), 8–9
Negative reactions to the diagnosis, 141–142. See also
    Diagnosis
Negative thoughts, 218. See also Automatic thoughts
Network involvement, 142–143
Neurodiversity, 10
Neurological disorders, 68
"Neurotypical (NT)" term, 4
Nomothetic formulation, 154–155
Nonconfrontation, 85–88
Nonsocial information processing. See Processing
    of nonsocial information
Nonverbal body language, 55, 93t, 260–261
Normalcy, 129–131
Norms, 161–168
Not-to-do lists, 177

Observing behavior, 92, 93t
Observing the self, 45, 109. See also Processing
    information about the self; Self-assessment
Obsessional focus, 4–5, 35, 38, 82
Obsessions, 38–39
Obsessive–compulsive disorder (OCD)
    assessment and, 100
    differential diagnosis and, 36, 38–39
    motor problems and, 68
    processing of information in nonsocial domains
        and, 69
Obsessive–compulsive personality disorder, 105, 218
Occupational functioning
    independence and, 25
    intake and, 81
    mental health needs of adults with ASD and, 4–5
    as an obstacle to treatment, 265–266
    overview, 276–277
    self-assessment of deficits and, 175
    vocational training and, 256, 276–277
Occupational therapy, 255
Older adults, 221
Olfactory system, 67t
Online community, 142
Organizational checklists, 176
Organizational skills
    compensatory strategies and, 175
    coping skills training and, 175, 176–177
    intake and, 83

Organizations, 142, 281
Orientation to treatment, 140, 145–153
Others, processing information about. *See* Processing information about others
Overgeneralization, 191*t*. *See also* Cognitive distortions

Pacing, 85, 149
Pain, 152, 218, 223
Panic disorder, 74, 99
Paranoia, 35
Paranoid personality disorder, 104
Paraphilia, 106
Patients, 148–149
Penn State Worry Questionnaire (PSW-Q), 65
Perceived social support (PSS), 72–73. *See also* Social support
Perception of information, 61–65, 88
Perception of internal states. *See* Alexithymia
Persistent depressive disorder (dysthymia), 103
Personality disorders (PD), 34, 40–41, 40*t*, 103–105
Personality features, 110
Personalization, 191*t*. *See also* Cognitive distortions
Perspective-taking skills, 169–171
Pervasive developmental disorders (PDD), 3, 13
Pharmacological treatment
    as an adjunctive therapy, 254
    as an obstacle to treatment, 267–268
Phone calls, 89–91
Planning skills, 69, 70–71, 175
Polypharmacy, 267–268
Positive and Negative Affect Schedule (PANAS), 64
Positive psychology, 108
Positive reactions to the diagnosis, 141. *See also* Diagnosis
Posttraumatic stress disorder (PTSD), 74, 101–102, 263–264
Pragmatic communication disorder. *See* Social (pragmatic) communication disorder (SCD)
Pragmatic expressive language
    as an obstacle to treatment, 260–261
    risk for mental health problems and, 72
Pragmatics, social language and, 59
Premature termination, 273–274. *See also* Termination
Present focus, 218
Presentation of ASD in adulthood
    age and cohort issues, 20–22
    case examples illustrating, 22–33
    differential diagnosis and, 34–41, 40*t*
    gender/sex, 18–20
    myths about ASD and, 41–43, 41*t*
    overview, 18–33, 45
    presenting problems, 22–33
    race/ethnicity, 20
    symptoms and, 33–43, 40*t*, 41*t*
    See also Presenting problems
Presenting problems
    case examples illustrating, 22–33
    creating a problem list and setting preliminary goals for treatment, 111–112

intake and, 79–84
    presentation of ASD in adulthood and, 22–33
    See also Presentation of ASD in adulthood
Presupposition, 59, 60
Primary medical care, 254
Problem list, 111–112, 116, 123
Problem-solving skills
    collateral therapy for family members and, 252–253
    coping skills training and, 175, 178–182, 179*f*, 180*f*, 181*f*
    mental health needs of adults with ASD and, 4–5
Processing information about others
    core problems in ASD and, 48*f*, 49*f*
    overview, 47, 50–61, 78, 155
    schemas and, 76*f*
    See also Social cognition
Processing information about the self
    core problems in ASD and, 48*f*, 49*f*
    overview, 47, 61–68, 67*t*, 78, 155
    schemas and, 76*f*
Processing of nonsocial information
    core problems in ASD and, 48*f*, 49*f*
    overview, 47, 49, 69–71, 78, 155
    schemas and, 76*f*
Processing speed, 56
Procrastination, 82
Program for the Education and Enrichment of Relational Skills (PEERS®) for Young Adults (Laugeson), 169
Proprioceptive system, 67*t*
Psychoeducation
    about emotions, 226, 227*t*
    alexithymia reduction treatment (ART) manual and, 230
    case examples illustrating, 211
    compensatory strategies and, 175
    overview, 140–145, 144*f*, 153
    resources for, 281
Psychosis, 218
Psychotherapy
    as an adjunctive therapy, 250–254
    collateral therapy for family members and, 252–253
    mental health needs of adults with ASD and, 9
    social-interaction difficulties as challenges to, 258–261
Psychotic disorders, 34, 35

Quality of life, 224

Race, 20
Rapport, 84–85
Rationale for treatment, 151–153
Reading the Mind in the Eyes test, 54
Reappraisal strategies, 239
Receptive language processing problems
    compensatory strategies and, 175
    as an obstacle to treatment, 259–261

Record review, 93
Record-keeping practices, 146
Referral sources, 79
Referrals to other providers, 248–250, 272–273
Reflective statements, 149–150
Rehabilitation services, 254–255
Relationships
  mental health needs of adults with ASD and, 5
  myths about ASD and, 42
  overview, 157
  strengths and resiliency factors and, 109–110
Relaxation skills, 175, 182
Repetitive patterns of behavior, 38
Residential support, 256–257, 277
Resiliency factors
  assessment and, 108–111
  case examples illustrating, 127, 136
  case formulation worksheet, 127
  treatment plan and, 136
Resources, 142–143, 279–281
Respect, 87–88
Responses, 187–190, 188f, 189f
Responsibilities, 174–182, 179f, 180f, 181f
Restricted patterns of behavior, 38
Rigidity, 77f, 174–175
Risk factors, 5–6, 270–271
Ritvo Autism and Asperger's Diagnostic Scale—14
  Screen (RAADS-14 Screen), 95t, 97
Ritvo Autism and Asperger's Diagnostic Scale—
  Revised (RAAD-R), 95t, 96–97
Routine adherence, 35
"Rude" behavior, 49
Rules
  case examples illustrating, 199–206, 202f, 203f,
    205f
  increasing the fund of social knowledge, 161–168
  recognizing and modifying intermediate beliefs
    and, 198–206, 202f, 203f, 205f
  See also Intermediate beliefs

Satisfaction, 129–131
Schedules, 176–177
Schemas
  activity schedule and, 199–201, 202f, 203f
  case examples illustrating, 125–126, 137, 207–209,
    210–213, 212f
  case formulation worksheet, 125–126
  cognitive model and, 74–77, 75f, 76f, 77f, 189f
  modifying, 206–213, 207t, 212f
  overview, 184
  treatment plan and, 137
  See also Core beliefs
Schizoid personality disorder, 40, 104
Schizophrenia
  differential diagnosis and, 35
  processing of information in nonsocial domains
    and, 69
  therapeutic relationship and, 84–85
Schizotypal personality disorder, 40, 104

Seeking to share enjoyment, 35
Self, processing information about. See Processing
  information about the self
Self as context, 218
Self-acceptance, 11
Self-assessment, 175, 226. See also Processing
  information about the self
Self-care issues, 83
Self-evaluation, 45
Self-management problems
  cognitive model and, 77f
  core problems in ASD and, 48f, 50
  overview, 155
  schemas and, 75, 76f
  skills training and, 156
Self-observation, 45, 109
Self-report, 80–81
Sensory system
  cognitive model and, 77f
  compensatory strategies and, 175
  daily tasks and responsibilities and, 174–175
  differential diagnosis and, 35
  as an obstacle to treatment, 259
  overview, 66–68, 67t
  risk for mental health problems and, 72
Sensory-based mindfulness strategies, 242. See also
  Mindfulness-based strategies
Sensory-motor processing, 65–68, 67t
Service eligibility appeals, 257
Severity level, 15
Sex, 18–20, 276
Sexual disorders, 106
Sexual dysfunctions, 106
Sexual problems
  adjunctive therapies and, 251
  assessment and, 105–107
  intake and, 83–84
Sexually offensive behaviors, 106
"Should" statements, 191t. See also Cognitive
  distortions
Skills deficit, 155
Skills training
  comorbid mental health problems and, 184
  dialectical behavior therapy (DBT) and, 221,
    222–223, 226
  habilitation for core problems and, 155–157
  improving emotion regulation skills, 236–243
  overview, 11, 155, 182
  See also Coping skills training; Interventions;
    Social skills training
Sleep problems
  adjunctive therapies and, 254
  differential diagnosis and, 39
  intake and, 81, 83
Sleep–wake disorders, 107
The Smart but Scattered Guide to Success (Dawson &
  Guare), 176
Social (pragmatic) communication disorder (SCD),
  34

Social anxiety disorder (SAD), 36–39, 98–99. *See also* Social phobia
Social cognition
  cognitive model and, 77*f*
  overview, 5–6, 50–61, 157
  schemas and, 75
  skills training and, 168–174, 172*f*, 173*f*
  See also Processing information about others
Social Communication Questionnaire (SCQ), 68
Social consequences
  core problems in ASD and, 48*f*, 49
  overview, 155
  schemas and, 75, 76*f*
  skills training and, 156
Social contexts, 59–60, 60. *See also* Context
Social developmental disorders (SDD), 55
Social functioning
  anxiety and, 37–38
  differential diagnosis and, 39
  myths about ASD and, 42
Social inference, 51–58, 198. *See also* Social cognition
Social information, 52, 56
Social knowledge, fund of, 161–168
Social language, 52, 58–59
Social Literacy (Cohen), 169
Social narrative, 165–168
Social norms, 161–168
Social perception, 53–54
Social phobia, 74, 98–99. *See also* Social anxiety disorder (SAD)
Social problems, 4–5
Social reciprocity, 35
Social Responsiveness Scale, Second Edition (SRS-2), 95*t*, 97
Social Responsiveness Scale (SRS), 65
Social situations, 59–60, 80
Social skills deficits
  cognitive model and, 77*f*
  core problems in ASD and, 48*f*, 49
  intake and, 88
  interventions and, 157–174, 172*f*, 173*f*
  orientation to treatment and, 150–151
  risk for mental health problems and, 72
  schemas and, 75, 76*f*
  social inference and, 52–53
  See also Social skills training
Social skills training
  case examples illustrating, 158–161, 163–165, 166–168, 169–171
  dialectical behavior therapy (DBT) and, 222–223
  improving assertive communication skills, 174
  improving social cognition, 168–174, 172*f*, 173*f*
  increasing instrumental skills, 158–161
  increasing the fund of social knowledge, 161–168
  overview, 156, 157, 182
  worksheets for, 171
  See also Skills training; Social skills deficits
Social Stories™ approach, 165, 168
Social Stories™ (Gray), 168

Social support
  core problems in ASD and, 48*f*
  as an obstacle to treatment, 264
  overview, 155
  risk for mental health problems and, 72–73
  schemas and, 76*f*
  strengths and resiliency factors and, 110–111
Sociocultural factors, 19–20
Socioeconomic status, 20, 265–267
Socioemotional processing disorder, 55
Specific phobia, 98
Speech, 59
Speech therapy, 255
Speech-language pathologists, 58–59
State–Trait Anxiety Inventory (STAI), 65
Stereotyped motor mannerisms, 35
Stereotyped patterns of behavior, 38
Strategy instruction, 11. *See also* Skills training
Strategy use, 108–109
Strengths
  assessment and, 108–111
  case examples illustrating, 136
  case formulation worksheet, 127
  compensatory strategies and, 175
  overview, 43–45, 44*f*
  personality disorders and, 104
  treatment plan and, 128, 136
Stress
  acceptance and commitment therapy (ACT) and, 218
  core problems in ASD and, 48*f*
  intake and, 88
  overview, 5–6, 275
  risk for mental health problems and, 72–73
  schemas and, 76*f*
  strengths and resiliency factors and, 109
  treatment plan and, 128
  See also Chronic stress
Stress inoculation model, 174–175
Stressor-related disorders, 101–102
Structure, responsiveness to, 45
Substance abuse, 84, 264. *See also* Substance use disorders (SUD)
Substance use disorders (SUD)
  acceptance and commitment therapy (ACT) and, 218
  adjunctive therapies and, 251–252
  assessment and, 107
  dialectical behavior therapy (DBT) and, 221
  See also Substance abuse
Suicidality, 84, 108, 221
Support groups, 253–254
Support service models. *See* Disability services
Symptoms
  in adults, 33–43, 40*t*, 41*t*
  case examples illustrating, 125, 136–137
  case formulation worksheet, 125
  classification systems and, 14–18, 16*t*, 17*t*
  presentation of ASD in adulthood, 18–33

Symptoms *(cont.)*
  psychoeducation regarding the diagnosis and, 141
  treatment plan and, 136–137

Tactical withdrawal, 85, 88
Tactile system, 67*t*
Talents of the patient, 110
Talk Blocks, 234–236, 234*t*, 235*f*
Task organization, 72, 176–177
Telehealth modalities, 146
Termination
  before goals of treatment are met, 271–274
  when the goals of treatment have been met,
    269–271
Terminology, 3–4
Theory of mind (ToM), 54, 78. *See also* Processing
  information about others
Therapeutic relationship
  intake and, 84–85
  orientation to treatment and, 146–151
  respect and, 87–88
  social-interaction difficulties as challenges to,
    258–261
Therapists
  accessibility of between sessions, 146
  overview, 2–3
  role of, 147–148
  social-interaction difficulties as challenges to
    treatment and, 258–261
Thinking about You Thinking about Me (Winner), 169,
  170
Thinking in Pictures (Grandin), 198
Thought records, 185–190, 188*f*, 189*f*, 190*f*, 192
Thoughts
  acceptance and commitment therapy (ACT) and,
    218
  cognitive model and, 74–75, 75*f*
  psychoeducation regarding, 228*f*
  See also Automatic thoughts; Cognitions
Tic disorders, 68
Time management skills, 175, 176–177
To-do lists, 176, 177
Tolerance of uncertainty, 238–240
Toronto Alexithymia Scale (TAS-20), 63, 64, 65
Tower of Hanoi test, 70–71
Transdiagnostic mental health problems, 5–6, 218
Trauma history, 263–264. *See also* Posttraumatic
  stress disorder (PTSD)
Trauma-related disorders, 101–102
Treatment
  adjunctive therapies and, 250–257
  comorbid mental health problems and, 183–184
  ending when the goals of have been met, 269–271

executive functions and homework completion
  and, 261
family issues that interfere with, 262–263
financial obstacles to, 265–267
interruption of before goals are met, 271–274
motivation and, 262
obstacles to, 138–139, 258–268
orientation to, 140, 145–153
presenting problems, 22–33
social-interaction difficulties as challenges to,
  258–261
working relationships and, 146–151
See also Adjunctive therapies; Cognitive-
  behavioral therapy (CBT); Interventions
Treatment plan
  case examples illustrating, 131–139, 132*f*–135*f*
  case formulation worksheet, 113*f*–114*f*, 131–139,
    132*f*–135*f*
  overview, 128–139, 132*f*–135*f*, 139
  preparing for and preventing potential obstacles,
    138–139
  See also Case formulation
Trichotillomania, 101, 219
"Typical" term, 4

Uncertainty, tolerance of, 238–240
Unconventional views, 43
Unexpected events, 174–175
Unlovable core beliefs, 207*t*. *See also* Core beliefs

Validation, 150
Values, 218, 243–247, 245*f*
Values Card Sort, 244–247, 245*f*
Vestibular system, 67*t*
Visual aids, 176, 188, 190*f*
Visual downward arrow technique, 192–198, 194*f*,
  195*f*, 196*f*
Visual system, 67*t*
Visual–social information, 53
Vocational training, 256, 276–277. *See also*
  Occupational functioning
Voice, 52, 55, 59–60

Wisconsin Card Sorting Test (WCST), 69–70
Withdrawal, 82
"Word-perfect" accuracy, 85–87
Working memory, 69
Working relationships, 146–151. *See also* Therapeutic
  relationship

Yale–Brown Obsessive Compulsive Scale (Y-BOCS),
  38
Youth with ASD, 5–6